Geriatrics and Ageing in the Soviet Union

Geriatrics and Ageing in the Soviet Union

Medical, Political and Social Contexts

Edited by
Susan Grant and Isaac McKean Scarborough

BLOOMSBURY ACADEMIC
LONDON • NEW YORK • OXFORD • NEW DELHI • SYDNEY

BLOOMSBURY ACADEMIC
Bloomsbury Publishing Plc
50 Bedford Square, London, WC1B 3DP, UK
1385 Broadway, New York, NY 10018, USA
29 Earlsfort Terrace, Dublin 2, Ireland

BLOOMSBURY, BLOOMSBURY ACADEMIC and the Diana logo are
trademarks of Bloomsbury Publishing Plc

First published in Great Britain 2023
Paperback edition first published 2024

Copyright © Susan Grant and Isaac McKean Scarborough, 2023

Susan Grant and Isaac McKean Scarborough have asserted their right under the Copyright,
Designs and Patents Act, 1988, to be identified as Editor of this work.

Cover image: © Isaac McKean Scarborough

This work is published open access subject to a Creative Commons Attribution-NonCommercial-NoDerivatives 3.0 licence (CC BY-NC-ND 3.0, https://creativecommons.org/licenses/by-nc-nd/3.0/). You may re-use, distribute, and reproduce this work in any medium for non-commercial purposes, provided you give attribution to the copyright holder and the publisher and provide a link to the Creative Commons licence.

Open access was funded by the Wellcome Trust [Grant No.: 209842/Z/17/Z]

Open access funding was also provided by Liverpool John Moores University, UK.

Bloomsbury Publishing Plc does not have any control over, or responsibility for, any third-party websites referred to or in this book. All internet addresses given in this book were correct at the time of going to press. The author and publisher regret any inconvenience caused if addresses have changed or sites have ceased to exist, but can accept no responsibility for any such changes.

Every effort has been made to trace the copyright holders and obtain permission to reproduce the copyright material. Please do get in touch with any enquiries or any information relating to such material or the rights holder. We would be pleased to rectify any omissions in subsequent editions of this publication should they be drawn to our attention.

A catalogue record for this book is available from the British Library.

A catalog record for this book is available from the Library of Congress.

ISBN: HB: 978-1-3502-7379-5
PB: 978-1-3502-7383-2
ePDF: 978-1-3502-7380-1
eBook: 978-1-3502-7381-8

Typeset by Integra Software Services Pvt. Ltd.

To find out more about our authors and books visit www.bloomsbury.com
and sign up for our newsletters.

Contents

List of figures	vii
List of table	viii
Glossary	ix
Note on transliteration	x
Notes on contributors	xi
Acknowledgements	xiv
Introduction: Ageing in a Soviet context	1
Part 1 Soviet gerontology: Ageing as a field of scientific study	**15**
1 The legend of Gilgamesh: Attempts at its realization in Soviet gerontology *Vladislav Bezrukov and Yurii Duplenko*	17
2 Medical propaganda: Fairy tales and miracles of surgery *Maria Tutorskaya*	35
3 Winding up the clock of life: Soviet research into infant 'mortality' in the context of ageing bodies *Anna Ozhiganova*	51
Part 2 Care for older persons: Soviet geriatrics, spatial organization and social support	**71**
4 Ageing minds and bodies: Caring for older patients at a Soviet psychiatric hospital *Aleksandra Marta Brokman*	73
5 A comfortable old age: Designing care homes for older Soviet persons *Susan Grant*	91
6 Age and the city: Older persons in Soviet urban milieu and thought in the 1970s and 1980s *Botakoz Kassymbekova*	113
Part 3 Narratives of ageing, public and private	**129**
7 The modern babushka: Rethinking older women in late socialism *Danielle Leavitt-Quist*	131

8   The right to a permanent collection: Archiving the lives of Soviet
    pensioners *Alissa Klots and Maria Romashova*   149

9   Soviet life cycle and ageing: Through the lens of museums of
    medicine *Katarzyna Jarosz*   165

Part 4 International contexts   183

10 The burden of old age: The fate of older people in the People's Republic
    of Poland *Ewelina Szpak*   185

11 Ageing and gerontology in Britain after 1945: The 'menace' of an
    ageing population *Pat Thane*   207

Epilogue: Socialist ageing in a global context *James Chappel and
Isaac Scarborough*   225

Select bibliography   239
Index   244

Figures

2.1 Poster: the cultivation of public health is the work of the working class 39
2.2 Photo montage: science in the service of building socialism 42
3.1 Ilya Arshavsky and Igor Charkovsky oversee babies' water training. Moscow, 1980s. Photo by Alexander Grashchenkov. 63
7.1 Cover of the satiral magazine *Krokodil*: 'Don't bother me, babushka!' 144
9.1 Reconstructed birthing room, Latvian Medical Exhibition, Latvia 170
9.2 Diorama of dying soldiers, Azerbaijan's Museum of Medicine 176

Table

11.1 Number of institutions and homes of various types in England and Wales 214

Glossary

BMA	British Medical Association
Delo (d.)	Folder in an opis'
EHRC	Equality and Human Rights Commission (England and Wales)
Fond (f.)	archive holding/collection
GAPK	State Archive of Perm Region
GARF	State Archive of the Russian Federation
GDR	German Democratic Republic (East Germany)
Giprogor	Russian Institute for Urban Planning and Investment Development
Gos/grazhdanstroi	State Committee for Construction Affairs
Gosstroi	Ministry of Construction and Architecture
KCPZPR	Central Committee of the Polish Union Workers' Party
List (l.)	Page (if followed by 'ob' [*oborot*'], then the reverse side of the page)
LPZP	Forest Park Protection Zone
MOIP	Moscow Society of Naturalists
Narkomzdrav	People's Commissariat of Public Health
NEP	New Economic Policy
NHS	National Health Service (United Kingdom)
NKVD	People's Commissariat of Internal Affairs
Opis' (op.)	fond subgroup
PGR	State Agricultural Farm (People's Republic of Poland)
RGASPI	Russian State Archive of Socio-Political History
RSFSR	Russian Soviet Federative Socialist Republic
TsDAVO	Central State Archive of the Supreme Organs of Government and Administration of Ukraine
TsDKFFA	Central State Film, Photograph and Phonography Archive of Ukraine
TsGAM	TsGA Moskvy or the Central State Archive of the City of Moscow
TsNIIEP zhilishcha	Central Scientific Research and Design Institute of Standard and Experimental Accommodation Design
VIEM	All-Union Institute of Experimental Medicine
WHO	World Health Organization
WVS	Women's Voluntary Service (UK)
ZhEK	Housing Maintenance Office

Note on transliteration

We have followed the Library of Congress system for Russian transliteration. In addition, we transliterate from Russian when referring to cities, towns and individuals located in the USSR (for example, Kiev instead of Kyiv), in order to retain the contemporaneous spelling and pronunciation of these toponyms, notwithstanding post-1991 changes. In the case of well-established English-language versions of names, these have been used in place of more direct transliteration (Yeltsin, for example, in place of El'stin).

Notes on contributors

Prof. Vladislav Bezrukov (Doctor of Medical Sciences) is Director of the Institute of Gerontology in Kyiv, where he has worked since 1965. An academic of the National Academy of Medical Sciences of Ukraine, Prof. Bezrukov has published extensively in the fields of physiology and social gerontology.

Aleksandra Brokman is an independent scholar working on the history of psychiatry in the Soviet Union. She has been a part of the 'Growing Old in the Soviet Union, 1945–1991' project at Liverpool John Moores University and has previously published on the development, theory and practice of psychotherapy in the Soviet Union.

James Chappel is Gilhuly Family Associate Professor of History at Duke University. An intellectual and social historian of Europe and the United States, his research has focused on the Catholic Church in modern European history, as well as the history of ageing across the Atlantic. Recent publications include *Catholic Modern* (Harvard University Press, 2018) and 'On the Border of Old Age: An Entangled History of Eldercare in East Germany', *Central European History* 53 (2020).

Prof. Yurii Duplenko (Doctor of Medical Sciences) was until his retirement Head of the Department of Informational Analysis of the Institute of Gerontology in Kyiv. One of the first employees of the Institute, Prof Duplenko is also the author of the first published history of Soviet gerontology, entitled *Starenie: ocherki razvitiia problemy*, which was issued in 1985.

Susan Grant is Professor of Russian and Soviet History at Liverpool John Moores University. She is the author of *Soviet Nightingales: Care under Communism* (2022) and *Physical Culture and Sport in Soviet Society: Propaganda, Transformation and Acculturation in the 1920s and 1930s* (2012). She holds a Wellcome Trust grant for the project 'Growing Old in the Soviet Union, 1945–1991'.

Katarzyna Jarosz is Assistant Professor at the International University of Logistics in Wrocław (Poland). Her research interests include the relationship between science and society, archaeology, politics and the mechanisms of cultural heritage protection, and museum studies. Dr Jarosz has published on memory and museum studies in the post-Soviet sphere; her most recent publication is *The Development of Museums of Pharmacy in Post-Soviet Countries* (2021).

Botakoz Kassymbekova is Postdoctoral Fellow at the University of Basel, Switzerland. She was previously a Wellcome Trust postdoctoral fellow and is currently researching a social and cultural history of ageing in the post-war Soviet Union. She is the author of *Despite Culture: Early Soviet Rule in Tajikistan* (2016).

Alissa Klots is Assistant Professor at the University of Pittsburgh in the Department of History. Her research focuses on gender and labour history. She is currently completing a manuscript on the history of domestic service in the Soviet Union. She is also collaborating with Maria Romashova on a project on older public activists in late Soviet society.

Danielle Leavitt-Quist is a PhD candidate in the History Department at Harvard University. Her research interests focus on ideas about age in the Soviet Union and Eastern Europe, gender and intergenerational family life.

Anna Ozhiganova (PhD) is a medical anthropologist and Senior Researcher at the Institute of Ethnology and Anthropology of the Russian Academy of Sciences. Her research interests concern the intersections of religion, health, reproduction and alternative social movements. She is currently studying the late and post-Soviet Russian homebirth movement and alternative practices of infant development. Dr Ozhiganova is the author of *New Religiosity in Modern Russia: Teachings, Forms and Practices* (2006) and of over fifty articles and book chapters on the Russian New Age and alternative health movements.

Maria Romashova is the director of Perm State University History Museum and research fellow at the Centre for Comparative History and Political Studies at Perm State University, Russia. Maria Romashova holds a PhD in Russian history from Perm State University (Russia) where she is currently teaching. She serves as the director of Perm State University History Museum and research fellow at the Centre for Comparative History and Political Studies at Perm State University. Her current project on ageing in the Soviet Union, on which she is collaborating with Alissa Klots, examines the role older public activists played in the late Soviet society.

Isaac McKean Scarborough is Assistant Professor of Russian and Eurasian Studies, Institute for History, Leiden University (The Netherlands). His research covers the socio-economic development of the post-war Soviet Union. He graduated from the LSE with a PhD in International History in 2018, and was previously a Wellcome Trust Postdoctoral Research Fellow on the 'Growing Old in the Soviet Union' project at LJMU.

Ewelina Szpak is Assistant Professor at the Institute of History of the Polish Academy of Sciences. Her fields of research include the social and cultural history of communism, social history of medicine, environmental history and history of biopolitics. She is an author of four books including *A Man Is Sick when He Is in Pain: A Socio-Cultural History of Health and Illness in the Polish Countryside after 1945* (Warsaw: IHPAN 2016). She is currently writing a book on the social and cultural history of cancer in post-war Poland.

Pat Thane, MA (Oxford), PhD (London), FBA, is Visiting Professor in History, Birkbeck College, University of London. Publications include *Foundations of the Welfare State* (2nd ed. 1996); *Old Age in English History. Past Experiences, Present Issues* (2000); *The Long History of Old Age* (ed, 2005); *Women and Ageing in British Society since 1500* (ed with Lynn Botelho, 2001); *The Long History of Old Age* (ed, 2005); *Britain's Pensions Crisis. History and Policy* (ed with Hugh Pemberton and Noel Whiteside, 2006); and *Divided Kingdom: A History of Britain 1900 to the Present* (2018).

Maria Tutorskaya is Senior Researcher in the Russian Medical Museum at FSSBI 'N.A. Semashko National Research Institute of Public Health' in Moscow, Russia. Her research interests are focused on the history of medicine, medical museums and the history of medical education in the Russian Empire and the USSR. She has published on Russian medical museums' history and medicine and literature. Her most recent paper *Fighting for the History of Medicine* (2021) deals with the medical humanities role in the development of modern medical curricula.

Acknowledgements

We are greatly indebted to many organizations and individuals who helped guide this volume to completion. Most of the contributions that follow were presented at two conferences as part of the Wellcome Trust-funded project 'Growing Old in the Soviet Union, 1945–1991'. The first of these events took place at Liverpool John Moores University in December 2019 and the second took place online, after some delay due to the Covid-19 pandemic, in May 2021. We would like to thank those who presented and participated. These include Stephen Lovell, Pat Thane, Donald Filtzer, Claire Hilton, Andrea Belehradova, James Whitehead, James Crossland, Tom Beaumont, David Clampin, Elena Zdravomyslova, Susan Pickard, Alissa Klots, James Chappel, Aleksandra Brokman, Botakoz Kassymbekova, Nikolai Krementsov, Pavel Vasilev, Anna Ozhiganova, Vladislav Bezrukov, Anastasia Belaeva and Yurii Duplenko. We are grateful to James Brocklesby for his stellar administrative assistance in organizing these events. Our colleagues at Liverpool John Moores University have encouraged and supported this research at all stages and we are very grateful to them. We are also indebted to the LJMU Library, especially Katherine Stephen, Cath Dishman and Maria Follett, who helped to make the chapters not funded by the Wellcome Trust available to all through Open Access. None of this research would have been possible without the generous funding and support from the Wellcome Trust, which funded the entire project, conferences and Open Access.

Several colleagues who work on ageing and gerontology have also been instrumental in our discussions and research at various stages of the project. These include Alissa Klots, Maria Romashova, Elena Zdravomyslova, Danielle Leavitt-Quist, Elena Bogdanova, Vladimir Anisimov, Lidiya Khoroshinina, Vladislav Bezrukov and Viktor Kholin. Our 'Growing Old' *kruzhka*, together with Aleksandra Brokman and Botakoz Kassymbekova, has been an important space for discussing conference ideas, concepts of ageing and works in progress. In Kyiv, the Institute of Gerontology proved to be a congenial place to do research, and we both have fond memories of our time in Kyiv and at the Institute. We hope that even in the present circumstances the committed and wonderful staff at the Institute will continue to produce excellent research, provide care for older patients and preserve the history of Soviet gerontology in its wonderful library.

At Bloomsbury we had the pleasure of working with Rhodri Mogford and Laura Reeves. Our anonymous reviewers provided excellent food for thought and we appreciate their constructive feedback. We hope to have managed to address all their comments and suggestions, which have no doubt helped to make this volume all the better. We thank Susan Certo at Mark Your Words for providing such a thorough index for the volume. Finally, we would like to thank our families and friends for their ongoing support. Much of this manuscript was prepared during lockdown conditions, in which the presence of family members and their encouragement helped to sustain and support us.

***

Funding acknowledgement

This research was funded in whole, or in part, by the Wellcome Trust [Grant No: 209842/Z/17/Z]. For the purpose of open access, the author has applied a CC BY public copyright licence to any Author Accepted Manuscript version arising from this submission.

Open access funding was also provided by Liverpool John Moores University, UK.

Introduction: Ageing in a Soviet context

This book is about ageing in the Soviet Union: the medical practices of geriatrics, the science of gerontology and the experience of growing old. Chapters in the volume focus on concepts and themes that examine Soviet ageing in its medical, political and social contexts, in both the Soviet Union and internationally. Compared to most sciences, gerontology is pitifully underfunded; geriatrics is amongst the least prestigious branches of medicine; and while the world's population is growing undeniably older, great disagreement remains over what can and should be done in response. This volume's chapters speak directly to some of these concerns. The epilogue also brings together some of the key issues addressed in the chapters and examines them in an international context, comparing the Soviet Union to the British and US experience. Initially, however, we introduce some of the main themes in the volume and contextualize the Soviet case. These include demographic trends; science, medicine and the place of the individual; women and ageing; and attitudes to and perceptions of ageing.

Demographics

As the USSR aged over the decades, so too did its populace. Like populations across the world during the twentieth century, moreover, the Soviet people seemed to age faster than the passage of years would attest. A statistically young nation in the 1920s – only 6.7 per cent of the population was over sixty in 1926 – by the 1960s the USSR found its populace aligning with the broader 'demographic shift' observed across Europe and elsewhere, where an increasingly large proportion of populations had crossed the mark of 'old age'. By 1975 approximately 13 per cent of the Soviet Union was now older than sixty.[1] As elsewhere, this demographic shift had been caused by a combination of factors, from declining birth rates to increased standards of living and improving healthcare. Yet whatever the causes, it was undeniable that the USSR was starting to grey around the temples.

Ageing is universal: one of the few aspects of human existence that can, at least today, be expected and shared across class, national and geographic borders. This is in many ways something to be celebrated, since, as the American geriatrician Louise Aronson has put it, hardly anyone would choose the alternative to growing old.[2] But for individuals and societies alike, the unavoidable toll of the years brings with it challenges and the need for change. Ageing bodies require individuals to confront the feeling of 'circles growing smaller until they cease' that the poet Donald Hall noted, while states are faced with reductions in working populations, lowered tax receipts and the need to provide additional services.[3] The chapters in this volume show both the reduction in personal circumference experienced by older Soviet (and socialist) citizens and the state's attempts to balance the needs of older citizens with its own ideological and economic priorities. As both Botakoz Kassymbekova and Danielle Leavitt-Quist show in their chapters, older Soviet citizens often found that their worlds were partially reduced as a result of this attempt at balance, with state demands for pensioners' unpaid childcare provision or 'efficient' housing outside of city centres conflicting with older person's own attempts to remain active and social as they aged. On the other hand, as Susan Grant and Aleksandra Brokman describe, many Soviet doctors, psychiatrists, architects and other experts were continuously at work trying to ascertain the needs of the ageing Soviet population and researching how to facilitate older person's access to resources, services and amenable housing.

Even as the population of Soviet citizens over the age of sixty grew with the decades, however, the provision of services lagged far behind. As Susan Grant highlights in her chapter, although the total number of Soviet citizens aged sixty and older had reached 28.5 million by 1970, less than 240,000 or less than 1 per cent of the total were living in state-run nursing or care homes. The vast majority remained in their own homes, or in the homes of relatives, a point brought into important comparison by both Ewelina Szpak and Pat Thane, whose respective chapters on Poland and Britain in the same post-war period demonstrate the similarity of many countries' response to similar demographic shifts. The USSR's struggles to balance the statistical ageing of its population against the needs of particular older individuals mirrored that of the West. As 'critical' gerontologists have argued in regards to the latter, this frequently aligned with the position that older and not infrequently infirm pensioners were at essence a 'problem' or 'crisis' to be solved: an existing or expected lack of workers or budget funding or a massive outlay of expenditure on rising medical costs. This sense of 'crisis', these critical voices have highlighted, has stopped many Western countries from addressing the demographic shift of the twentieth century as a space of opportunity or possible change – that is, a chance to rethink economy structures and even 'work' around the newly growing older population.[4] Instead, as the Russian philosopher Anatoly Baranov has said, the focus has remained on the outdated concept of industrial labour and the idea that after sixty-five most workers are no longer a positive asset on the balance sheet.[5]

This calculative consideration, as Baranov also points out, seems to have been alive and well in the USSR, reflected in this volume's discussion of the limitations on programmes meant to benefit the older population. Instead of moving large-scale funds into geriatric medicine, moreover, the USSR continued to focus, as Katarzyna Jarosz's chapter demonstrates, on preventative medicine and reproduction: on the health and re-creation of younger worker cohorts. At the same time, the universality of ageing was clearly undeniable, as were the biological processes underlying it – biological processes that could be modified, and in accordance with Soviet materialist ideology, as Maria Tutorskaya points out, *should* be modified. This proved an amenable entry point to the biological study of ageing, in which Soviet scientists came to hold a leading international role, from those biologists and visionaries in Moscow described in Anna Ozhiganova's chapter, to the established school of Kievan gerontology outlined by two of its leading practitioners, Vladislav Bezrukov and Yurii Duplenko. While the USSR's demographic shift did not lead to a significant change in social practice, it seems, it did spur significant interest in the biology of ageing as a clear space for Soviet science to show its drive for visionary struggle.

Science, medicine and the place of the individual

Science is just one of many possible perspectives that can be used to tell the story of ageing: a view out from under the microscope, teeming with cellular life and death, cycles of systems function and collapse, and an infinite variety of spiralled and spiralling nucleonic acids. This was a form of narrative that Soviet bio-gerontologists excelled at telling, but it was incomplete, and often little relevant to the lives of millions of older Soviet citizens, whose existences were spent not in laboratories, per se, but in the broader laboratory of late Soviet social existence. Visionary science and the hopes for the future expounded by biologists, cytologists or trainers of future generations' 'dolphin children' needed to be balanced against the mundane necessities of daily life. Like in other twentieth-century societies, Soviet medicine was in theory meant to fill in this gap: to bring the knowledge and achievements of science to the vast stretches of the Soviet Union and its hundreds of millions of citizens.

Geriatrics may never have reached the peaks of medical priority in the USSR, but as the chapters in this volume show, the influence of gerontology as a science and geriatrics as a medical discipline was able to reach many of the Soviet Union's citizens in a variety of social spheres. As Susan Grant and Botakoz Kassymbekova write in their chapters, detailed research was conducted about the housing and home care needs of older Soviet citizens – research that then found application in the development of nursing homes and projects for housing that would accommodate different generations' needs. These projects drew in part on existing gerontological research from the Institute of Gerontology in Kiev, as well as the network of geriatric medical specialists across the USSR. As Aleksandra Brokman shows in her chapter, moreover, scientific research into ailments more common in older age – whether physiological or psychological – formed the basis of many medical interventions aimed to help older Soviet citizens live healthy and productive lives.

As services were provided and medical research applied, however, the Soviet state inevitably found itself applying what Timothy Mitchell and others have termed 'state effects': practices of flattening citizens into standardized and malleable 'norms' to which services can be more efficiently provided.[6] As Brokman demonstrates, however, this process left many older Soviet citizens with debilitating mental illness outside of the remit of medical provision; Kassymbekova equally shows how the housing needs of certain older citizens (and primarily women) did not always find a place in the state's standardized models. In her chapter, Grant shows similar limits to the nursing home projects developed by Soviet architects, while also highlighting the medicalizing aspects of the flattening state effect, whereby services provided to older citizens often became standardized into the realm of the medical to the detriment of individuals' social needs.[7] Throughout, these chapters (as well as those by Ewelina Szpak and Pat Thane on similar processes in the international context) demonstrate the limits that the state application of medical research had in terms of encompassing the full breadth of older citizens' needs in the late Soviet period.

While limiting, however, the state's practices of defining old age and its place in society created a field of contention for those older people pushing to define their own space in the Soviet Union. As Danielle Leavitt-Quist and Alissa Klots and Maria Romashova show in their chapters, older Soviet citizens took it upon themselves to rewrite the social definitions around themselves. Grandmothers, Leavitt-Quist writes, redefined themselves as 'modern babushkas', engaged workers, social activists and local Communist Party leaders. Older party members and those who lived through the October Revolution and the building of socialism, Klots and Romashova write, were particularly focused on developing their historical place within the state's flattening narrative. Instead of accepting the existing unitary story of old age presented by the Soviet state, in which certain older figures (often men) were heralded and others (often women) were forgotten, Klots and Romashova's protagonists inserted themselves into the story of old age in the USSR.

Women and ageing

Many of the narratives of old age that we see in the Soviet Union are gendered and feminized. In the twentieth century women tended to outlive men everywhere,[8] but this differential was exacerbated in the Soviet Union by the loss of a generation of men during the Great Patriotic War (as the Second World War is called in Russia), which saw some 27 million citizens perish. The growing gender disparity in the population was borne out by statistics. In 1959 women constituted 55 per cent of the Soviet population, compared to 52.1 per cent in 1939.[9] Wartime population losses were met by an emphasis on reproduction and pro-natalism, exemplified by Nikita Khrushchev's proposal on the 1944 Family Code, which rewarded fertility.[10] Khrushchev, who at the time was First Secretary of the Communist Party of Ukraine, suggested a tax for the childless and infertile.[11] Women were expected to bear children irrespective of whether they were married. Demographic challenges evidently preoccupied the Soviet government after the war, and it was women who were singled out to help compensate for the millions of men who had died. Of course, the Soviet Union was not alone in its concern with the declining birth rate and demography: many other countries also worried about these problems during the twentieth century. Pat Thane's chapter, for example, captures British anxiety about population decline in the 1940s and 1950s and the measures put in place to keep older people working for longer.

The number of women in the Soviet population increased in the 1960s. Differences remained particularly pronounced in rural areas where women 'remained tied to the land'.[12] A growing trend of predominantly older people living in the countryside was also visible in post-war Poland, as Ewelina Szpak's chapter shows so convincingly. Women in the late Stalinist and Khrushchev years were engaged in both paid and unpaid labour to fill the gaps left in the job market. Before the Great Patriotic War in 1941 about 40 per cent of paid workers in the

Soviet Union were women; this increased to 55 per cent immediately after the war and stood at 49 per cent in 1964.[13] Middle-aged and older women were well-represented in these post-war figures, with women over forty returning to work after their children had reached adulthood.[14] In contrast to the Stalinist years, Khrushchev (and later Leonid Brezhnev) attempted to raise the Soviet standard of living through welfare reforms. Although many Soviet citizens continued to contend with problems such as a lack of housing, a less than efficient healthcare service or low salaries, living conditions generally improved.[15] This was to an extent reflected in life expectancy rates, which increased for women after 1955 and remained at about seventy-three years between 1960 and 1986.[16]

But when people reached old age, their meagre pension (if they had one) meant that they often had to remain in work or were dependent on their families for support. This was despite the pension reforms that Khrushchev introduced in the mid-1950s. 'Age relations', as sociologist Toni Calasanti notes, 'constitute an axis of inequality, and thus old age disadvantages both men and women.'[17] Despite the disadvantages of age, some Soviet pensioners pushed back against traditional expectations related to growing old. Older men and especially older women became involved in activist work and joined groups such as pensioners councils or women's councils (*zhensovety*). As both Leavitt-Quist and Klots and Romashova show, older women refused to be marginalized because of their age and were eager to continue their work as builders of communism.

Indeed, the 1960s witnessed the emergence of a politically engaged, self-monitored 'public woman', made legible through autobiographical text.[18] As Leavitt-Quist shows in her chapter, the 'modern babushka' represented a stark contrast to the traditional image of Russian and Soviet grandmothers. The post-war era saw women and grandmothers assert themselves at the local level through their involvement in the community. This activism reflected the trend of a rising number of women who were also members of the Communist Party.[19] Still, as successive Soviet generations grew older and increasingly infirm, the physical disadvantages of old age became evident. The need for medical and social support often set limitations on old people's independence, as we see in Szpak's discussion of one eighty-year-old woman in 1970s Poland. Older women were also more likely to be more materially disadvantaged, as Kassymbekova argues in her chapter, a fact that no doubt had implications for their long-term health. Various paradoxical depictions and images of older women are evident in this book – a sign that there is no standard for how women, or indeed men, should behave as they grow old, or how they experience their old age.

Attitudes to and perceptions of older people

In her book on old age, the writer and philosopher Simone de Beauvoir captures many of the negative attitudes that society harbours towards old age, and especially towards ageing women. She describes the societal expectations placed on old people, who are held up as virtuous or mocked if they deviate from this image; either way, 'they stand outside humanity'.[20] Although harshly negative, de Beauvoir's reflections find place in both Soviet history and, indeed, contemporary society. Western society's ongoing attempts to prevent and slow down the ageing process, whether through exercise, rejuvenation or medication, reflect people's discomfort with old age.

In his work on constructing and deconstructing old age, the sociologist and social anthropologist Haim Hazan writes about several 'traps' when it comes to the representation of old age. These include social, cultural, personal and theoretical traps, all of which often prove difficult to avoid when writing about ageing and older people.[21] Society, for example, might attribute certain stereotypes and labels, such as wisdom or senility, to older people and thus perpetuate a specific imagery around ageing.[22] Older people can also be trapped by the roles that family and society assign to them.[23] In the Soviet context, we can see this happening through the role of the *babushka* (grandmother), as described by Leavitt-Quist in her chapter. But as Leavitt-Quist shows, such stereotypes of the wise, old, homely babushka were not representative of many older women in late Soviet society. Similarly, in her chapter on psychiatry, Brokman shows that Soviet expectations about healthy persons left little space for older people living with mental illness or dementia. Whether in the hospital or in the home, older people were commonly confronted with ideas and images that did not reflect their reality.

Society's attitudes towards older people and the ageing process are reflected in the pursuit of youth and immortality. These appear extreme in the early Soviet period when rejuvenation captured the imagination of scientists and the public. In showing how ageing and death were represented and approached in early Soviet society, Tutorskaya's chapter leaves us in no doubt that science and medicine have 'magical' qualities that can influence perceptions of ageing. Attempts to halt the processes of ageing were not limited to the early Soviet period: we also see examples of scientists seeking to improve longevity and health in old age in Ozhiganova's chapter. Infants and children, rather than older adults, became the subjects of experimentation to improve their immune systems and life expectancy, essentially achieving 'physical maturity'. We continue to see similar attitudes to delaying old age or pursuing cultural expectations of physical health in contemporary society, where scientists and medical practitioners in many countries in the Western world advertise various sorts of 'anti-ageing' treatments. In Russia the pursuit of immortality is still visible in the form of cryonics, the science of freezing and later reanimating the dead.[24]

Apparent in this fascination with ageing is the importance of narratives and discourse and how the state (and its various organs of power in the case of the Soviet Union), media and society shape perceptions of ageing and old age. Many of the chapters in this book refer to 'stories' of some kind, such as the legend of Gilgamesh in Bezrukov and Yurii Duplenko's chapter, the museum narratives and stories in Jarosz's chapter or the fairy tales described in Tutorskaya's chapter. Our attitudes and understanding of ageing, whether we realize it or not, are shaped by a range of factors that promote certain ideas around ageing, whether positive or negative. The crafting of narratives is an ongoing symbiotic process between state and society. We see this kind of creation of public and private narratives quite explicitly in the chapter by Klots and Romashova.

Older people writing about their own lives and ageing is perhaps one of the best ways we can understand old age. But as Hazan has acknowledged, there is a dearth of scholarship 'dedicated to deciphering the world of old people as subjects, and even less of this work attempts to understand the ways in which knowledge about ageing is produced and reproduced'.[25] Although Soviet gerontologists produced a vast literature on older people, and did much to advance our understanding of ageing, there is still much that we can learn. In this volume scholars from various disciplinary backgrounds discuss a range of themes and issues about ageing to better understand contemporaneous society and the world of older people.

Chapter synopses

This book is divided into four sections, generally focused on biological gerontology, medical and social care for older persons, narratives of ageing and the international context in which ageing in the Soviet Union existed. The first section opens with a chapter by two leading Soviet and Ukrainian bio-gerontologists, Vladislav Bezrukov and Yurii Duplenko. Using their extensive first-hand experience and unique access to institutional history, Bezrukov and Duplenko describe the development of Soviet biological gerontology – the study of the underlying mechanisms of ageing – from its inception in the 1920s through its heyday in the 1970s and 1980s. By the latter decades of the Soviet period, as Bezrukov and Duplenko describe, the USSR was at the forefront of many scientific debates in the field of gerontology, with important international influence in a number of subfields. From the central Institute of Gerontology in Kiev, Ukraine, moreover, Soviet scientists directed a wide network of research centres across the USSR.

While Bezrukov and Duplenko describe the history of Soviet biological gerontology spanning from the 1920s to 1980s, Maria Tutorskaya's chapter focuses on the 1920s as a period of especial vibrancy in the history of Soviet gerontology. From the research projects conceived and pursued to the level of social interest in ageing research, Tutorskaya writes, the 1920s demonstrated a push for 'visionary science' in the field of ageing. This was in line with the broader Bolshevik agenda to remake the physical work as part of their drive to build communism; it was also aligned, Tutorskaya writes, with the traditional Russian view of medicine as miracle-work. With the early twentieth century having gifted humanity with flight and the moving image, she suggests, it was hardly far-fetched for early Bolshevik scientists to begin thinking about 'apples of youth' as well.

Completing the first section, Anna Ozhiganova's chapter also touches on the intersection of visionary belief and hard science through a description of the work of Ilya Arshavsky and its relation to human development and ageing. Arshavsky, as Ozhiganova writes, conducted unique research on the processes early in life – the so-called winding up the clock of life – that had positive effects much later. This body of research came to emphasize the importance of physical activity and controlled physical stress in childhood, which in turn inspired a range of semi-scientific or even pseudo-scientific efforts to harness these effects. This included 'cold treatments' for infants or the extensive 'aquaculture' programme of Igor Charkovsky; Ozhiganova demonstrates how these programmes served to support Arshavsky's conclusions just as his body of work had inspired their creation.

The second part of the book examines different aspects of eldercare, specifically mental health and the living needs of older people. Aleksandra Brokman analyses psychiatric care for older people in the post-war Soviet Union, using patients in Moscow's Clinical Psychiatry Hospital No. 4 named for P. B. Gannushkin as a case study. Psychiatrists and medical workers in the hospital were preoccupied with the care of the body and meeting the physical needs of older patients. Here Brokman pays particular attention to the mind/body nexus in the Soviet context. Soviet psychiatrists, argues Brokman, focused on an image of the 'ideal' Soviet person and emphasized the importance of working on oneself to keep healthy. This discourse had negative implications for people who became old and sick and thus stood outside of Soviet society and its conceptions of continuous improvement. As Brokman shows, infirm older people often came to inhabit a liminal space between life and death. The chapter raises questions about mental health in old age as well as the tendency of medical institutions to see older people as 'bodies' requiring only physical care. How do hospitals 'manage' older people? What is a good old age, and according to whom?

In her chapter on ageing and the city, Botakoz Kassymbekova assesses how the urban environment worked for older Soviet citizens in the 1970s and 1980s. Although focusing on three European Soviet cities – Moscow, Leningrad and Kiev – the experience of urban ageing that Kassymbekova describes seems representative of the Soviet urban environment *in toto*. We learn that urban planners took a 'familial' approach to accommodating older people, with multi-generational families living with or close to one another. As Kassymbekova shows, older persons often preferred to live in communal housing rather than the new style of individualized living that became more commonplace after Stalin. As well as detailing the kind of housing that older people lived in, Kassymbekova also examines how urban planners and sociologists discussed improving the accommodation options for older people in the city. These debates about ageing in a city speak to a larger discussion about the humanization of Soviet society. Why did sociologists want to make new urban neighbourhoods more 'human' for older people? What does this quest for greater 'humanization' tell us about Soviet society in the 1970s and 1980s?

Susan Grant's chapter on care homes for older people in the late Soviet Union demonstrates how Soviet attempts to design and build multifunctional homes eventually became subservient to the simple demand of accommodating growing numbers of older people in need of medical care. Cold war politics, Grant argues, also played a role in influencing Soviet architectural thinking on living conditions for older people. Architects and urban planners looked abroad to Europe and the United States for ideas about designing homes for older people. Drawing on best practices abroad, they then transposed these ideas to socialist experience and collective living. Grant focuses on general (*tipovye*) types of homes to show how Soviet utopian visions of the nursing home developed and were realized in the late Soviet period. These visions had to contend with numerous limitations, including construction priorities and budgets, as well as the built environment. The chapter raises questions about how care home design, whether in the USSR or elsewhere, is able to meet the changing needs of older people.

The modern *babushka* is the subject of Danielle Leavitt-Quist's chapter. In analysing representations of the 'classic babushka', Leavitt-Quist debunks myths related to older women in Soviet society. She argues that debates about the modern babushka had serious implications for ideas of communist morality, care and socially useful work. The changing needs and desires of babushkas in the late Soviet period led to intra-generational tensions. Older people who had contributed to building communism after the 1917 revolution wanted to continue their pursuit of socially useful work, often to the chagrin of their children who expected their mothers to assume the role of de facto nanny. This new scenario, as Leavitt-Quist also shows, led to sociological debate about the modern babushka. Drawing on magazines, film and archival sources, Leavitt-Quist's chapter asks several important questions about paid and unpaid labour in old age, social expectations around grandmothers and the representation of older women.

In the third section of the book, two chapters emphasize the importance of narrative and storytelling in the process of ageing. In their chapter, Alissa Klots and Maria Romashova describe the process of self-making undertaken by a series of older activists in the city of Perm in the latter decades of the USSR. These individuals – primarily women – had been part of the Soviet project since the beginning, teaching at Soviet schools, volunteering in literacy and atheist campaigns, and engaging in the committee work that underpinned much of the Soviet state's development project. They had not, however, been part of the Soviet state's official narrative of socialism's building: they had not fought in the Revolution, nor had they held important state posts. When given the opportunity to engage with the history of the USSR and their own history as ageing Soviet citizens, however, these activists came to see their own important place in the larger narrative, literally writing themselves back into the files and story of the ageing Soviet state.

Klots and Romashova's chapter on individual narratives is complemented by the next chapter by Katarzyna Jarosz, which compares and contrasts nine post-Soviet medical museums, with a focus on how these museums describe the process of ontogenesis – the process of life from birth to development to death. Overwhelmingly, Jarosz finds that the latter processes of life – ageing and death – are left out of this narrative – or are dealt with in a very limited fashion. Instead, she writes, the focus throughout the former Soviet sphere in medical museums remains on childbirth, childhood and preventative medicine, the hallmarks of the Soviet medical system and more or less the same discourse that can be found in the late Soviet period. Perhaps out of place in the visionary conception of socialism or the high modernity of the present, Jarosz writes, the prosaic nature of old age and death from chronic illness is simply not to be found.

In the final, international section of the volume, several themes already considered are examined in different contexts. Gender, representation and eldercare are addressed in Ewelina Szpak's chapter, where she assesses the burden of old age in Poland after the Second World War. Szpak analyses official discourse and older people's experiences to determine the accuracy of images of destitute pensioners in Polish society. Her analysis includes a close consideration of economic and welfare policies, as well as urban and rural contexts – and provides important insight into the woefully inadequate Polish pension system. With many pensioners in dire financial straits, Szpak assesses some of the sociological and medical discourses around social responsibility and care for older people. Szpak looks at how these issues played out in rural and urban settings and pays particular attention to problems of financial dependence and housing options. This chapter asks important questions about the structures that states can put in place to prevent older people from falling into poverty.

The last chapter turns to ageing and gerontology in the UK. Pat Thane discusses many pertinent issues around old age, including labour, pensions, discrimination, family, social welfare and representations of older people. As Thane's chapter shows, Britain in the mid-twentieth century was at the forefront of scholarship on ageing and older people, and this included studies of older people at work, geriatric medicine, as well as sociological research. As Thane notes, the emergence of geriatrics in Britain in the mid-1930s marked a move towards 'more positive thinking about old age'. This young field developed in subsequent decades, although it lacked prestige. Growing interest in ageing, as well as improved access to healthcare after the establishment of the NHS, benefited older people but did not eradicate inequalities or age discrimination. Thane also examines representations of old age and gender, arguing that older women were more likely to live in poverty, and that wealthier older people were (and are) less likely to fall into age-related stereotypes. Thane's chapter captures much of the progress made over the last one hundred years – but also shows how older people are still confronted with a myriad of challenges, including the age-related discrimination that remains endemic in many environments.

Notes

1 For statistics and analysis of the USSR's changing demographics in the mid-twentieth century, see I. Kaliniuk, 'Starenie naseleniia SSSR', in D.I. Valentei et al. (eds.), *Pozhilye liudi v nashei strane. Vypusk 19* (Moscow: Statistika, 1977), 16.
2 Louise Aronson, *Elderhood: Redefining Aging, Transforming Medicine, Reimagining Life* (New York: Bloomsbury, 2019), 400.
3 Donald Hall, 'Out the Window: The View in Winter', *The New Yorker*, 23 January 2012.

4   For leading voices in this critical body of literature, see Kavita Sivaramakrishnan, *As the World Ages: Rethinking a Demographic Crisis* (Cambridge: Harvard University Press, 2018); Stephen Katz, *Disciplining Old Age: The Formation of Gerontological Knowledge* (Charlottesville: University Press of Virginia, 1996).

5   A. Baranov, 'V god smerti moego pokoleniia', in M.B. Khodorkovskii (ed.), *Postchelovechestvo* (Moscow: Algoritm, 2006), 270–301.

6   Timothy Mitchell, 'Society, Economy, and the State Effect', in Timothy Mitchell and George Steinmetz (eds.), *State/Culture* (Ithaca: Cornell University Press, 2018), 76–97; also see James C. Scott, *The Art of Not Being Governed: An Anarchist History of Upland Southeast Asia* (New Haven: Yale University Press, 2009).

7   For a broader critique of the medicalization of ageing, see Carroll L. Estes and Elizabeth A. Binney, 'The Biomedicalization of Aging: Dangers and Dilemmas', *The Gerontologist* 29, no. 5 (1989): 587–96.

8   Phyliss Moen, 'Gender, Age, and the Life Course', in Robert H. Binstock and Linda K. George (eds.), *Handbook of Aging and the Social Sciences* (San Diego; London: Academic Press, 1996), 171–87.

9   Melanie Ilic, 'Women in the Khrushchev Era: An Overview', in Melanie Ilic, Susan E. Reid and Lynne Attwood (eds.), *Women in the Khrushchev Era* (Basingstoke and New York: Palgrave Macmillan, 2004), 7.

10 Mie Nakachi, 'Population, Politics and Reproduction: Late Stalinism and Its Legacy', in Juliane Fürst (ed.), *Late Stalinist Russia: Society between reconstruction and reinvention* (London and New York: Routledge, 2006), 23–44.

11 Nakachi, 'Population, Politics and Reproduction', 30; 40. Many of Khrushchev's proposals were accepted and the 1944 Family Code remained in place until the late 1960s.

12 Ilic, 'Women in the Khrushchev Era', 7.

13 Ibid. For more on female labour in the Khrushchev period, see Donald Filtzer, 'Women Workers in the Khrushchev Era', in Melanie Ilic, Susan E. Reid and Lynne Attwood (eds.), *Women in the Khrushchev Era* (Basingstoke and New York: Palgrave Macmillan, 2004), 29–51.

14 Barbara A. Anderson, 'The Life Course of Soviet Women Born 1905–1960', in James R. Millar (ed.), *Politics, Work, and Daily Life in the USSR* (Cambridge and New York: Cambridge University Press, 1987), 203.

15 These kinds of improvements have been attributed to the rise of the welfare state in the twentieth century. See Christine L. Fry, 'Age, Aging, and Culture', in Robert H. Binstock and Linda K. George (eds.), *Handbook of Aging and the Social Sciences* (San Diego and London: Academic Press, 1996), 117–36.

16 Barbara A. Anderson and Brian D. Silver, 'The Changing Shape of Soviet Mortality, 1958–1985: An Evaluation of Old and New Evidence', *Population Studies* 43, no. 2 (1989): (243–54), 246. The authors note the inaccuracy of Soviet population statistics, particularly among certain age cohorts.

17 Toni Calasanti, 'Gender and Ageing in the Context of Globalization', in Dale Dannefer and Chris Philipson (eds.), *The SAGE Handbook of Social Gerontology* (London: SAGE Publications Ltd., 2010), 137–50, quote on 142, DOI: http://dx.doi.org/10.4135/9781446200933.n10, accessed 30 June 2015, 137–50.

18 Marianne Liljeström, 'Monitored Selves: Soviet Women's Autobiographical Texts in the Khrushchev Era', in Melanie Ilic, Susan E. Reid and Lynne Attwood (eds.), *Women in the Khrushchev Era* (Basingstoke and New York: Palgrave Macmillan, 2004), 131–45.

19 For statistics, see Gail Warshofsky Lapidus, *Women in Soviet Society: Equality, Development, and Social Change* (Los Angeles and London: University of California Press, 1978), 210.

20 Simone de Beauvoir, *Old Age*, trans. Patrick O' Brian (Middlesex: Penguin Books, 1985 [1970]), 10.

21 Haim Hazan, *Old Age: Constructions and Deconstructions* (Cambridge: Cambridge University Press, 1994), 13–52.

22 Hazan, *Old Age*, 28–32.

23 Hazan, *Old Age*, 40–5.

24 For discussion of the history and contemporary state of Russian cryonics, see Anya Bernstein, *The Future of Immortality: Remaking Life and Death in Contemporary Russia* (Princeton: Princeton University Press, 2019).

25 Hazan, *Old Age*, 3.

Part One

Soviet gerontology: Ageing as a field of scientific study

1

The legend of Gilgamesh: Attempts at its realization in Soviet gerontology

Vladislav Bezrukov and Yurii Duplenko
Translated by Isaac Scarborough

Dating to the second millennium BCE, the Accadian legend of Gilgamesh tells of the posthumously deified ruler of the Sumerian state of Uruk (located in modern-day Iraq). Gilgamesh is considered the contemporary of the biblical Abraham. The mythological Gilgamesh is said to have ruled for a period of 126 years. Tales of Gilgamesh have reached our days in the form of an epic poem, rewritten or recorded in the seventh or eighth century BCE under the title of 'Gilgamesh, Enkidu, and the Netherworld'. In the poem, Gilgamesh first recognizes his own mortality while mourning his friend Enkidu. He seeks and finds the only individual, Uta-Napishti, to have received the gift of immortality from the gods; from Uta-Napishti he learns of the secret Flower of Eternal Youth. Having retrieved the Flower, Gilgamesh loses it to a thieving snake, leaving him without the possibility of putting to use its miraculous magical power.[1]

This legend reflects humanity's ancient dream to extend life and return youth. History tells of innumerable attempts – sadly, all in vain – to acquire immortality or overcome ageing. Consider the alchemists' search for the 'philosopher's stone' or later anti-ageing blood transfusions. But there have been more grounded attempts made by naturalists, scientists and doctors to fulfil this human dream. One striking example of such work can be found in the history of Soviet gerontology, which aimed to illuminate the mechanisms of ageing and begin to feel out ways of extending human lifespan and health-span.

We have attempted here to analyse the central schools of thought that developed in Soviet gerontology's subdisciplines of biological and physiological studies, as well as to clarify the influence of earlier scientists' progressive views on later stages of the development of gerontological conceptions. Finally, we suggest some future possibilities for the discipline. We believe this work is timely and topical: the authors of previous generalizing works on the history of gerontology have not focused attention on the particularities of gerontological concepts in the USSR.[2] In Soviet literature, on the other hand, there were until the final quarter of the twentieth century little more than short historical supplements to bibliographical bulletins of national works on developmental physiology, biochemistry, or morphology. This historical analysis of Soviet gerontology is of particular importance, however, insofar as the USSR's school of gerontological science led research in the twentieth century across many aspects of human ageing. Rationally predicting future areas of development in the discipline is possible only through a close investigation of the historical succession of ideas across time and geography.

Soviet gerontology's biological pre-history

Soviet gerontology's first glimmerings could be observed in the 1920s and were due to an application of the results achieved from the generally accepted (at the start of the twentieth century) physical-chemical approach to physiological studies of ageing processes. This approach, in turn, would have been inconceivable without the work of A. Weisman, I. Mechnikov, E. Maupas, Ch. Minot, N. Kholodkovskii and V. Shimkevich in the 1880s–90s; their research provided the evolutionary and cytological basis needed for the formation of gerontological concepts. Physical-chemical ideas about the processes of ageing were developed in the USSR by A. Blagoveshchenskii, A. Kizel and E. Bauer. Their ideas were part and parcel of the broader worldwide contemporaneous discussions about the roots of ageing, including 'protoplasmic hysteresis' (imbalanced cellular and chromatin development), 'the maturation of colloids' in live tissues and their flocculation (coagulation), and the tendency of molecules towards ring formation over the course of ontogenesis (lifespan). It is worth noting that N. Gaidukov and V. Lepeshkin made interesting observations about colloidal changes associated with the onset of death as early as 1911–13.[3] In 1925–35, moreover, A. Blagoveshchenskii connected these physical-chemical changes with reductions in an organism's energy potential, reactionary capacity and ability to withstand change.[4] Later Blagoveshchenskii wrote that as ageing progressed, 'more and more importance is taken on by exothermic reactions, leading to the build-up of the long-lasting by-products of specialized cellular processes'.[5] According to experimental work conducted by A. Kizel, increased age notably lessened the solubility of proteins. He emphasized the definite relationship between the rate of protein ageing and the length of normal life expectancy for one or another life form.[6] These ideas about the connections between ageing and molecular changes were quite progressive for their time; they were later confirmed by experimental data. Early Soviet research into the physical-chemical parameters of metabolic function and ageing was also highly appraised at the time by A. Nagornyi, the future founder of one of the Soviet Union's leading schools of gerontological thought – the Kharkov school of developmental physiology and biochemistry.[7]

E. Bauer took a more unusual approach to the study of ageing's molecular processes. In his discussions about 'molecules of live matter', he built off of the concept of 'live protein', which had been suggested by E. Pfluger and later developed by M. Rubner. The logic of contemporaneous natural science led him to a generally colloidal-chemical framework for age-related changes. Working in a laboratory together with V. Ružička, Bauer also took part in experiments with V. Bergauer meant to research processes of protoplasmic hysteresis. The results of these experiments were publicized in a series of articles under the heading of 'Towards the Causes of Ageing', in which Bauer aimed to clarify the physical underpinnings of those changes observed at the basis of cellular hysteresis (imbalanced development caused by structural damage).[8] In these articles Bauer connected cellular hysteresis with ageing-related changes in electric charges of the protoplasm's molecules. Later Bauer worked to consider the processes of ageing-related molecular changes more broadly. Conducted in Moscow, his work was driven by a desire to find an explanation for certain phenomenon he had observed in living organisms; as he put it, 'in the particular condition of that molecular structure that is characteristic for living matter'. He operated with the foundational concept (as he postulated) of the 'stable imbalance of living systems', which provides the capacity for life.

This imbalanced state, in Bauer's view, was defined by a molecular structure – the 'deformed state of molecules' or 'the activation of molecules' – and was expressed in the free energy that was particular to this structure ('the system potential'). Bauer's theory of an organism's naturally increasing limitations on growth was based on that organism's reaching a maximum 'system potential' (or 'assimilation limit'). Theoretically investigating the levels of a system's free energy over time, he came to the conclusion that this energy 'must decrease following the attainment of the assimilation limit. In this way, an organism's ageing is unavoidable'.[9] This theory helped Bauer arrive at morphogenetic mechanisms of ageing. He equally emphasized the close connection between mechanisms of ageing and cancer growth. This overlap allowed him to conclude that changes in metabolism, which naturally occurred during ageing, were also characteristic for organisms experiencing cancerous growths. At the same time, he also concluded that such conditions as come together in an ageing organism are conducive to cancer growth. This formulation was in concordance with the spirit of Bauer's age: an attempt to shed light on many common aspects amongst different physical processes.

In his theoretical work, Bauer noted a well-defined mutual supervenience between metabolic intensity, the speed of ageing processes and the length of expected lifespan. The modern development of gerontology provides some evidence of Bauer's influence. Today, the concept of a 'specific metabolic level' particular to one or another lifeform is used in gerontological theory to define ageing levels and the limits of expected lifespan. This appears to point to Bauer's early work as an important step towards modern conceptions of ageing.

Another of the initiators of Soviet gerontology and the founder of one of its central schools, Aleksandr Bogomolets, also based his work over the course of 1926–39 on the physical-chemical characteristics of cellular bio-colloid ageing. In 1932 Bogomolets wrote that cellular colloids' ageing process 'brought cells, by way of their aged micelles [colloid particles] to a condition of standstill much earlier than the capacity for cellular plasma to regenerate itself chemically is extinguished'.[10] Put another way, long before the mechanisms of protein biosynthesis were mapped, Bogomolets was insisting on the importance of age-related changes in protein molecules for broader mechanisms of ageing. Considering his arguments from the position of modern gerontology, which tends to divide age-related changes in the synthesis of protein molecules and post-translational molecular changes – the so-called molecular ageing – it is worth noting that Bogomolets aimed to describe the latter process and its links to processes of self-renewal. Later on, this research trajectory would be developed further by A. Nagornyi.

Having begun working in the field of developmental physiology and biochemistry in 1922, Nagornyi quickly grew interested in gerontology, giving a series of public lectures at Kharkov University on the physiology of periods of change and preparing a theoretical monograph published in 1923 under the title of 'Life, Ageing, and Death'.[11] In 1926–7, moreover, he conducted a series of experiments investigating the hysteresis of gelatinous tissues. Nagornyi's ideas and work brought together a group of students and like-minded researchers, whose collective work over many years led to the formation of a respected scientific school – the Kharkov school of developmental physiology and biochemistry. Together, experiments conducted in Kharkov under Nagornyi's oversight formed the basis for a new conception of the mechanisms of ageing and the driving factors of ontogenesis.[12] This conception was first outlined in Nagornyi's 1940 monograph *The Problem of Ageing and Longevity*.[13] One of the central elements of Nagornyi's approach to the study of ageing was analysis of an organism as an indivisible whole of chemical activity, structure and function. This led to the conclusion that age-related changes would be synthesized chemically, physically-chemically, morphologically and functionally. The framework for an individual live organism's patterns of ontogenesis and growth was outlined in his 1940 monograph. In it, Nagornyi operated from the conception that 'during its development over the course of a life, the metabolism is the cause of the occurrence of conditions in the organism, which in early stages aid metabolic processes, but which at later stages, in contrast, complicate and slow them down'.[14]

Nagornyi's ideas demonstrate the further development – and molecular documentation – of the fruitful concept previously discussed by I. Shmalgauzen in the USSR and J. Bidder in the West:[15] namely, the effects of a certain regulatory mechanism, active over the course of an individual organism's lifespan, which initially plays a progressive (developmental) role, but later leads to restrictions on biological activity, bringing about a limit on individual existence. In later decades (1958–75), this idea was transformed by Vladimir Dilman into the modern concept of the 'elevational ageing mechanism'.[16] (Dilman, based in Leningrad, was the central figure in the Leningrad school of gerontology.) For his part, Nagornyi concluded that the main cause of an individual organism's ontogenesis and particular path of development could be found in the slow loss of that organism's capacity for regeneration. This idea of waning regenerative capacity was embedded by Nagornyi at the centre of his work on the mechanisms of ageing.

Parallel to Nagornyi and others' work on the structural processes of ageing, moreover, early Soviet scientists were also investigating the control mechanisms behind these processes. As early as the second half of the nineteenth century work began on the idea of physiological self-regulation. In the beginning of the twentieth century, further development of physiological ideas related to the regulation of metabolism and cellular function led to research on homeostasis and modern concepts of neurohormonal regulation.[17] This provided the basis on which to conduct experiments into mechanisms of ageing from the perspective of age-related changes in the neurohormonal system. In the 1920s N. Belov, a student of A. Reprev (Kharkov University) and the colleague of V. Bekhterev at the Institute for the Study of the Brain, first proposed studying ageing as a result of disequilibrium, unavoidably occurring over time through the complex mutual interactions of human organs and internal systems. In 1922 Belov published a chapter from a previous manuscript under the title of 'Age-related Variability as a Result of the Laws of Mutual Interaction of Organismal Elements'. In this work Belov attempted to apply his previously formulated conception of 'parallel-crossed organismal construction' – that is, negative reflexive linkages in regulation – in order to explain individual levels of variation and age-related organismal changes.[18]

Belov's was one of the first attempts to develop a mathematical model covering an organism's age-related changes. By researching these changes, Belov posited, it would be possible to analyse the 'overall schematic of organized structures' in order to characterize the 'general conditions accompanying the lifecycle of living creatures'. He concluded that the system of organismal regulation holds within itself mechanisms that would unavoidably undermine that very system; it was this process of degradation that represented ageing and led to organismal death. Belov's systemic approach to ageing was developed further by A. Bogdanov (Malinovsky), who outlined his views on the mechanisms of ageing in the book *The Fight for Life and Health*, published in 1927.[19] This was an attempt to understand the processes of ageing from the perspective of Bogdanov's own theoretical framework, 'tektology' (*tektologiia*) – a framework that found influence in the latter half of the twentieth century in the development of systems theory and cybernetics.[20] Applying his theories to ageing, Bogdanov argued that loss of life capacity over time was the basis for age-related change, while activity that counteracted ageing should be understood as the creation of 'conditions for the greatest possible life activity'. His work hinted at later understandings of 'vitality minimums', which occur during ageing, as well as their importance as limitational steps in biological systems that lead to the development of age-related changes. This was also the basis for Bogdanov's view that blood transfusions during the ageing process could act as a method 'to equalize the most weakened element' – and, equally, his broader views on blood transfusion.[21]

The adaptational theory of ageing

Already by the 1940s, the broader development of the biological sciences led to a realization that greater research into the processes of life activity and ontogenesis on the molecular level was necessary. Leading scientific discoveries were mobilized in the search for ageing's molecular mechanisms. Nagornyi's students, I. Bulankin and V. Nikitin, made an important contribution towards developing their teacher's concepts. Their research into the age-related changes involved in the synthesis and metabolism of proteins over the course of ontogenesis provided for a series of new discoveries, which were included in the second edition of *The Problem of Ageing and Longevity*, published in 1963. Here they noted that, first, as an organism's age increases, so increases the frequency of observable changes in proteins on the supramolecular level.[22] Second, their work demonstrated that ageing was the result of cellular and tissue differentiation: as cells aimed at optimal regenerative results, they eventually reached a limit. As part of this broader work, V. Nikitin proposed the idea that with increased age came the growing 'pessimization' (degradation in form) of gene structure and a cell's protein synthesis, which in turn were defined as the deciding factor in an organism's process of ontogenesis, molecularly or biologically speaking. This was particular true of DNA and its formation in the chromatin.[23]

During the same period (1960–9) B. Goldshtein, working at the Institute of Gerontology in Kiev, also argued that DNA should be the central focus on research into the driving mechanisms of biological ageing. Goldshtein held that DNA was one of the most frequently regenerating structures in a cell, as well as the factor that defined the biosynthesis of proteins. He underlined the importance of qualitative changes in DNA structure. In particular, Goldshtein emphasized the role of DNA fragmentation, triggered by the build-up of chelated iron in a molecule, which then affected the process of DNA replication – in turn influencing changes in the structure of DNA.[24] He was one of a few scientists at the time working to connect age-related changes in molecular mechanisms to particular changes in DNA, which had been indirectly confirmed through experiments – changes that were reflected in changes to the functional capacity of a cell's genetic material. In later years (1965–81), Vladimir Frolkis, continuing Goldshtein's work at the Institute of Gerontology, argued for a genetic-regulatory theory of ageing. According to this theory, the central focus of research into ageing ought to be not only structural changes in DNA molecules, but also shifts in the realization of genetic information, in other words in the regulation of the overall process of DNA transcription.[25]

In later years Frolkis and his students at the Institute of Gerontology established a systematic approach to research into the mechanisms of ageing, which included analysis at all systemic levels, from the molecular and genetic to the organismal. The basis for this approach was the adaptational-regulatory theory of ageing, which Frolkis developed over the course of 1960–81. Its roots, however, reach back into the history of gerontology; Frolkis's theory would have been inconceivable without preceding research. Amongst the works already mentioned above and others, we can highlight a number of studies that provided particular foundational support for Frolkis's theories. These included Shmalgauzen's research into the natural laws of growth (1926), Bauer's conception of 'stable imbalance' in living organisms (1935–6), A. Dogel's research on age-related changes in sympathetic ganglia (1922),[26] M. Milman's neurotrophic hypothesis (1926),[27] the experiments conducted by S. Voronov (1924–7),[28] the development of an endocrinological theory of ageing by N. Shereshevskii and M. Zavadovskii (1924–41),[29] work conducted on the physiology of ageing by the students of I. Pavlov (1912–55)[30] and, finally, research programmes targeting organismal reactivity under the oversight of A. Bogomolets (1926–39). It was Frolkis's approach to the study of ageing and its underlying mechanisms, building upon the work of his predecessors in the field, that proved to be the most promising in terms of crafting a comprehensive theory of an organism's (human or animal) ontogenetic development – and pointing towards solutions for the challenge of extending life and health-spans.

The Institute of Gerontology

Everything described here demonstrates that by the end of the 1930s the USSR – as other countries of the world – was observing the consolidation of gerontology as a scientific discipline.[31] Those scientists working on gerontology began to form 'schools' of thought and scientific collectives came together. Around this time the first scientific conferences on gerontology were convened: one of the first in the world was the All-Union Conference on Ageing, the Genesis of Old Age and Preventing Premature Ageing, which was held in Kiev in 1938.[32] This conference was organized by A. Bogomolets, at the time the president of the Ukrainian Academy of Sciences. Thanks to his particular efforts, the growth of Soviet gerontology began to acquire certain aspects of administrative development as well. The 1938 conference aided the formation of collectives within the young discipline of Soviet gerontology. This began for the USSR the modern period of gerontology's development, which differed in terms of its unity: it was characterized by many parties' efforts to arrive at an optimal balance of scientific workers and materials and their coordination to solve the discipline's complex problems.

Further optimization occurred with the opening of a specialized institute, called upon to focus on the challenges of gerontology. Later on, this institute would serve as the basis for an All-Union Task Force, subsequently changed to the Scientific Council on Gerontology and Geriatrics of the Academy of

Medical Sciences of the USSR. Together with the Soviet Academy of Sciences' 'Biological and Social Foundations of Ageing' section, this Scientific Council coordinated gerontological research across the country. Finally – and this was a new, completely modern form of scientific organization – these research centres were brought together under a long-term all-union comprehensive scientific programme implemented from 1978 under the title of 'Extending Life'.[33]

The Soviet Union's Institute of Gerontology was founded as an element of the Soviet Academy of Medical Sciences in 1958 in Kiev. The choice of Kiev as the geographical basis for the institute was completely justified, given that the development of Soviet gerontology had been traditionally connected with Ukraine. This included Ilya Mechnikov's work at the Novorossiiskii University in Odessa; Shmaulgauzen at Kiev University; Nagornyi in the Institute of Biology at Kharkov University, and Bogomolets' expansive work in Kiev. The Institute's founding was also timely: towards the middle of the twentieth century the demographic situation in the USSR, much as in other economically developed countries, began to be defined more and more by the so-called ageing of its population. There was a notable shift in the absolute number – and to an even greater degree, the relative percentage – of individuals falling into older age categories. These demographic changes have occurred in different forms in different parts of the planet, but by and large the 'demographic shift' to an older population has been constant – and likely to continue in the future.

The founders of the Institute of Gerontology took into consideration the experience of previously established foreign centres of gerontological research. These included the Gerontology Branch of the National Institutes of Health, which had developed a close relationship with Baltimore City Hospital in the United States, and the Bucharest Institute of Geriatrics in Rumania. The Soviet Union's own institute (initially called the Institute of Gerontology and Experimental Pathology) was organized over the course of May–June 1958 under the medical-biological division of the Academy of Medical Sciences. Nikolai Gorev, a student of Bogomolets, was appointed as its first director. The Institute's initial Scientific Council included representatives of experimental science, including Gorev, a pathologist, and P. Marchuk, an immunologist, as well as clinicians, such as the internist D. Chebotarev and the neurologist B. Mankovskii. All four had previously worked in the Institute of Clinical Physiology of the Academy of Sciences of the Ukrainian SSR, of which Bogomolets had been the director. The Council also included the hygienists G. Shakhbazian and L. Medved. The participation of this wide spectrum of specialists in the creation and development of the new research centre in many ways helped to define the further path taken by Soviet gerontology. The Institute's staff thereafter began to slowly but consistently grow, as leading specialists in many different fields were invited to Kiev.

From its initial steps, the work of the Institute and its employees was clearly delineated into three central trajectories. The first scientific trajectory was research into the mechanisms of ageing and organismal capacity, as well as the role of regulatory processes. The second trajectory included a comprehensive package of research into the particulars of pathogenesis (disease development), diagnostics, clinical practice, treatment and disease prophylactics, all within the frame of those conditions and diseases most common in older and aged populations. The third trajectory was represented by research into the role of hygienic and social-hygienic factors in ageing and longevity. These three scientific programmes had been defined by the objectives set for the Institute of Gerontology by a Session of the Academy of Medical Sciences of the USSR held in Minsk in April 1958, which had laid the groundwork for the Institute and its activities.

Under Gorev's leadership the Institute underwent its period of growth: it grew stronger in both a scientific and organizational sense and gained many new and well-qualified scientists in its employ. The overall structure of the Institute came together, and its scientists formed networks with other collectives working on gerontology across the USSR. After 1961 the Institute of Gerontology was transferred administratively to the Clinical Medicine Division of the Academy of Medical Sciences, while D. Chebotarev became the Institute's director. Chebotarev's arrival as director of the Institute was fitting: the Institute was now led by a clinician with a wide medical profile and background, and opportunities were created for additional research into the processes of organismal ageing. It was of importance that the new director had worked for the famous clinicians N. Strazheskii and V. Ivanov, and that Bogomolets had also had a notable influence on his scientific work, bringing him to work after the Second World War in the Kiev Institute of Clinical Physiology of the Academy of Sciences of the Ukrainian SSR.

After 1961 the Institute's development was influenced by two organizational factors: first, Chebotarev placed particular importance on fundamental research in gerontology, first and foremost the biology of ageing and clinical-physiological aspects of gerontological studies. At the same time, Chebotarev was equally dedicated to finding comprehensive approaches to gerontological problems – to organically combine experimental, clinical, hygienic and social aspects of the study of ageing. Today, Chebotarev is known in the USSR as one of the founders of geriatrics as a new division of Soviet medicine, as well as one of the central figures in the organization of medical and social care for older persons. He was instrumental as well in the creation of the USSR's first Department of Gerontology and Geriatrics in the Kiev Institute of Medical Post-Diploma Education.

One of the more effective methods of coordinating scientific work in the field of gerontology proved to be through the organization of conferences, symposiums and congresses. Most frequently, the initiator for such events – and their host – was the Institute of Gerontology in Kiev. The Institute's first conference was convened in 1961, an event which attracted attention from a wide swath of the medical and scientific public. Biologists, morphologists, biochemists, physiologists and clinicians took part in this conference, arriving in Kiev from Moscow, Leningrad, Kharkov, Tbilisi, Baku, Tashkent, Kuibyshev, Tartu and other Soviet cities. This was just the first of many similar conferences and symposiums to be held at the Institute. These events were dedicated to the study of the mechanisms of ageing, the particularities of neurohormonal regulation, mobility during ageing, social-hygienic issues (lifestyle and ageing, and clinical problems), internal and psychological diseases amongst older persons, and similar topics. Conferences and symposiums were also held in Moscow, Leningrad, Tbilisi, Gorkii, Stavropol, Sukhumi, Kharkov and elsewhere.

One symposium that would come to have significant importance for the later development of Soviet gerontology was held in June 1962 in Leningrad. This symposium was dedicated to the development of classifications and terminology for periods of ageing and old age itself, as well as methods of establishing age-related limits.[34] Another important symposium – the All-Union Symposium on 'Neurohormonal Regulation in Ontogenesis' – was convened in May 1964 in Kiev. This event was attended by scientists from many institutes within the Soviet Academy of Sciences system, including those participating in the Scientific Council on 'Human and Animal Physiology' and from the Institute of Physiology named for Bogomolets in Kiev. One further notable step along the path to firmly establishing links between the country's gerontologists came with the formation of the All-Union Society of Gerontologists and Geriatricians. This occurred in Kiev in 1963 at the Society's Founding Conference, which was dedicated to functional and morphological signs of ageing. The Conference elected Chebotarev to be Chairman of the new Society, and from then on continuously organized scientific conferences and congresses, many of which included foreign participation.

The symposium 'The Reactive Capacities of the Ageing Organism', held in Kiev in 1967, particularly stands out in importance. This event saw the participation of leading international gerontologists: F. Verzar (Switzlerand), N. Shock (USA), A. Comfort (UK), W. Ries (GDR) and D. Mateev (Bulgaria). Soviet gerontologists also took active part in European and international congresses and symposiums. Yet the most notable confirmation of Soviet gerontology's increasing authority in the world came as the result of the International Association of Gerontology's (IAG) decision to hold the 9th International Congress of the IAG in the USSR, which was duly held in Kiev in 1972. Chebotarev became president of the congress – and thus for the next three years the president of the IAG. (At the risk of moving too quickly forward, we should also mention that Chebotarev wished upon his retirement to pass the leadership of the Institute to someone equally influential on the world stage. Preparing to retire in 1988, he proposed V. Bezrukov, a student of Frolkis and a specialist in the hypothalamic regulation of autonomic functions during ageing.[35] In those years, Bezrukov was working for the UN in Vienna, promoting social gerontology across the world. Today, having returned to the Institute in 1988, Bezrukov remains its director in modern independent Ukraine.)

Over the course of its history, the Institute of Gerontology grew into a major scientific-research organization: the centre of research in the USSR on the complex challenges of ageing and active longevity, as well as the coordinative headquarters for research collectives across the country, brought together as part of the Institute's work on gerontology and geriatrics. With the goal of improving the administration of related scientific research, the All-Union Task Force on gerontology was reformed by the Presidium of the Academy of Medical Sciences of the USSR in 1976 into the Scientific Council on Gerontology and Geriatrics of Academy of Medical Sciences of the USSR. This Council included eight smaller task forces, which covered a wide range of topical issues in biological gerontology, clinical practice and social-hygienic aspects of ageing. The country's gerontological community now was able to coordinate its research through this Scientific Council together with the 'Biological and Social Bases of Ageing' division of the Scientific Council on Applied Human Physiology of the Academy of Sciences of the USSR. This coordination of research projects brought together around 100 institutes and organizations, all of which were part of networks overseen by the Academy of Medical Sciences, the Ministry of Healthcare of the USSR, the Academy of Sciences of the USSR and the Academies of Sciences of various union republics.

The great volume of research conducted at the Institute, together with its organizational and administrative experience coordinating the work of the Scientific Council, provided the opportunity in 1978 to move to an even higher level of oversight on gerontological research: to the objective-management method of planning.[36] The all-union comprehensive programme 'Extending Life' was developed and confirmed by the central Soviet government, providing a platform to organize the work of many different specialists. This included biologists, physicists, chemists, physiologists, clinicians, hygienists and sociologists. The central objective of the programme was to study mechanisms of organismal ageing and on this basis develop methods and materials to preserve the health of ageing persons and extend their lifespan. The programme's implementers, its themes and its concrete activities were defined in coordination with the collectives of leading scientific-research institutes across the USSR.[37] The programme was put into reality by ten institutes from the Academy of Sciences of the USSR, ten from the Academy of Medical Sciences of the USSR, seven from the Academies of union republics, thirty-seven from the Ministries of Healthcare of the USSR and the republics, twelve universities and a variety of other institutes and state agencies.

The research planned for inclusion in the 'Extending Life' programme could be distinguished by a number of scientific foci. Research was focused on establishing causal relationships between metabolic and functional shifts during ageing; on the elucidation of key stages in ageing mechanisms; on the search for optimal methods of influencing these mechanisms. In other words, clarification of the fundamental mechanisms of ageing was set as the basis of the programme – and, within the programme, as the basis for its search for methods of extending lifespans and assisting persons to achieve active and healthy longevity.

The programme was initially planned to last for more than ten years, and included controls to verify programme implementation and, as necessary, introduce corrections. In order to track broader tendencies in the development of Soviet gerontology vis-à-vis global research in the field, efforts were undertaken from the perspective of science studies and scientometric analysis, as well the collection of expert opinions. Qualitative and quantitative analyses of worldwide publications demonstrated that the strongest and most promising of Soviet research tracks were those focused on research into genetic and regulatory mechanisms of ageing, especially neurohormonal. More than half of all Soviet publications (of those published internationally) were about topics of fundamental research and focused on neurohormonal mechanisms of ageing and metabolic and functional manifestations of ageing and old age. At the same time, this analysis discovered increasing focus within the internationally published Soviet research on genetic and molecular-biological tracks of enquiry.

According to the aggregated opinions expressed in the expert survey, research into the physiological mechanisms of ageing had developed in the USSR in alignment with the growth of their importance for gerontology. A total of eleven research tracks were analysed; of these, the following demonstrated a high or statistically significant level of correlation between development and discipline importance: research on the neurohormonal mechanisms of ageing, the immunology of ageing and functional-metabolic gerontological research. The statistical analysis and analysis of expert opinions demonstrated the factually existing tendencies in Soviet gerontology's development at the time. It further confirmed future perspectives for development, elucidated by extrapolating from current tracks of research, which had been followed throughout the comparative analysis. The specifics of the research front clarified through this analysis served as the foundation for particular recommendations that were provided to the leaders of the 'Extending Life' programme in order to further improve its implementation.

By and large, we can conclude the following: the history of Soviet gerontology analysed here demonstrates that the study of ageing followed a complex scientific path in the Soviet Union from a scattered field of separate ideas, opinions, values, suggestions and guesses to the formulation of strictly defined research trajectories, the foundation of scientific 'schools' and research collectives that together developed a comprehensive approach to the study of ageing and longevity. Together, researchers in the field developed an understanding that without elucidation of the underlying mechanisms of ageing and limitations to lifespan it would be impossible to completely clarify the shape and length of life. Controlling ageing mechanisms – one of the central aims of gerontology – this research has suggested, will open up opportunities for the extension of life.

Notes

1. Numerous versions of the Gilgamesh legend have been found and translated since the epic's rediscovery in the mid-nineteenth century. For an overview of the versions, controversies and underlying legend, see Michael Schmidt, *Gilgamesh: The Life of a Poem* (Princeton: Princeton University Press, 2019).
2. For histories of gerontology that avoid much reference to Soviet gerontology, see W. Andrew Achenbaum, *Crossing Frontiers: Gerontology Emerges as a Science* (New York: Cambridge University Press, 1995); Kavita Sivaramakrishnan, *As the World Ages: Rethinking a Demographic Crisis* (Cambridge: Harvard University Press, 2018); Stephen S. Hall, *Merchants of Immortality: Chasing the Dream of Human Life*

Extension (Boston: Houghton Mifflin, 2003); Sue Armstrong, *Borrowed Time: The Science of How and Why We Age* (London: Bloomsbury, 2019).

3   See V.V. Lepeshkin, 'O stroenii protoplazmy', *Trudy Sankt-Peterburgskogo obshchestva estestvoispytatelei* 42, nos. 1–2 (1911): 6–16; W.W. Lepeshkin, 'Death and Its Causes', *Quarterly Review of Biology* 6 (1931): 167–77; N.M. Gaidukov, 'Ul'tramikroskopicheskie issledovaniia', *Trudy Sankt-Peterburgskogo obshchestva estestvoispytatelei* 43, no. 1 (1912): 1–136. Colloids are dispersions of insoluble particles in a medium. In the body, blood is one of the most endemic colloids.

4   A.V. Blagoveshchenskii, 'K voprosu o napravlennosti protsessa evoliutsii', *Biulleten' Sredne-Aziatskogo gosudarstvennogo universiteta* 10 (1925): 17–33; A.V. Blagoveshchenskii, 'Biokhimicheskie osnovy evoliutsii organizmov', *Sotsialisticheskaia rekonstruktsiia i nauka* 5 (1935): 10–21.

5   A.V. Blagoveshchenskii, 'Biokhimiia individual'nogo razvitiia rastenii vo vzroslom sostoianii', in A.V. Blagoveshchenskii, *Biokhimicheskaia evoliutsiia tsetkovykh rastenii* (Moscow, 1966), 177–87.

6   A.A. Kizel, 'O roli razvitiia miksomitsetov i ob ego al'buminoidnom kharaktere', *Zhurnal eksperimental'noi biologii i meditsiny* 5, no. 15 (1927): 279–88.

7   See A.V. Nagornyi, *Problema Stareniia i dolgoletiia* (Kharkov, 1940).

8   E. Bauer, 'Beitrage zum Studium der Protoplasmahysteresis und der hysteresischen Vorgange (Zur Kausalitat der Alterns)' and 'Die physikalischen Voraussetzungen der hysteretischen Veranderungen', *Arch. mikroskop. Anat. Entwicklungsmech* 101 (1924): 483–8. In modern cellular biology, hysteresis is a process by which DNA is impacted by external factors, changing the shape of the chromatin, which is the packed spiral of DNA that contains instruction for the production (or suppression) of proteins, enzymes and basic cellular function. Hysteresis can imply either persistence notwithstanding external factors or imbalance, as external damage changes the chromatin and thus the expression of DNA. More recent research, while eschewing the term 'hysteresis', has emphasized the importance of a cell's history of change, damage and rebuilding on the chromatin, and the chromatin's impact on cellular function during ageing. On this point, see V.Kh. Khavinson, *Peptidnaia reguliatsiia stareniia* (St. Petersburg: Nauka, 2009); David A. Sinclair with Matthew D. LaPlante, *Lifespan: Why We Age – and Why We Don't Have To* (London: Thorsons, 2019).

9   E.S. Bauer, *Teoreticheskaia biologiia* (Moscow, 1935). Bauer's ideas of living systems' 'stable imbalance' seem strikingly similar to those posited in later decades: for example, James Lovelock's famous concept of life being an 'ordered disequilibrium' (see James Lovelock, *Gaia: A New Look at Life on Earth* (Oxford: Oxford University Press, 2000)), or NASA's concept of life as being 'a self-sustaining chemical system capable of Darwinian evolution' or, simply put, change. For the latter definition, see Philip Ball, 'Are Aliens Hiding in Plain Sight?' *The Guardian*, 5 September 2020.

10 As reprinted in A.A. Bogomolets, *Izbrannye trudy, v 3-x tomakh* (Kiev, 1956), v. 1. Micelles are the particles suspended in a colloid medium; Bogomolets emphasized the breakdown of these particles within the colloid as leading to disbalanced cellular function.
11 A.V. Nagornyi, *Zhizn', starost' i smert'* (Kharkov, 1923).
12 Ontogenesis is the history of the development of an individual organism, from the earliest stages through maturation to death.
13 Nagornyi, *Problema Stareniia i dolgoletiia*.
14 Ibid. This is remarkably similar to the modern gerontological conception of the 'disposable soma', by which it is meant that evolution has provided for biological systems that help bring an organism to maturation, but which in the process may lead to long-term structural imbalances that play out in later life. For modern versions of this theory, see Armstrong, *Borrowed Time*, 20–4.
15 I.I. Shmalgauzen, *Problema smerti i bessmertiia* (Moscow, 1926); I.I. Shmalgauzen, *Rost zhivotnykh* (Moscow, 1935), 8–84; G.P. Bidder, 'Senescence', *British Medical Journal* 2 (1932): 583–5.
16 Vladimir Dilman's idea of 'elevational ageing mechanisms' argued that over an organism's lifespan, cells' barriers to reactivity became elevated. In other words, cells reacted to low dosages of hormones early in life; the level of hormone necessary to elicit a reaction became elevated over time. With hormone levels remaining constant or decreasing over the course of ontogenesis, this meant cells became in practice less reactive with age, leading to a loss of regenerative and developmental capacity. See V.M. Dil'man, 'O vozrastnom povyshenii deiatel'nosti nekotorykh gipotalamicheskikh tsentrov', *Trudy Instituta fiziologii im. I.P. Pavlova* 7 (1958): 326–36; V.M. Dil'man, 'Elevatsionnyi mekhanizm razvitiia, stareniia i vozrastnoi patologii. III. Aktseleratsiia razvitiia i vozrastnaia norma', *Fiziologiia cheloveka* 1, no. 2 (1975): 352–8; M. Dilman, *Chetyre modeli meditsiny* (Leningrad: Meditsina, 1987). For a brief biographical sketch, see V.N. Anisimov, *Gody priveredlivye* (St. Petersburg: Eskulap, 2014), 49.
17 Neurohormonal regulation refers to the centralized biological systems, linked to the central nervous system in humans, which regulate the release and re-uptake of hormones.
18 N.A. Belov, 'Vozrastnaia izmenchivost'' kak sledstvie zakona vzaimodeistviia chastei organizmov', *Voprosy izucheniia i vospitaniia lichnosti* 4–5 (1922): 600–24.
19 A.A. Bogdanov, *Bor'ba za zhiznesposobnost'* (Moscow, 1927). For more on Bogdanov's life and work, see Nikolai Krementsov, *A Martian Stranded on Earth: Alexander Bogdanov, Blood Transfusions, and Proletarian Science* (Chicago: University of Chicago Press, 2011).
20 'Tektology' was the term Bogdanov used to describe his broader intradisciplinary research into systems of organization amongst and between the sciences. His work later found reflection in mid-twentieth-century 'cybernetics' (the study of

control and communication systems in complex networks) and 'systems theory' (the broader study of complex networks and their internal relations). Direct links to Bogdanov's 'tektology', however, are ambiguous. For overviews of cybernetics and systems theory in the Soviet context, see Slava Gerovitch, *From Newspeak to Cyberspeak: A History of Soviet Cybernetics* (Boston: MIT Press, 2003); Egle Rindzeviciute, *The Power of Systems: How Policy Sciences Opened Up the Cold War World* (Ithaca: Cornell University Press, 2016).

21 Bogdanov was one of the world's first haematologists and founded the first Institute of Blood Transfusion in Moscow in 1926. He also believed that the blood of biologically younger individuals would have rejuvenating effects on older individuals and engaged in experiments to test this hypothesis, partially on himself. He died in 1928 as the result of such an experiment, his work occurring before the full description of blood typing (antigens and Rh factors) and the incompatibility between various types. Recently, the idea of 'rejuvenating' old organisms through blood transfusions from old organisms has received renewed interest, albeit with inconclusive results; on this count, see Armstrong, *Borrowed Time*, 167–76.

22 A.V. Nagornyi, V.N. Nikitin, and I.N. Bulankin, *Problema stareniia i dolgoletiia* (Moscow, 1963), 585–621. In other words, in the larger structures or colloids that include multiple molecules that may or may not be covalently bonded (bonded by electron chain).

23 For the importance of chromatin's form and damaged state in modern theories of ageing, see footnote 8.

24 Chelation is a binding process between ions, generally between metallic and non-metallic ions. In the case of DNA, it refers to the build-up of extraneous metallic ions (iron atoms) that distort the shape of the DNA structure (chromatin). For Gol'dshtein's work, see B.I. Gol'dshtein, 'Vozrastnye izmeneniia molekuliarnykh struktur kletki', in D.F. Chebotaryov, N.B. Man'kovskii and V.V. Frol'kis (eds.), *Osnovy gerontologii* (Moscow, 1969), 38–49.

25 For a selection of Frolkis' work, see V.V. Frol'kis, 'Geno-reguliatornaia gipoteza stareniia', in D.F. Chebotaryov and V.V. Frol'kis (eds.), *Gerontologiia i geriatriia. 1977 Ezhegodnik. Geneticheskie mekhanizmy stareniia i dolgoletiia* (Kiev, 1977), 7–18; V.V. Frol'kis, 'Rol' protsessov regulirovaniia i prisposobleniia v mekhanizme stareniia (adaptatsionno-reguliatornaia teoriia)', in *Vedushchie problemy sovetskoi gerontologii* (Kiev, 1972), 55–85; V.V. Frol'kis, *Starenie: Neirogumoral'nye mekhanizmy* (Kiev, 1981).

26 A.C. Dogel, *Starost' i smert'* (Petrograd, 1922). Ganglia are neural-cell constructions that allow an organism's nervous system to spread and receive information. The sympathetic ganglia are those ganglia located within the sympathetic nervous system, a network largely structured (in humans) around the spinal cord that provides neurohormonal signalling across many organs and organismal frameworks.

27 M.S. Mil'man, *Uchenie o roste, starosti i smerti* (Baku, 1926).
28 S.A. Voronov, *Starost' i omolazhivanie* (Moscow, 1927).
29 I.A. Shereshevskii, 'Starost' i endokrinnaia sistema', in I.V. Bazilevich, P.D. Marchuk and N.B. Medvedeva (eds.), *Starost': Trudy konferentsii po probleme geneza starosti i profilaktiki prezhdevremennogo stareniia organizma. Kiev, 17-19 dekabria 1938 g* (Kiev, 1939), 31–8; M.M. Zavadovskii, *Vozmozhna li bor'ba so starost'iu?* (Moscow, 1924); M.M. Zavadovskii, *Dinamika razvitiia organizma* (Moscow, 1931).
30 For example, see: L.A. Andreev, 'Materialy k izucheniiu funktsional'nykh starcheskikh izmenenii tsentral'noi nervnoi sistemy (1924)', *Trudy fiziologicheskoi laboratorii im. akad. I.P. Pavlova* (1953): 74–82.
31 On the comparative development of Soviet and Western gerontology over the twentieth century, see Isaac Scarborough, 'A New Science for an Old(er) Population: Soviet Gerontology and Geriatrics in International Comparative Perspective', *Social History of Medicine*, forthcoming.
32 See I.V. Bazilevich, P.D. Marchuk and N.B. Medvedeva (eds.), *Starost': Trudy konferentsii po probleme geneza starosti i profilaktiki prezhdevremennogo stareniia organizma. Kiev, 17-19 dekabria 1938 g.* (Kiev, 1939).
33 For more on this programme, see D.F. Chebotarev, 'Kompleksnaia nauchnaia programma "Prodlenie zhizni"', in D.F. Chebotarev and V.V. Frolkis (eds.), *Gerontologiia i geriatriia. 1979 ezhegodnik. Prodlenie zhizni: prognozy, mekhanizmy, kontrol'* (Kiev, 1979), 5–10.
34 This classificatory system of periods of ageing was later codified in Kiev at the Institute of Gerontology and spread internationally by the WHO.
35 The hypothalamus is an important part of the diencephalon: the brain region that also includes the thalamus. It plays an important role in the regulation of autonomic (vegetative) functions, such as hemodynamics (the organization of the cardiovascular system), endocrine secretions, sexual behaviour, food and water consumption, thermoregulation and cellular metabolism, which occur in the background of most other biological processes.
36 The 'objective-management method of planning' (*programmno-tselevoi metod planirovaniia*) was a Soviet-era formulation used to classify centrally directed state projects, where programmes of action were built around final goals to be achieved. For a structural overview and application in modern Russia, see Z.B. Luk'ianenko and N.V. Iugova, 'Programmno-tselevoi metod v gosudarstevennom upravlenii biudzhetnoi sferoi', *ARS Administrandi* 2 (2014): 72–8.
37 The 'scientific-research institute' (*nauchno-issledovatel'skii institut* or *NII*) was a Soviet institution in which scientific research was focused on a particular sub-field of enquiry. Researchers at one or another NII did not teach, but were full-time researchers; the institution was endemic across the USSR.

2

Medical propaganda: Fairy tales and miracles of surgery

Maria Tutorskaya

In the Soviet Union of the 1920s, birth and death, contraception, sexuality and rejuvenation all became popular subjects in specialized literature as well as in novels and newspaper accounts, and even radio broadcasts. Communist cultural reconstruction presupposed the all-inclusive reorganization of society – from its social mechanisms to the physiology of its members. Themes of the body and corporeality were widespread in Soviet culture, the cultural revolution and the discourse of the New Man.

In this chapter, I rely on the collections of the Museum of the Institute of the Sanitary Enlightenment, which the Russian Medical Museum in Moscow inherited in 2015.[1] The history of this collection is worthy of a separate study. The nucleus of the collection was formed from the property of the Commission for the dissemination of hygienic knowledge of the Society of Russian Doctors in memory of N.I. Pirogov.[2] The chairman of the commission, almost throughout its existence, was Alfred Molkov (1870–1947), a hygienist and medical educator in the Russian Empire and then later the conceptual developer of 'social hygiene' and a Soviet medical professor. He handed the collection over to the People's Commissariat of Public Health in 1918. At that point a new institution – the Museum of Social Hygiene (1919–23) – was founded with Molkov as its director. In 1923 the museum was reorganized into the State Institute of Social Hygiene with Molkov again its chairman. The museum, and then the Institute, laid claim to ideological leadership in medical education in the USSR, coordinating the work of most medical museums, exhibitions and houses of health education throughout the country. The collection from this museum covering questions of rejuvenation includes educational publications, minutes of meetings, journals and brochures. In contrast to national libraries' collections, which were compiled through the acquisition of all published materials sent to the Book Chamber (legal deposits), the collection of the Museum of the Institute of Social Hygiene was hand-picked and selective. The collection that the Russian Medical Museum inherited today holds the materials that visitors to earlier museums interested in problems of ageing could explore in the 1920s. These are the materials that current museum staff have selected as 'must reads' for re-constructing the rejuvenation narrative of the time – and which constitute the basis for this article as well.

It is worth adding that the collection of the Russian Medical Museum combines these materials with collections from certain other former Soviet medical museums closed in 1990s, for example, the Pharmacy Museum and the Museum of the Sklifosovsky Institute. The museum's total collection contains more than 300,000 objects, including medical propaganda matters of all types, books and paintings, documents and private papers, instruments and equipment, correspondence, and case notes of medical practitioners and scientists. Although only a small number of items held by the museum have been catalogued – not to mention that Museum lacks a permanent exhibition – the Museum presents its collections via temporary exhibits on a wide range of subjects. In recent years, the exhibits 'Healthcare of Russia – 1917' (2017–18) and 'Cultivating National Health' (2018–present) have been on view at the museum. These exhibitions, along with participation in large-scale events elsewhere, have allowed the Museum to share some of its extensive holdings.

In terms of the early Soviet period, printed materials from the museum vault, including leaflets and brochures on ageing and rejuvenation and the nature of death, go hand in hand with materials on the importance of healthy living and preventative medicine. In this chapter, I will showcase the duality of the concept of ageing in the 1920s in Soviet Russia and its representations in professional literature and popular science publications. This duality mirrors the emphasis in early Soviet Russia on founding an 'ideal' society that would at the same time be accessible to the masses: to bring into reality the words of a popular song from that time – 'We were born to make the fairy tale come true'[3] by all the means that enquiring minds could offer.

The place of rejuvenation, 'radical' science and the interaction between the new Bolshevik rulers and scientists pursuing physiological research has recently received increased academic attention. The historical accounts of the origins and early progress of Soviet endocrinology were uncovered by historian Nikolai Krementsov in his paper 'Hormones and the Bolsheviks: From Organotherapy to Experimental Endocrinology, 1918–1929'.[4] In *Revolutionary Experiments: The Quest for Immortality in Bolshevik Science and Fiction*,[5] Krementsov further illustrates how the global (as well as Soviet) trends of the first quarter of the twentieth century led to an experimental revolution in the life sciences, a revolution of scale, which made science a mass profession. He also shows how the revolution in sciences' public visibility got crossed with the Bolshevik revolution and the 'death decade' in Russia, during which 'some fifteen to twenty million people out of a population of 140 million in Russia died'.[6] Krementsov focuses on the institutional development of endocrinology in that period as well as personal interactions between the main actors and their reflection in literary works.

Perspectives on the social measures for rejuvenation in the 1920s are presented in Tricia Starks's book, *The Body Soviet: Propaganda, Hygiene, and the Revolutionary State*.[7] Starks shows that social change in Russia was seen as an effective remedy to care for the sick in particular and for public health in general from the late nineteenth century. Starks refers to the work of Dr Kagan, who, writing in the 1920s, believed that rejuvenation could be achieved through an improvement in labour legislation. Weekends and breaks during the working day could purify workers of the 'poisons of fatigue'[8] – argued Dr Kagan. Starks also provides the later gerontologists' idea that 'the crudest and most merciless enemy of human longevity is a society in which man is exploited by man'.[9] Starks emphasizes that the discourse of health and the medicalized gaze were a part of the Bolsheviks pursuit of socialist success.

Furthermore, regarding the ageing and rejuvenation discourse in 1920s, it is impossible not to mention research related to the concept of death of that time. Philosopher and anthropologist Anna Sokolova's[10] work on the problem of the 'new' Bolshevik world and 'old' (unchanged) death has focused on how death was represented in the public sphere, reflected in new rituals, and the place funeral institutions should have in new exemplary socialist cities. She considers Soviet planners and architects developing projects for cities in which there are no cemeteries, along with the creation of new types of residential spaces, such as communal houses, and projects for garden cities. Rejecting the traditional attributes of death such as cemeteries and burial, the Bolsheviks attempted to establish 'a way of life that formed communist consciousness and values among residents'.[11] There should have been no visible evidence of the existence of death in these rituals.

The newly created Soviet state called for believing in ambitious goals: world revolution and the triumph of communism. Longevity and immortality, as well as victory over death, were pieces of these highflying social projects. However, rejuvenation research in the 1920s in Russia was being waged on many different fronts. It followed routes outlined long before the revolution, including increasing life expectancy through the reduction of infant and child mortality, as well as improving working and living conditions. In the meantime, it relied on the latest scientific discoveries and developments in microbiology, surgery and pharmacy. The orthodox belief in the immortality of the soul and eternal life was shaken by atheistic ideas. In this regard, rejuvenation drew inspiration from science and looked to miracles that could be performed by scholars, not saints.

Narkomzdrav, and its head Nikolai Semashko, proclaimed the idea of disease prevention as the basis of Soviet healthcare. Medical propaganda prescribed discarding unhealthy habits, following hygiene requirements and undergoing regular check-ups for a long and healthy life. 'The cultivation of public health is the work of the working class' (Figure 2.1), noted one of the widespread slogans of this period, neatly capturing the state's proclivity to shift responsibility for the health of citizens onto themselves. Consequently, health education and the elimination of health illiteracy were inescapably embedded into the public campaigns to eliminate more general illiteracy (*likbez*). The decree 'On the elimination of illiteracy in the RSFSR' was adopted in 1919. The Department of Public Health Enlightenment under the People's Commissariat for Health was established during the same year. Not coincidentally, the recommended basic phrases and sentences included in the 'toolkits' provided to the liquidators of illiteracy related to both politics and healthcare. For example, in a lesson plan for a study group learning to read, students were meant to learn the unsurprising phrase 'We were slaves of capital'. This was followed, however, by lessons dedicated to medical phrases: 'Give children milk from healthy cows'; 'Weak children need more sunlight'; and 'There are many consumptives among the workers. The Soviet state gave the workers free treatment'.[12] State officials had made it clear that health illiteracy and sanitary hygiene were at the centre of its healthcare system.

At the same time, however, Narkomzdrav also established new institutions and supported research on invasive methods that suggested an explosive and forward-facing approach to medicine: blood transfusion, the injection of crushed animal glands and transplantation. The Institute of Blood Transfusion, headed by the old Bolshevik, utopist and physician-writer, Alexander Bogdanov, is a vivid example of such institutions. Bogdanov was an ideologist of 'physiological collectivism' – the exchanging of blood through transfusion.[13] This blood exchange, from Bogdanov's point of view, would not only promote comradery, but also help to cure ageing: the old could receive strength and energy from young in this way, establishing communist links not only in their ideological, but also physiological, existence.

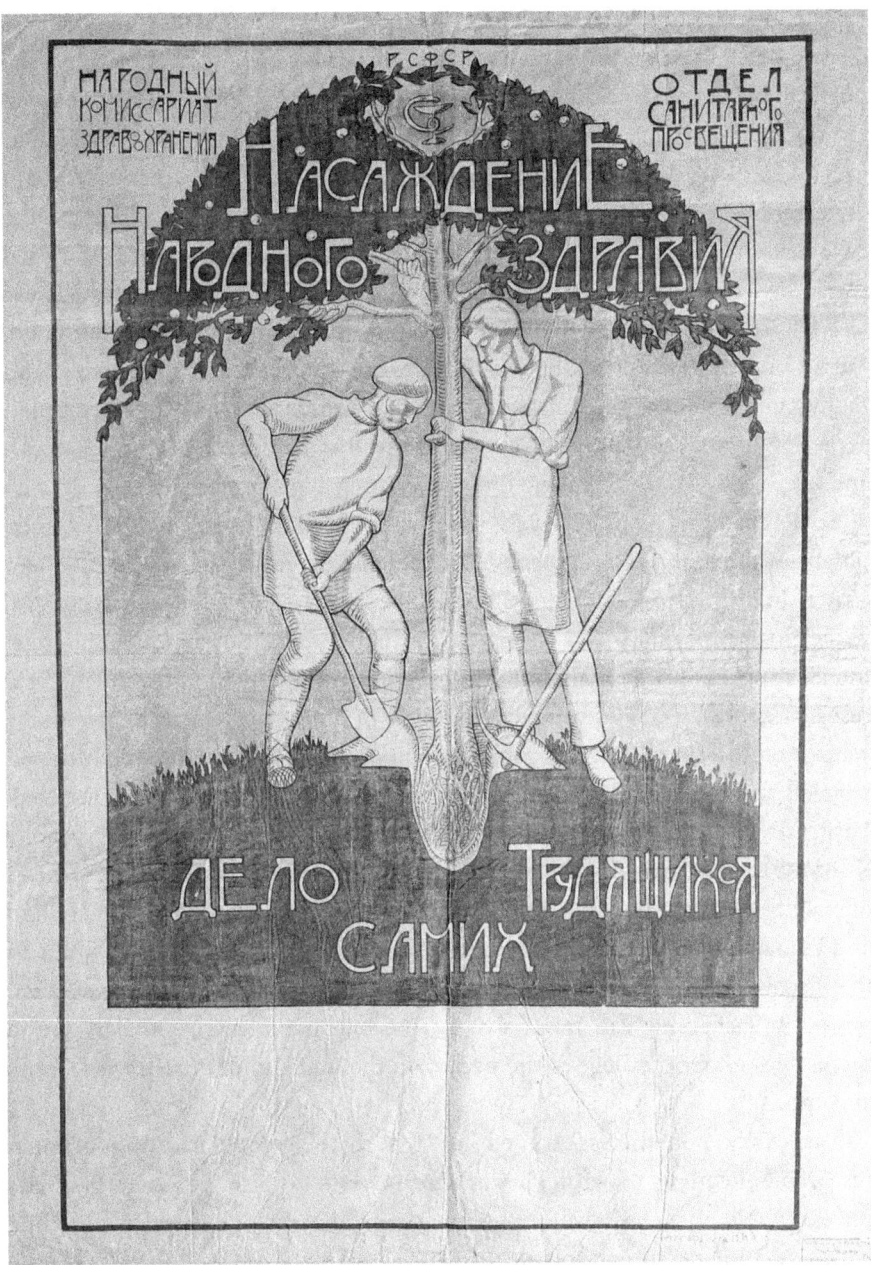

Figure 2.1 Poster: the cultivation of public health is the work of the working class.
Source: Image from the collections of the Russian Medical Museum, Moscow, part of the FSSBI 'N.A. Semashko National Research Institute of Public Health'.

The idea that medicine could act like magic – in a flash – to solve chronic disease or even extend life was tempting for state officials, scientists and the public. This particular concept of magic originated from two opposite sources. On the one hand, medical professionals aspired to find 'magic bullets', similar to Paul Ehrlich's discovery of chemical cures for syphilis and other diseases in the early twentieth century. Ehrlich's Nobel lecture[14] in 1908 and address to the Seventeenth International Congress of Medicine in London in 1913 promised the audience a 'radical cure of the body by means of a single injection'.[15] These views were widely represented in the medical community. On the other hand, there were widespread folk beliefs that treatment should be simultaneous and momentary, rather than painstaking, gradual and progressive. New drugs and surgeries promised a miracle of technology that could get back one's youth and were seen as something like the rejuvenating apples of fairy tales.

Soviet medical researchers were also aware of both the promises and potential pitfalls of this futuristic approach to medicine. Lev Vasilevsky, a physician and writer, in the introduction to a popular science essay *Rejuvenation* (1927), wrote that immortality and eternal youth had always been amongst the most intoxicating desires of mankind. He drew parallels between current medical research and the earlier search for 'the elixir of life' by alchemists or the 'living water'[16] of Russian fairy tales. From his point of view, these questions, which had worried scientific minds for thousands of years, were close to being resolved. Vasilevsky in particular emphasized the studies being conducted by Nikolai Kravkov, the pharmacologist, experimentalist and researcher of vital properties of tissues preservation, and his followers on the extraction of testicular fluid and its injection for the purposes of rejuvenation. Vasilevsky compared this to the discoveries of Eugene Steinach[17] and Paul Ehrlich. For all of their success, however, Vasilevsky also saw risks: on the one hand, these pioneers found themselves under the siege of the needy, on the other, under fire from sceptics and critics.[18]

Vasilevsky nonetheless argued for the further popularization of such research. Of course, he wrote, it was inadmissible to raise the general public's unreasonable and excessive hopes for a cure that 'at one blow' could cope with any ailment, disease or old age. Yet Vasilevsky did not agree, as some of his contemporaries argued, that controversial scientific discoveries that affected the interests of the general public should not be made public until they were fully formulated and established. Vasilevsky called this approach the 'caste arrogance' of science hierophants. He insisted that it was instead necessary to formulate the modern doctrine of rejuvenation in such a way as to bring readers closer to understanding what humanity could expect from this academic field in the future.

Vasilevsky's insights were a reflection of existing scientific debates. The matter under discussion was a new branch of medical science: endocrinology. This was a science that studied the functioning of the endocrine glands, such as the testes and ovaries, the thyroid gland, the pancreas and the pituitary gland – all of which were thought to play some role in ageing. The first issue of the *Herald of Endocrinology*,[19] which was published in January 1925, pointed to the need for scientific and educational literature on the topic, as well as popular talks and lectures and the establishment of an Endocrinological Museum for both specialists and the public. In the same years, the newly founded Institute of Experimental Endocrinology, which had been set up in 1925 under the directorship of V.D. Shervinsky, one of the Herald of Endocrinology's editors, succeeded in the production of anti-thyroid serum, as well as the production of adrenaline and pituitrin. These institutions also considered the ideas of setting up a special clinic or polyclinic, conducting training courses for doctors, and systematically studying the influence of various factory and technical industries on diseases of the endocrine glands (Figure 2.2).

The first issue of the *Herald of Endocrinology* contains the particularly interesting and polemical report 'Some observations on the transplantation of endocrine glands',[20] which concerned rejuvenation, and was written by Alexander Prokin.[21] This report depicted surgeries conducted in the Surgical Clinic of the 1st Moscow Medical University. Prokin wrote that, despite the determination of the Soviet scientists' research, the fact remained that any heteroplastic transplantation (from animals to humans) was doomed to failure. Serge Voronoff's and Max Thorek's transplantations of genitals and other glands, Prokin wrote, reported the complete success of transplantation surgeries without indicating why or how such brilliant results were obtained. In reality, Prokin suggested, the results of such experiments were much more ambiguous, and perhaps even worrisome. The concerns raised by these experiments were endemic at the time, it should be said, and were made not only in specialized medical journals. Mikhail Bulgakov, the popular physician-writer, published the novella The *Heart of a Dog (Sobachee serdtso)* that very same year, in 1925. Bulgakov warned readers and colleagues that the transplantation of animal organs could have unpredictable results.

For his part, Prokin provided an analysis of the endocrine gland transplantations made to twenty-one patients at the Moscow University Surgical Clinic. These patients had sought endocrinological treatment for senility (7),

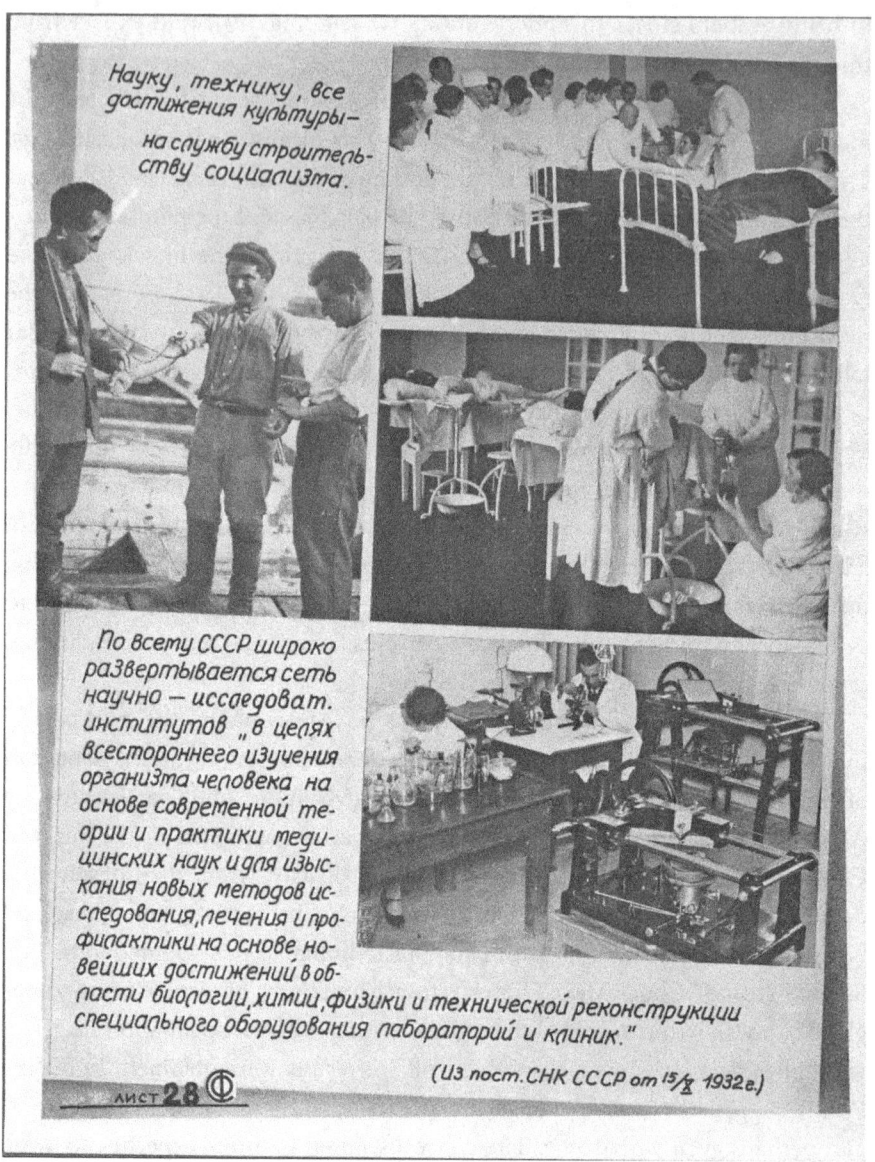

Figure 2.2 Photo montage: science in the service of building socialism. Source: Image from the collections of the Russian Medical Museum, Moscow, part of the FSSBI 'N.A. Semashko National Research Institute of Public Health'.

infantilism (1), homosexuality (1), schizophrenia (2), hypothyroidism (3), Basedow's disease (3), Addison's disease (1), multi-glandular insufficiency (1) and spontaneous gangrene (1). Prokin noticed that all the patients who sought treatment for senility were mostly of advanced age; only one patient was relatively young – he was forty-seven years old, when the average age of this all-male patient group was sixty-four years.

All seven patients treated for senility were intellectuals and had arrived knowledgeable about rejuvenation work. Everyone was waiting for positive results from the testicle transplantation. An immediate positive effect was observed in four out of the seven patients after the transplantation. All four of these patients noted increased physical vigour; however, there were no changes in their sexual potency in the postoperative period. Long-term results were received from five out of seven patients: one patient reported that he had resumed his scientific research, while another began to conduct intensive social work. One, who had completely grey hair, gradually developed a lot of black hair in his beard. In three patients, the improvement of the general condition was maintained. Only one patient felt worse than before the transplantation – after the surgery, his general condition was very good but then quickly deteriorated.

Based on these observations, Prokin drew some conclusions. While mentioning that the *influence* of the transplanted gland had been detected, he noted that had not been any verification of graft attachment. In those cases where a specific effect was noted, it eventually disappeared. The length of time that patients experienced improvements in their conditions after surgery lasted from two to nine months, but the reasons for the longer or shorter duration of effects remained unclear. Moreover, Prokin claimed that the patients who had sought endocrinological treatment for their senility had arrived with high expectations about the surgery and that the psychological aspect of high expectations and a belief in success could have created something of a placebo effect. The results obtained, Prokin wrote, should be evaluated with great caution.

Patients' high expectations had been formed under the influence of numerous popular publications distributed in the Soviet 1920s, including 'Transplantation of Tissues and Organs' by professor E. S. London and doctor I. I. Kryzhanovsky (Petrograd, 1923); 'What Is Old Age and Rejuvenation', by V. S. Muralevich, a biology lecturer in the Communist University of the Working People of the East in Moscow (Moscow, 1923); 'Old Age and Rejuvenation: The Popular Presentation of the Question of Old Age and Rejuvenation', by A. Gobert (Moscow, 1923); the collection of essays 'Rejuvenation in Russia' (Leningrad, 1924); 'Is It Possible to Fight Old Age', by M. M. Zavadovsky (Moscow, 1924); and the popular science essay 'Rejuvenation', by the doctor L.M. Vasilevsky (Moscow, 1927). Many other books and pamphlets were published by a wide variety of publishing houses and departments, demonstrating the growing social interest in biological ageing. Nikolai Krementsov has linked this interest to 'three revolutions' occurring in science at the time (the experimental revolution in the life sciences, the revolution of scale and the revolution of the sciences' public visibility[22]) and with the horrifying experience of the 'decade of death'. I would argue that the search for the possibility of extending life was also associated with the desire for a new faith in eternal life and miracles. This is faith that is not based on religion, but on belief in science and the capabilities of scientists. This new form of belief found wide application in the sciences, especially the medical sciences. In his book *Ivan Pavlov: A Russian Life in Science*,[23] Daniel P. Todes has shown how the life and career of the most recognizable Russian and Soviet scientist, the Nobel Prize winner Ivan Pavlov (1849–1936), represents the broader acclaim of science in the first decades of the USSR. For scientists and citizens alike, Science in the early Soviet era was a symbol of the new, modern Russia that was being built. It was a source of understanding for humanity: the 'surest path to human progress, to human beings' rational control over themselves and society'.[24]

Those in the field of ageing research and rejuvenation continued to attribute an important role to endocrinology. Here we turn to the role played by Vasily Shervinskiy (1850–1941), who is considered the founder of Soviet clinical endocrinology. By the 1920s, the medical community knew and respected Vasily Shervinskiy as an authority figure.[25] He managed to prove himself in many aspects of clinical practice and medical research, and effectively consolidated the medical community. He was Professor of the Medical Faculty of Moscow University from 1884 until 1911 and the Director of the Faculty's Therapeutic Clinic. Shervinskiy was also an active member of the Pirogov's Congresses, and a founder of the Moscow Therapeutic Society in 1894. He was elected Chairman of the Society in 1899, thereafter holding that post for a quarter-century. After 1917, Shervinskiy became a member of the Scientific Medical Council of the People's Commissariat of Public Health of the RSFSR. Most of his efforts during the post-Revolution decade were directed towards the formation of endocrinological institutes and studies – an area in which he had been passionate since the early 1910s, giving talks and publishing on various approaches to the treatment of diseases of the endocrine glands.

In the medical textbook *Fundamentals of Endocrinology*, Vasily Shervinskiy pointed out in his introduction that over the last decades of the nineteenth century and up to 1929, experimental and clinical studies aimed at elucidating the functions of the endocrine glands had continuously appeared in increasing numbers. He noted: 'If you were to draw a curve representing the number of research papers over the past 50 years dedicated to the studies of these organs, it would demonstrate a continuous and steadily upward trend'.[26] Interest continued to grow, including in Shervinsky's own textbook.

The *Fundamentals of Endocrinology* was an important educational and scientific publication meant for the professional community. In a section entitled 'Transplantation of the Endocrine Glands', Vladimir Rozanov[27] provided a brief overview of the existing methods of transplantation: auto-transplantation, homo- and hetero-transplantation.[28] His conclusions were similar to Alexander Prokin's view that even though microscopic analysis showed that transplantations of tissues from donors of the same species, and even more from other species, were generally doomed to failure, clinical analysis of such operations did not allow for categorical conclusions in one direction or another. While histological examination showed that the engraftment of transplanted organs was not successful – glands had become necrotic and were not functioning as organs of internal secretion – the clinical picture and general condition of the patients provided reasons to believe that graft tissues had temporarily served as a source of hormones missing in the body. Rozanov refers to the work of Vladimir Oppel and his argument that 'next to the microscopic criterion for the suitability of a graft, it is currently necessary to put forward a chemical criterion'. Oppel had suggested detailed laboratory tests for identifying a patient's 'endocrine formula'. His point was that the shortcomings of existing medications could serve as the basis for research into ways to get rid of pharmaceutical preparations and 'to move the cure inside the patient for a more or less long and constant use of it'.[29] At the same time, Rozanov was both sceptical about the results achieved by doctors like Voronoff and full of hope for future achievements.

Shervinsky also pointed out that some scientists were sceptical and asserted an ongoing crisis in endocrinology. The editor of the *Fundamentals of Endocrinology* was referring to the work of Aleksandr Bogomolets and his *The Crisis of Endocrinology*, which had been published in 1927. Bogomolets, a pathophysiologist, drug developer and specialist in life extension, wrote that the goal of his book was to liberate the reader from the holy faith in endocrinology, which had 'turned into modern cabalism'.[30] Bogomolets lamented the huge number of unsubstantiated hypotheses, fantastic theories and schemes in endocrinological science, which had revolutionized biology – but proposed to go too far in many cases, promising to reveal many aspects of biology that were as of yet unknowable. All this undermined the authority of modern endocrinology, 'but a crisis does not mean death'. Bogomolets argued that endocrinology's difficulties could be resolved through improvements made to its methodological base, the development of a critical attitude to the facts and the rejection of the dominant position of endocrinology over other aspects of physiology and pathology. Following the underlying provisions of Soviet social hygiene, Bogomolets stated that 'The success of an individual struggle for normal longevity can only be ensured by the success of public hygiene and prevention' and suggested that endocrinology should adhere to the larger Soviet medical programme. Social hygiene (*sotsialnaya gigiena*) was given significant import by Nikolai Semashko, the founding People's Commissar of Public Health (directed 1918–30) and architect of the Soviet healthcare system, and he also encouraged the concept to be interpreted as broadly as possible. Social hygiene was defined as 'science which studied the influence of the economic and social conditions of life on the health of the population and the means to improve that health'.[31] Semashko contended that 'Social hygiene stands on the shoulders of general experimental hygiene'.[32] In support of this programme, Bogomolets did not insist that endocrinology should rise to the top, but instead work towards the broader achievement of public health and hygiene.

Nikolai Koltsov, a Soviet biologist and one of the founders of the Russian school of experimental biology and genetics, on the contrary, sought ways to increase the prestige of and societal faith in the young scientific field of endocrinology and to recruit loyal supporters. He used radio broadcasting to popularize his perspectives and beliefs. In 1925, Koltsov read radio lectures on behalf of the Moscow House of Scientists. These lectures were then published as a book, *The Wonderful Achievements of Science*.[33] Koltsov began his radio talk about endocrinology and rejuvenation with lyrical descriptions of his early years, when there had been no automobiles, telephones or streetlights. The talented speaker made allusions to popular fairy tale wonders that had become reality because of the rapid development of science. He compared magic carpets with airplanes, magic mirrors with cinematography and mythical 'submariners' with current underwater explorers. He emphasized at the beginning of his radio broadcast that the talk was not so much for townspeople and students, but for the residents of remote rural areas. Koltsov had never practised in a local village commune, but he was undoubtedly informed that such 'magical' scientific discoveries seemed to be the most attractive to peasants. According to the book *Russian Folk Medicine*, which had been published by Gavriil Popov in 1903, the 'peasant is a great practitioner by nature'.[34] Materials collected through a survey of villagers indicated that peasants did not like to lie down during illness, worked until the last minute and, having become ill, looked for means to recover as soon as possible. They firmly believed that there was a special medicine for each disease and that it would act almost magically: one just needed to find it.

If a drug prescribed by a doctor acted slowly, the troubled sufferer simply drank the entire 'potion' immediately. The only 'disease' that was seen by peasants as a legitimate cause of illness and rest was old age. In these cases, treatment was completely unnecessary and 'died of old age' was even used in church metrics. Offering the possibility of healing this incurable disease, Koltsov won a new loyal audience for himself and endocrinology.

The mid to late 1920s were the brightest years of the endocrinology-driven rejuvenation discourse in Russia, including discussion on a wide range of scientific programmes and means of promoting health enlightenment alike. Rejuvenation proved to be one of the more popular themes of medical propaganda employed by the People's Commissariat of Public Health – the institution that came to direct medical affairs in the early USSR. Popular brochures were written, lectures were given and radio broadcasts were prepared on the science of ageing and the possibilities for 'rejuvenation'. Contributors to these efforts included biological researchers, medical practitioners and writers, as well as people at the crossroads of these fields, such as Mikhail Bulgakov.

Daring experiments in medicine were associated not only with recent scientific discoveries and breakthroughs in surgery, chemistry and genetics but also with the spirit of the times, the avant-garde, which during these years captured many areas of art and everyday life, not excluding science. The collections of the Russian Medical Museum document the formation of the time's secular mythology. Brochures, leaflets and photographs all reflect the idea of rejuvenating the old world and sculpting a new human being by any and all means necessary. As the materials of the time show, this would include the prevention of infectious and chronic diseases, wondrous surgical interventions and a promised bright future.

Notes

1. For more information about the museum, see its website: http://medmuseum.ru/ru/.
2. The Society of Russian Doctors in memory of N.I. Pirogov or, as frequently referred to, the 'Pirogov Society' was founded in 1881 to celebrate the fiftieth anniversary of Nikolay Pirogov's medical practice. The Pirogov Society had branches across Russian Empire, organized congresses and regularly published reports on its activities; it gradually ceased its activities after the revolution.
3. This is the first line of the song 'The March of the Pilots', written by Pavel Herman and first published in 1923.

4   Nikolai Krementsov, 'Hormones and the Bolsheviks: From Organotherapy to Experimental Endocrinology, 1918–1929', *Isis* 99, no. 3 (2008): 486–518.
5   Nikolai Krementsov, *Revolutionary Experiments: The Quest for Immortality in Bolshevik Science and Fiction* (Oxford: Oxford University Press, 2013).
6   Nikolai Krementsov, 'Off with Your Heads: Isolated Organs in Early Soviet Science and Fiction', *Studies in History and Philosophy of Science Part C: Studies in History and Philosophy of Biological and Biomedical Sciences* 40, no. 2 (2009): 87–100.
7   Tricia Starks, *The Body Soviet: Propaganda, Hygiene, and the Revolutionary State* (Madison: University of Wisconsin Press, 2009).
8   Ibid.
9   Ibid.
10 Anna Sokolova, 'Novyi mir i staraia smert': sud'ba kladbishch v sovetskikh gorodakh v 1920-1930-x godov', *Neprikosnovennyi zapas* 1 (2018): 74–94.
11 Ibid.
12 *V pomoshh' likvidatoru negramotnosti* (Moscow: Glavlit, 1928).
13 See Alla Morozova, 'Neleninskii bol'shevizm' A. A. Bogdanova i 'vperedovtsev': idei, al'ternativy, praktika (Moscow: Nestor-Istorija, 2019) and Nikolai Krementsov, *A Martian Stranded on Earth: Alexander Bogdanov, Blood Transfusions, and Proletarian Science* (Chicago: University of Chicago Press, 2011).
14 Ehrlich received the Nobel Prize in Physiology or Medicine 'in recognition of their work on immunity' in 1908 (shared with Ilya Mechnikov).
15 Paul Ehrlich, 'Address in Pathology, on Chemotherapy, Delivered before the Seventeenth International Congress of Medicine', *BMJ* 2, no. 2746 (1913): 353.
16 The *Encyclopaedic Dictionary* of Brockhaus and Efron (St. Petersburg, 1890–1907) identifies 'living water' as a subject presented in the folk tales of all Indo-European peoples. One of the most popular examples is a German fairy tale 'The Water of Life', which was collected by the Brothers Grimm. In Russian folklore living water returns life to the dead and sight to the blind.
17 Steinach's practice of rejuvenation was built around a partial vasectomy, which was meant to stimulate the production of testosterone ('male sex hormone'). This was a variation on earlier attempts, such as by the French surgeon Serge Voronoff, to stimulate hormones through genital transplants. See Nils Hansson, Matthis Krischel, Per Södersten, Friedrich H. Moll, and Heiner Fangerau, '"He Gave Us the Cornerstone of Sexual Medicine": A Nobel Plan but No Nobel Prize for Eugen Steinach', *Urologia internationalis* 104, no. 7–8 (2020): 501–9.
18 Lev Vasilevsky, *Omolozhenie: Nauchno-populjarnyj ocherk* (Moscow: Zhizn' i znanie, 1927).
19 *Vestnik Endokrinologii*, edited by N.I. Korotnev, A.V. Martynov, O. A. Stepun, Ya.A. Tobolkin, M.N. Shaternikov, V.D. Shervinsky. no. 1. Moscow: State Institute of Experimental Endocrinology, 1925.

20 Alexander Prokin, 'Nekotorye nabliudeniia pri peresadke endokrinnykh zhelez', *Vestnik endokrinologii* 1 (1925): 23–31.
21 Alexander Prokin was a surgeon and a senior assistant of the Clinic's Director and the Dean of the Faculty of Medicine at Moscow State University (1919–22), Prof L. V. Martynov, one of the editors of *The Herald of Endocrinology*.
22 Krementsov, 'Off with Your Heads'.
23 D.P. Todes, *Ivan Pavlov: A Russian Life in Science* (New York: Oxford University Press, 2014).
24 Ibid.
25 G.A. Mel'nichenko, V.I. Kandror, N.P. Makolina, and N.D. Ivanova, 'K istorii endokrinologii v Rossii. V.D. Shervinsky', *Problemy endokrinologii* 58, no. 1 (2012): 74–6.
26 V.D. Shervinsky and G.P. Sakharov (eds.), *Osnovy endokrinologii: uchenie o vnutrennei sekretsii i klinika zabolevanii gormonotvornogo apparata* (Leningrad: Prakticheskaia meditsina, 1929).
27 Vladimir Rozanov (1872–1934) graduated from the Medical Faculty of Moscow University in 1896. In 1910 he founded and directed the surgical department at the Soldatenkovskaia hospital in Moscow. Rozanov operated on Lenin in 1918. In 1929 he became director of the Kremlin Hospital's surgical department.
28 Auto-transplantation implies the transplantation of a person's own glands. Rozanov mentions that this type of transplantation is quite rare and is usually the result of an accident, e.g., when removing the thyroid gland if the parathyroid glands were also accidentally removed. In this case the parathyroid glands should be immediately implanted back. Homo-transplantation implies transplantation from and between individuals of the same species, generally meaning human and human glands. Hetero-transplantation implies animal glad transplantation to humans: e.g., glands taken from monkeys, goats or cats. Today the term used is 'xenotransplantation'.
29 Vladimir Rozanov, 'Transplantatsiia zhelez vnutrennej sekretsii', in V.D. Shervinsky and G.P. Sakharov (eds.), *Osnovy endokrinologii: uchenie o vnutrennei sekretsii i klinika zabolevanii gormonotvornogo apparata* (Leningrad: Prakticheskaia mediitsina, 1929), 581–93.
30 Aleksandr Bogomolets, *Krizis endokrinologii* (Moscow: Moszdravotdel. 1927), 14.
31 Susan Gross Solomon, 'Social Hygiene and Soviet Public Health, 1921–1930', in Susan Gross Solomon and John F. Hutchinson (eds.), *Health and Society in Revolutionary Russia* (Bloomington: Indiana University Press, 1990), 175–99.
32 Ibid.
33 Nikolai Koltsov, *Chudesnye dostizheniia nauki* (Moscow: Rabotnik prosveshcheniia, 1927).
34 Gavriil Popov, *Russkaia narodno-bytovaia meditsina: po materialam etnograficheskogo biuro kniaza V.N. Tenisheva* (St. Petersburg: Tipografii A. S. Suvorina, 1903).

Winding up the clock of life: Soviet research into infant 'mortality' in the context of ageing bodies

Anna Ozhiganova

Introduction: The Soviet science of ageing as visionary biology

Early Soviet gerontology considered ageing to be a disease that could be cured and a problem that could be solved by cutting-edge science. At the first conference on ageing held in Kiev in 1938, one of the founders of Soviet gerontology, academician Alexander Bogomolets, urged his colleagues to act decisively:

> Soviet science has, in fact, long ago declared war on everything that shortens human life. At our conference, the war is declared openly. We, representatives of Soviet medicine and biology, are throwing the glove to such seemingly invincible enemies as old age and death![1]

In this battle, it became very important for Soviet gerontologists to differentiate the concepts of *normal*, or physiological ageing that was not complicated by disease, and *premature*, or pathological ageing, caused by severe diseases. The concept of premature ageing was initially proposed by Russian physiologist Ivan Tarkhanov in 1891[2] and widely used by Russian and Soviet scientists such as Ivan Pavlov, Elie Metchnikoff, Alexander Bogomolets, Lev Komarov and others.[3] Research in Soviet gerontology was carried out not only on the functioning of various organs and physiological systems of older people, but primarily on the factors underlying human longevity. A striking example was the research of the prominent zoologist and microbiologist, Elie Metchnikoff, who created a theory which attributed ageing to the 'poisoning' of the organism with toxins produced by bacteria inhabiting its intestines. Metchnikoff suggested that considerable prolongation of human life could be achieved by replacing the noxious bacteria with the healthy lactic acid bacteria present in yoghurt.[4] Later, in the 1960s–70s, the Soviet gerontologist and biologist Lev Komarov engaged in laboratory experiments aiming towards the radical extension of human life: he proposed methods of influencing the ageing process that included hypothermia, the use of electric and magnetic fields, and vitamin therapy (large doses of ascorbic acid and other, rarer, supplements).[5] Over the decades, Soviet gerontology developed various experimental approaches to increasing life expectancy, including dietary changes, the use of bio-stimulants, neurohumoral factors, physical activity and immunotherapy.[6]

After the First World War there was a rise of interest across the world in anti-ageing and rejuvenation remedies, inspired by the new experimental biology and medicine. Societal faith in the omnipotence of science and its ability to change human destiny by solving the 'eternal' issues of ageing and death, opposition to religion and 'old' myths, and searches for a new vision of the future all gave this research the features of a 'new' or 'visionary' biology.[7] However, the case of Russia was also unique due to the revolutionary dreams of a 'new world' and the militant atheism and materialism, which permeated the country after the Bolshevik Revolution. As Nikolai Krementsov has noted in his research on early Soviet revolutionary experiments on immortality, 'experimental means of control over life, death, and disease made evident that humans were no longer passive subjects to God's will or Nature's inexorable laws: armed with new scientific knowledge, they could "conquer Nature" and become masters of their own individual fates and communal destinies'.[8] Since the Bolshevik project itself was an experiment on a grand scale, experimental biology and medicine were transformed into an influential cultural resource. Many radical projects of human enhancement originated in the early Soviet period: Alexander Bogdanov's experiments with blood exchanges, aimed at the creation of a 'physiological collective', which would rejuvenate and unite its members; Nikolai Fedorov's (and his followers') attempts to freeze humans in liquid nitrogen; and Alexey Zamkov's 'gravidan' therapy, which was supposed to provide for rejuvenation and an increase in vitality thanks to the use of *gravidan*, a special medicine made from the urine of pregnant women.[9]

In his work, Krementsov has connected the emergence of visionary science in Soviet Russia – primarily biology and medicine – with two main factors: the development of experimental science ('the very word experimental in the Russian language has connotations of something new, never before attempted, and untried') and the active popularization of scientific research.[10] Scientists themselves were engaged in the popularization of their works, becoming the authors of publications in which they could more freely operate with the data obtained during experiments by placing it in broad cultural contexts. Their pioneering ideas were taken up by journalists and authors involved in the popularization of science, including life extension, which always aroused the keen interest of the general public and state officials. Thus, there was a process of 'continuous cross-examination, cross-pollination, and hybridization of various ideas', and, in some cases, even the intertwining of actual and fictional experiments, in which a variety of actors were involved: visionary biologists, officials, journalists, popular writers and the general public.[11]

Bolshevik visionary science flourished not only during the immediate post-revolutionary period. We can find signs of its development in various studies across Soviet history, although they, for the most part, were not as radical as those experiments conducted in the 1920s. It is important to consider these studies in a broad context, taking into account the efforts of the scientists themselves to popularize their work and the public reception of their ideas. For one such example of visionary science, we can consider the research of Professor Ilya Arshavsky (1903–90) on the positive influence of various stress factors, such as reduced caloric intake, moderate hypoxia and exposure to cold experienced at the early stages of ontogenesis – in the prenatal period and early infancy – on the lifespan of mammals, including humans. In his search for answers, he employed both his own laboratory research on animals and studies conducted on of the experience of alternative projects for infant care and development that arose in the late Soviet Union.

Ilya Arshavsky and his research into developmental physiology: *The Energy Principle of Skeletal Muscles*

Professor Ilya Arshavsky was one of the few students of the outstanding Russian physiologist Alexei Ukhtomsky (1875–1942). In 1935, Arshavsky founded the laboratory of developmental physiology at the All-Union Institute of Experimental Medicine (VIEM), which he ran for many years until 1980. After the reorganization of VIEM in 1944, Arshavksy's laboratory moved to the newly created Academy of Medical Sciences. According to some evidence, the real initiator of the VIEM project was Maxim Gorky, who, under the influence of Bertrand Russell's book *The Scientific Outlook* (1931), had dreamed of creating a unique academy for the comprehensive study of human health in the Soviet Union.[12] VIEM, founded in 1931, was supposed to become the largest scientific centre for the 'integrated study of the human body', as well as solving the more practical problems of radical life extension and the fight against the most dangerous diseases, such as cancer, typhus and tuberculosis.[13]

Arshavsky had a wide range of scientific interests: he studied the physiological mechanisms of individual development, as well as the activities of the nervous, respiratory, cardiovascular, musculoskeletal and digestive systems. Arshavsky emphasized that studies of ontogenetic patterns could not be limited to any particular period of life, but should cover the whole lifespan, from fertilization to the ageing and death of an organism. He was known as a gerontologist as well as a specialist in intrauterine development and the physiology of infants. He authored popular books for parents and made a number of practical proposals for maternity hospitals, nurseries and kindergartens. Arshavsky was also an active proponent of early breastfeeding: in the 1950s, when the separation of mothers from their babies immediately after birth was a mandatory practice in Soviet maternity wards, he declared that newborns should instead be attached to their mothers' breasts within 30 minutes after birth, as this contributed to the successful formation of a child's immune system.[14]

In 1957, together with the well-known Soviet biologists Vladimir Alpatov, Lev Komarov and Zhores Medvedev, Ilya Arshavsky participated in the creation of the gerontological section of the Moscow Society of Naturalists (*Moskovskoe obshchestvo ispytatelej prirody – MOIP*), one of Russia's oldest scientific societies.[15] Arshavsky was also a regular participant at gerontological conferences. For example, he took part in an international symposium on the prospects of using physical activity to help ageing organisms, which was held by the Institute of Gerontology and Experimental Pathology in Kiev in 1969. The topic of the conference was highly relevant to Arshavsky's research on physical activity and its influence on ageing and life expectancy. In his paper at the conference, Arshavsky made one of his favourite comparisons: an organism, he said, was like a clockwork mechanism, wound and beginning its course at the moment of fertilization. At the same time, he rejected the contemporaneously popular idea that the body was like a machine: that the more it worked the sooner it would wear out, along with the associated assertion that a body in the process of life is gradually using up its genetically predetermined energy fund. Arshavsky put forward an alternative opinion, which was the key thesis of his theory of individual development:

> In the process of ontogenesis, the energy capabilities of the organism are constantly increasing to a maximum in adulthood, after which, the dissipation of energy starts to increase more and more. This energy loss is associated with the beginning of ageing and peaks in the age of senility.[16]

Arshavsky also contributed a chapter to the first Soviet manual on the biology of ageing, in which he proposed to study the 'true physiological mechanisms' that determined life expectancy in different animal species.[17] This became the main focus of his research, most fully described in the monograph *Physiological Mechanisms and Patterns of Individual Development*, in which he cited the data of comparative ontogenetic studies on different species of mammals carried out in his laboratory.[18] Arshavsky was continuing an ongoing dispute with the ideas of the German physiologist Max Rubner (1854–1932). Rubner had been one of the early proponents of the rate-of-living theory, which suggested that slow metabolisms would increase lifespans: in other words, larger animals would live longer than smaller ones.[19] Arshavsky tirelessly refuted Rubner's 'surface hypothesis':

> The data from our studies on rabbits and hares, rats and squirrels reaching the same weight and linear dimensions at adulthood, has made it possible to verify that the energy fund acquired in the process of individual development is the greater, the higher is the behavioral motor activity, and accordingly, the longer is the lifespan of the corresponding mammalian species.[20]

In place of Rubner's hypothesis, Arshavsky put forward the 'principle of skeletal muscles': 'Energy features and accordingly the level of physiological functions of different organ systems and the whole body are determined by the skeletal muscle characteristics in each age period.'[21] Turning to thermodynamics, Arshavsky argued that 'the amount of free energy in open living systems for each recuperation process following the period of activity increases in comparison with what took place in the initial state'. Explaining the physiological mechanism of redundant recovery, he draws attention first of all to the cellular metabolism process: 'the work of the muscular system leads to redundancy in anabolic processes, ensuring the growth and development of the body'.[22] He also analysed the connection between motor activity and the work of the cardiovascular, respiratory and nervous systems, paying particular attention to 'the emergence and successive change of dominant states that are formed in the nervous system'.

The social factors affecting human life expectancy also attracted Arshavsky's attention. Explaining why human energy funds are higher than that of other mammalian species, he referred to Engels's thesis that labour was an important factor in the evolution of humans as a species. In addition to reproductive functions, Engels wrote, humans have an important species mission: creative labour activity, which continues after the end of their childbearing period. Thus, labour should be considered as a factor in the induction of excess metabolism and an increase in free energy, and thus a factor that could help to ensure longer human life expectancies.[23]

Arshavsky's ideas about ageing were widely known in the Soviet Union, thanks to the efforts of journalists and popular authors who were engaged in the popularization of science[24] and healthy lifestyle.[25] The famous surgeon and academician Nikolai Amosov, also known as a promoter of active lifestyles and jogging, referred to the works of Arshavsky and in particular to his experiments with hares and rabbits as evidence of the positive effect of physical activity on life expectancy. 'The theory of I. A. Arshavsky shows us the real paths leading to an increase in life expectancy', Amosov wrote: 'If you give a domestic rabbit the physical activity of a hare, many of its metabolic indicators will become close to those of a wild hare. With physical activity life expectancy will also increase. We should emphasize: optimization of physical activity is the right way to improve health and, therefore, longevity.'[26]

Arshavsky's research into child development and physiology: The concept of 'infant immaturity'

Arshavsky's interest in the early stages of ontogenesis was driven by his research on the factors underlying life expectancy and the human body's energy capabilities. In his early works, he drew attention to changes in heart and respiratory rates occurring in the process of growth: an infant's heart rate is more than two times higher than that an adult's, while its respiration rate is four times higher.[27] Observing sick children who were unable to walk, he found that an increase in their body size in their case did not create a decrease in heart or respiratory rates. He suggested that the normal decrease was associated with physical activity and began at the moment when a child mastered the standing posture and began to walk – when the skeletal muscles came into play. These observations were continued in laboratory studies on baby mammals with different lifestyles, active and sedentary, for example, hares and rabbits. Unlike a hare, whose heart rate drops over the years of its lifespan and reaches 60 beats per minute in adulthood, while its breathing slows down by a factor of 4–5, in the case of a rabbit, both remain unchanged: 300 heart beats per minute in the first hours of life and about the same in adulthood, although its body size has grown 100 times larger. Comparing this data with the correlation that animals with a high heart and breathing rates do not live long – rabbits live four to five years and hares two to three times longer – Arshavsky turned the problem into an entire experimental field. If a lack of physical activity leads to premature ageing, would it be possible to influence life expectancy by increasing physical activity in the early stages of ontogenesis?

As a theoretical basis for his experiments, Arshavsky used the ideas of his teacher, A. Ukhtomsky, about the processes of excitation and inhibition in the nervous system by which the body continuously interacts with the environment. Ukhtomsky's theory of 'dominant focus' – the ability of living tissue to respond to stimuli with the maximum number of excitations per unit of time – helped Arshavsky to formulate the idea of a human body's 'potential lability'. In Arshavsky's laboratory, studies were carried out on various species of mammals in the process of ontogenesis to study their adaptive responses to changes in the level of motor activity. For example, it was found that if pregnant rabbits were exposed to moderate systematic hypoxia, the foetuses gave an adaptive response: there was an increase in total muscle mass, as well as the size of the heart, lungs and brain. Similar experiments with nutritional deficiencies and physical training demonstrated the same results. On the contrary, with an excess of oxygen and nutrients motor reactions decreased and even stopped, while growth and development were delayed.[28] These experiments confirmed Arshavksy's hypothesis about the high physiological adaptability of a foetus and allowed him to formulate the concept of a *gestational dominant* – a form of nervous-system regulation of endocrine support for a normal pregnancy, which ensured normal antenatal development.

Arshavsky claimed that all sorts of complications during pregnancy – any shift away from the *gestational dominant* – led to the birth of physiologically immature infants. He formulated the concept of *physiological immaturity* of newborns to denote the condition of newborns characterized by a physiological age lagging behind their calendar age, but different from the concept of true prematurity.[29] He noted that a physiologically immature child could have a normal gestational age, weight and body size, and on the surface appear no different from a healthy one. Among the main signs of physiological immaturity, however, Arshavsky referenced muscle hypotension, poor reflexes and underdeveloped thermoregulation.[30] He associated physiological immaturity with reduced immunobiological resistance and claimed that it was the main cause of pathologies and illnesses, as well as the cause of premature ageing. Arshavsky found signs of physiological immaturity in most newborns, noting later that their number had grown steadily and by the late 1980s had reached more than 80 per cent of all newly born children.[31]

At the same time, however, Arshavsky did not consider physiological immaturity to be a disease, as it could be fully compensated for through proper care and vigorous exercise. The concept of physiological immaturity was important for Arshavsky as a framework for directing research and, above all, as a search for ways to compensate for physiological lag. Accordingly, he was critical of the neonatal diagnostic method known as the Apgar Score, which had been proposed by the US physician and medical researcher, Virginia Apgar, in the 1960s and later recommended by the World Health Organization (WHO) and adopted in many countries, including Russia.[32]

In search of optimal ways to compensate for immaturity and restore normal muscle tone, Arshavsky applied to baby mammals such methods as increased physical activity, cold strengthening, calorie restriction and moderate oxygen starvation (hypoxia). As a result of these experiments, he managed to raise animals that differed markedly from ordinary representatives of their species on numerous parameters: they were larger and had greater muscle mass, better thermoregulation, consumed less oxygen and had high resistance to various types of toxic substances and bacteria. In addition, Arshavsky noted that such animals reached sexual maturity later, which he attributed to factors that positively affected life expectancy. Indeed, according to Arshavsky, the rabbits experimented on in his study lived three to six years longer than those from the control group.[33] In particular, he managed to raise a so-called muscle rabbit, which in many respects was close to the parameters of a hare.

Arshavsky argued that the animals experimented upon had improved not only their physical, but also intellectual development. He found that rats and rabbits raised 'under conditions of optimal musculoskeletal activity' had a greater relative and absolute mass of the brain and cerebellum; he concluded that the amount of received and processed information had also increased.[34]

As a result of his experiments, Arshavsky concluded that stress experienced at the early stages of ontogenesis was beneficial. If the intensity of stressful stimulation did not exceed the adaptive capabilities, he argued, the body acquired the ability to resist not only the influencing stimulus but also other stress factors.[35] Moreover, he argued that a specific phenotype, a kind of adaptive modification, was formed as a result of the stress response.[36] Experiments with baby mammals further allowed Arshavsky to make some recommendations about newborn baby care, which were supposed to compensate for their physiological immaturity. He recommended the delayed cutting of the umbilical cord and the joint stay of the mother with the newborn, early breastfeeding, cold strengthening and swimming. He also spoke out against tight swaddling and in favour of loose clothing for newborns, which would not restrict physical activity.

Arshavsky's interest in alternative practices of infant development: Cold strengthening, swimming and gymnastics

The general mistrust of doctors and medicine in the late and immediate post-Soviet period was especially strong in maternal and child health care.[37] In this atmosphere, a variety of alternative approaches to pregnancy, childbirth and infant development appeared among broad-minded parents. The Nikitins's child-rearing system, the 'Aquaculture' method of infant swimming created by Igor Charkovsky, and children's sports training and cold strengthening as per the work of Vladimir Skripalev all gained great popularity among supporters of healthy and active lifestyles. Formal Soviet medicine in general disapproved of these practices, but they were supported by well-known actors and journalists, as well as influential officials (for example, Zakharii Firsov, the Chairman of the Swimming Federation of the USSR) and scientists. Ilya Arshavsky was among the scientists who made important contributions to the support and popularization of these projects.

The family of teachers Boris and Elena Nikitin and their seven children became widely known in the 1970s and 1980s for their innovative methods of early childhood development. They focused on physical training: gymnastics on homemade sports equipment and cold strengthening (infants were carried outdoors naked or in light clothes in winter, while older children walked barefoot in the snow). The Nikitins believed that early physical activity allowed children to overtake their coevals both physically and intellectually; they put forward a 'creativity hypothesis', according to which creativity emerged during infancy and early childhood, so that it was critical to make effective use of this time.[38] The Nikitins also concluded that most childhood illnesses were created by adults and based on all sorts of prejudices: 'Illnesses are hidden in medical recommendations, manuals and instructions for obstetricians, [and in] popular lectures on radio and television.'[39] They wrote several books, which garnered immense popularity among Soviet parents and even abroad. Their house became a kind of pilgrimage place for parents from all over the country and the Nikitins themselves travelled throughout the country, promoting their experience and active infancy methods.

Ilya Arshavsky was among several Soviet scientists who supported the Nikitins's child-rearing practices. The first edition of the Nikitins's book *We and Our Children* (1979) was published with an interview with Arshavsky, in which he comprehensively supported their method. Since 1966, Arshavsky said, the laboratory he headed had been constantly monitoring the health and physical development of the Nikitins's children. Anna Nikitina recalled: 'They measured us, told us to do various physical exercises, recorded cardiograms ... – it was very serious.'[40] Arshavsky greatly valued the experience of the Nikitins, noting that they were able to compensate for the health problems of their children by finding techniques that could be used from the first days of life: 'All their children were born immature [...]. Nevertheless, in all cases, remarkable success was achieved.'[41] In turn, the Nikitins recommended Arshavsky's scientific and popular books to parents and themselves appealed to his works as a theoretical basis for their experiments. In their books, they also published Arshavsky's recommendations on reforming maternity hospitals and supporting breastfeeding in infancy.

Arshavsky's ideas about the energy potential of newborns, published in popular articles and brochures, inspired many parents to develop activities for their children, especially in cases when children had health problems. Amongst those inspired was the engineer Vladimir Skripalev, who designed his first home-made sports complex in 1971 to train his son, although doctors had said that he would never be able to walk normally. This experiment turned out to be very successful, and drawings of Skripalev's sports complex and training programme began to be published in a regular column entitled 'Stadium in an Apartment' in the popular magazine *Physical Culture and Sport* (*Fizku'tura i Sport*) over the course of 1977–8. Skripalev noted that Arshavsky's research and his *Energy Principle of Skeletal Muscles* had created the methodological basis for his engineering ideas and provided a particularly laconic version of Arshavsky's main idea: 'Life expectancy is longer the more a mammal moves during the period before puberty.'[42] In 1981, Skripalev's published a book with his ideas and training programmes, for which Arshavsky wrote an afterword: 'From the first minutes after birth, even during sleep, a baby periodically makes movements with his arms and legs. Their great importance is that they provide for the baby's further growth and development. ... That is why every apartment needs a sport complex similar to the one designed by V. Skripalev.'[43] In his book, Skripalev tells how Arshavsky, examining his son and observing his training, had spoken a phrase that Skripalev himself did not understand: 'Skripalev's children and the Nikitins' children had different genotypes, but the same phenotype.' It can be assumed that Arshavsky saw in these children, due to their increased physical activity, a special 'phenotype' or outward physical characteristic – 'a kind of adaptive modification, which was formed as a result of stress response' – which he had written about in connection with his experiments with baby mammals.[44]

The author of the most radical approach to infant training was the charismatic teacher and psychic Igor Charkovsky. In 1970–80, Charkovsky developed a method he called 'Aquaculture', which included the intensive training of pregnant women (swimming, diving, gymnastics and cold strengthening); giving birth in water (ideally, in the sea); baby yoga (a kind of neonatal manual correction) immediately after birth; parents helping the baby to swim and dive from the first day of life; babies breastfeeding, sleeping and playing in water; dynamic gymnastics with infants (a set of exercises that consisted of twisting, rotation and throwing), cold strengthening by bathing in ice holes and metaphysical connection with dolphins.[45] His ideas about infant swimming became widely known owing to numerous publications and documentaries about 'dolphin babies' who could swim and stay underwater for extended periods of time. One of these articles – 'Amphibian Girl' – about Charkovsky's water workouts with his newborn daughter was published as 'Swimming before Walking' in the magazine *Physical Culture and Sport*, which was edited in 1974–5 by the Chairman of the Swimming Federation of USSR, Zakhary Firsov.[46] In 1976, the All-Union Television channel released a documentary about infant swimming entitled 'Like a Fish in Water'. For a while, Charkovsky achieved international recognition thanks to a book by the Swedish journalist Erik Sidenbladh (1982)[47] and even became a kind of tourist attraction: famous foreigners, such as John Lilly, Jacques Mayol or Marsden Wagner, Director of the Women's and Children's Health Committee of the World Health Organization, met with Charkovsky during their visits to Moscow in the 1980s.[48]

In the 1970s and early 1980s Charkovsky worked as a research fellow at the Sports and Bio-mechanics Laboratory of the All-Union Scientific Research Institute of Physical Culture (VNIIFK). He conducted experiments with animals, participated in conferences and even prepared to defend a thesis. At the same time, Charkovsky gained further fame as a psychic (*ekstrasens*): he was engaged in healing and participated in various public events where psychics demonstrated their paranormal abilities. This mixture of academic science and esotericism was not exceptional for the time. Social interest in paranormal phenomena in the late Soviet period led to the emergence of a variety of hybrid forms: specially created laboratories even attracted psychics to study the physical mechanisms of extrasensory phenomena. One of the leading institutions conducting such research was the Academy of Sciences' Institute of Radio Engineering and Electronics. This institute undertook to investigate the healing power of the famous Soviet *ekstrasens* Eugenia Davitashvili ('Dzhuna').[49] This 'hybridity' was based on an ideological foundation: many Soviet scientists believed that paranormal phenomena, such as telekinesis, clairvoyance and extrasensory healing, had a material essence and saw their task in registering these phenomena through special devices and thus getting closer to understanding the nature of this abilities.[50]

In his laboratory, Charkovsky conducted endless experiments with land animals and insects – flies, cockroaches, hens, mice, cats and many others – trying to accustom them to life in the water: 'We tried to change the attitude of animals to the aquatic environment, to help them overcome their fear and inherited neurotic attitudes, and to increase their ability to solve a variety of problems in this environment.'[51] For example, animals had to dive or cross a water hazard to get food, raise offspring in the water, etc. Charkovsky argued that all creatures could swim and lead an aquatic life through special training; moreover, the trained animals could breed offspring in the aquatic environment and transfer their acquired skills. Charkovsky also claimed that if a mother experienced regular hypoxic conditions during pregnancy, she 'accustomed' her foetus to these states, which would have a positive effect because this experience increased brain volume and speeded up physical and mental development.[52] Clearly referencing Arshavsky, Charkovsky also claimed that the offspring would have greater vitality and life expectancy.[53] According to Charkovsky, a newborn's prolonged stay in water could save him from 'gravitational shock': due to the decrease in gravitational pull in water, the energy consumption of the body was reduced and an 'energy reserve' was created, which could be used for nursing weakened, injured and premature babies.[54]

Arshavsky was very enthusiastic about Charkovsky's Aquaculture methods: not only did he give positive comments about this 'innovative swimming training for babies' in the press, but he also wrote about Charkovsky's experiments in his popular books.[55] Charkovsky, in turn, argued that the Aquaculture method was based on a 'thorough knowledge of physiology', and, above all – on Arshavsky's research.

Arshavsky examined children who had been trained according to the Aquaculture system and positively evaluated the workouts, confirming that the 'amphibian children' were stronger than normal (Figure 3.1). He regarded infant swimming as a hardening practice and recommended dipping a baby in water for a few seconds several times a day. He also found it extremely beneficial to dip a child

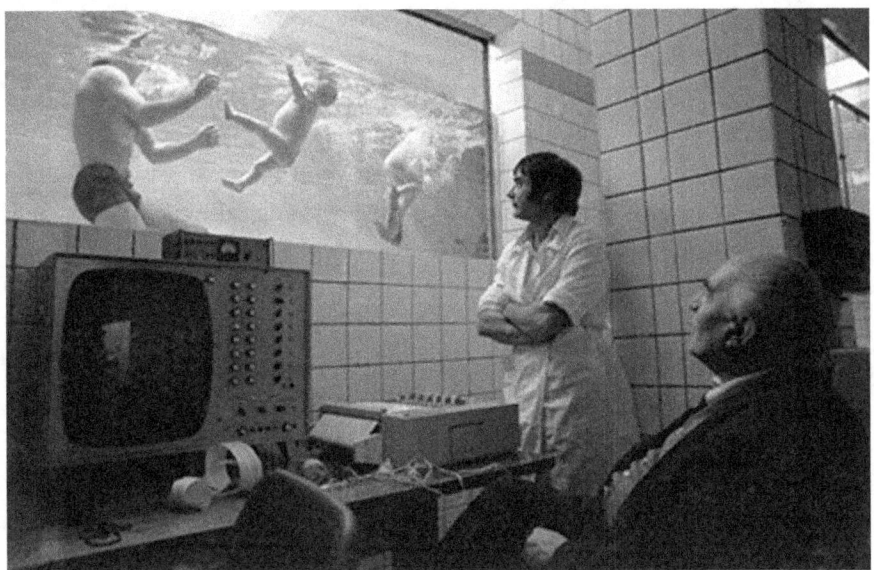

Figure 3.1 Ilya Arshavsky and Igor Charkovsky oversee babies' water training. Moscow, 1980s. Photo by Alexander Grashchenkov. Source: RIA Novosti.

at the age of several weeks in cold water or in an ice hole, and claimed that short-term oxygen deficiency was a good stimulant for the body.[56] At the same time, he did not share Charkovsky's idea that a child could swim from the very first days of life, because he believed that a child could not learn to coordinate swimming movements earlier than at the age of 2.5–3 years, and before that age could only stay on the water's surface.[57]

On the one hand, in creating his utopian project, Charkovsky was inspired by various para-scientific concepts: studies of human contacts with dolphins, studies of extrasensory perception and bioenergetics, the teachings of Porfiry Ivanov and others.[58] His project belonged to the late twentieth-century wave of esoteric, or para-scientific, teachings that shared a faith in hidden human potential and the ability to master it through special technologies. Thus, it belongs to the late Soviet New Age – its own sort of 'occult milieu'.[59] On the other hand, scientific research was also an important source of inspiration for Charkovsky: he found there the confirmation of his thoughts and believed that his experiments were based on scientific knowledge. There was a kind of two-way process between scientists like Arshavsky and practitioners like Charkovsky. Alternative projects served for Arshavsky as a source of data on the physiological parameters of children who had been engaged in early swimming, cold strengthening, etc., while Arshavsky's research worked as a scientific and theoretical basis for these alternative radical experiments. An important role in this cooperative relationship was played by the popularization of Arshavsky's works: quotes from his books were to be found in many publications on health issues in the 1980s and early 1990s,[60] and one of his expressions became particularly popular: 'A baby who was born physiologically mature not only cannot die but cannot even get sick.'[61]

Conclusion – Towards a 'new physiology': Arshavsky's contribution to the Soviet science of ageing and developmental physiology

Professor Ilya Arshavsky is remembered in today's Russia primarily for his recommendations on reforming maternal and child healthcare, as well as for his advice for parents. His efforts have contributed to progressive changes in maternity wards, children's hospitals, nurseries and kindergartens, and in general, to the perception of babies in society. However, his concept of *infant immaturity* has not received appreciable acceptance or implementation. In part, this was due to a mismatch between his suggestions and social expectation. Many of Arshavsky's ideas concerning infant care, in particular his views on cold strengthening, ran counter to the approaches promoted at that time in Soviet paediatrics. Although various 'strengthening' practices were quite popular in the Soviet Union and were actively promoted as a means of improving health, they had not been applied to small children. The well-known slogan 'Sun, air and water are our best friends' ('Solntse, vozdukh i voda – nashi lushchie druz'ia!') in reality took second place to a strict regulation of child healthcare: dietary habits, physical and mental development standards, and daily care routines that included obligatory tight swaddling, were all closely and strictly regulated.

One of the founders of Soviet physiotherapy and sports medicine, Ivan Sarkizov-Serazini, explained the standard mechanism according to Pavlov's theory of conditioned reflexes: 'Undoubtedly, with the systematic effect of temperature stimuli on the human body, the nature of the responses to these stimuli begins to change.'[62] For example, under the influence of frequent use of cold water, the body becomes accustomed to low temperatures and becomes immune to cold. However, Sarkizov-Serazini is not talking about hardening in general, that is, increasing the body's resistance to other environmental factors beyond cold. Moreover, he says that long breaks in hardening weaken the strength of adaptive connections, reduce and even negate the developed resistance to a certain stimulus.[63] Arshavsky had a slightly different understanding of the physiological mechanism of strengthening. He did not limit the positive benefits of cold training to the fact that it gave resistance to low temperatures: instead, he believed that, like any type of hardening, it would lead to an increase in the vitality of the body, including its adaptability to temperature changes. He based this claim primarily on his Energy Principle of Skeletal Muscles: any locomotor activity, including muscle contractions when exposed to cold, contributed to the production of excess energy, which was necessary for normal growth, development and health. Physical activity, including that experienced in the form of stressful conditions caused by a lack of nutrition and oxygen, as well as exposure to cold, was especially important during critical periods of life – at the early stages of ontogenesis. Arshavsky argued that the stress experienced in the prenatal period and early infancy hardened the body for life: that it literally 'winds up the clock of life'.

Arshavsky's works about the benefits of physical activity, cold strengthening and babies' swimming from the first days of life also inspired broadminded parents to experiment with such practices as early swimming, baby-yoga, ice-hole dipping, etc. His popular articles and brochures also greatly contributed to the legitimization of these practices. His personal support for Charkovsky contributed to the formation of the para-scientific concept of 'Aquaculture', and their informal cooperation could be seen as an example of hybrid projects of esoteric and scientific approaches and practices, aimed together at radical human enhancement. The phenomenon of late Soviet para-science, which includes belief in supernatural abilities, esoteric and para-religious beliefs, has already been covered in a number of studies,[64] but its connection with academic science, at both institutional and personal levels, remains unstudied. The very use of the concepts of 'para-science', 'pseudoscience' and 'alternative science' in this historical context is complicated, since it is not easy to draw a clear line between or around them. First, certain pseudoscientific trends actually found homes in formal academic institutions. Secondly, there existed the phenomenon of 'semi-alternative science': studies that did not contradict the canon of official science but were banned for ideological reasons.[65] As a result, many studies of the 'supernatural' were presented as 'cutting-edge science', which had simply not yet received recognition in the ideologized field of Soviet research. In fact, however, there was also an active popularization of parascience, both by researchers themselves and also by journalists. Altogether, there was a favourable environment for alternative modes of visionary science, including Arshavsky's vision of overcoming infant 'immaturity' or even Charkovsky's extension to overcoming the bounds of gravity on land.

Notes

1. Aleksandr A. Bogomolets (ed.), *Starost'. Trudy konferentsii po probleme geneza starosti i profilaktiki prezhdevremennogo stareniia organizma*, 17–19 December 1938 (Kiev: Publishing House of the Academy of Sciences of the Ukrainian SSR, 1939), 5.
2. Ivan R. Tarkhanov, 'Prodolzhitel'nost' zhizni zhivotnyh, rastenii i liudei', *Vestnik Evropy* 3, no. 6 (1891): 538–52; no. 9 (1891): 87–125.
3. The concept of *premature ageing* is widely used in contemporary works on ageing in the post-Soviet space in a variety of contexts. See, for example: M.S. Pristrom, S.L. Pristrom, and I.I. Semenenkov, 'Starenie fiziologicheskoe i prezhdevremennoe. Sovremennyi vzgliad na problem', *Mezhdunarodnye obzory: klinicheskaia praktika i zdorov'e*, 5–6 (2017): 40–64.
4. Nikolai L. Krementsov, *Revolutionary Experiments: The Quest for Immortality in Bolshevik Science and Fiction* (Oxford: Oxford University Pres, 2014), 11.
5. T.A. Belova and S.E. Borisov, 'Iz istorii radikal'nogo uvelicheniia prodolzhitel'nosti zhizni cheloveka: Lev V. Komarov', *Vestnik gerontologicheskogo obshhestva Rossiiskoi akademii nauk* 11–12 (December 2000): 33–4.
6. For an overview, see Vladimir V. Frol'kis (ed.), *Biologiia stareniia* (Leningrad: Nauka, 1982).
7. Mark B. Adams, 'Last Judgment: The Visionary Biology of J. B. S. Haldane', *Journal of the History of Biology* 33 (2000): 457–91, doi: 10.1023/a:1004891323595.
8. Krementsov, *Revolutionary Experiments*, 163.
9. Anya Bernstein, *The Future of Immortality: Remaking Life and Death in Contemporary Russia* (Princeton: Princeton University Press, 2019).
10. Krementsov, *Revolutionary Experiments*, quote on 186.
11. Ibid., 192.
12. Tatiana I. Grekova and Kirill A. Lange, 'Tragicheskie stranitsy istorii Instituta eksperimental'noi meditsiny (20-30-e gody)', *Repressirovannaia nauka* 2 (1994): 12.
13. Resolution of the Council of People's Commissars of the USSR of July 15, 1936. № 1272 'O rabote Vsesoiuznogo instituta eksperimental'noi Meditsiny imeni A. M. Gor'kogo pri SNK Soiuza SSR'.
14. Ilya A. Arshavsky, 'Fiziologicheskoe obosnovanie vskarmlivaniia grud'iu novorozhdennyh detei totchas posle rozhdeniia. (K preduprezhdeniu tak nazyvaemoi fiziologicheskoi poteri vesa)', *Voprosy okhrany materinstva i detstva* 5 (1952): 45–50.

15 Valery M. Novoselov, 'Vzgliad klinicheskogo gerontologa na istoriiu gerontologii mira i Rossii', *Doklady MOIP* 65 (2018): 11–16.
16 Ilya A. Arshavsky, 'Skeletnaja muskulatura i osnovnye zakonomernosti ontogeneza', in *Dvigatel'naia aktivnost' i starenie* (Kiev: Gerontologicheskoe obshchestvo, 1969), 50.
17 Ilya A. Arshavsky 'Vidovaia prodolzhitel'nost' zhizni mlekopitaiushhih', in V.V. Frol'kis (ed.), *Biologii starenii* (Leningrad: Nauka, 1982), 24–38, quote on 25.
18 Ilya A. Arshavsky, *Fiziologicheskie mehanizmy i zakonomernosti individual'nogo razvitiia: Osnovy negentropiinoi teorii ontogeneza* (Moscow: Nauka, 1982).
19 Stephan Rössner, 'Max Rubner (1854–1932)', *Obesity Reviews* 14, no. 5 (2013): 432–3. https://doi.org/10.1111/obr.12023
20 Arshavsky, *Fiziologicheskie mehanizmy*, 41.
21 Arshavsky, 'Skeletnaia muskulatura', 68; Arshavsky, *Fiziologicheskie mehanizmy*, 27.
22 Arshavsky, *Fiziologicheskie mehanizmy*, 32.
23 Arshavsky 'Vidovaia prodolzhitel'nost' zhizni mlekopitaiushhih', 36.
24 Alexander D. Popovsky, 'Trud i dolgoletie', *Nauka i zhizn* 7 (1962): 71–4.
25 Anatoly M. Chaikovsky and Steve B. Shenkman, *Iskusstvo byt' zdorovym* (Moscow: Fizkul'tura i sport, 1987); O. Franzen, 'Kovarstvo komforta' (Interview with I.A Arshavsky, recorded in the late 1970s), appendix in Boris Nikitin and Lena Nikitina, *My, nashi deti i vnuki*, vol. 1 (Moscow: Samokat, 2017), 189–215.
26 Nikolay M. Amosov, *Entsiklopediia Amosova: Algoritm zdorov'ia* (Moscow: AST, 2002), 225.
27 Ilya A. Arshavsky, *Nervnaia reguliatsiia deiatel'nosti serdechnososudistoi sistemy v ontogeneze* (Moscow: Biomedgiz, 1936).
28 Arshavsky, *Fiziologicheskie mehanizmy*, 92–3.
29 Ilya A. Arshavsky, *Ocherki po vozrastnoi fiziologii* (Moscow: Meditsina, 1967).
30 Arshavsky, *Fiziologicheskie mehanizmy*, 195.
31 Ilya A. Arshavsky, *Vash rebenok. U istokov zdorov'ia* (Moscow, 1992), 25.
32 Ilya A. Arshavsky, *Vash malysh mozhet ne bolet'!* (Moscow: Sovetskii sport, 1990).
33 Ilya A. Arshavsky, 'Osnovy vozrastnoi periodizatsii', in V.N. Nikitin (ed.), *Vozrastnaia fiziologiia* (Leningrad: Nauka, 1975).
34 Arshavsky, *Fiziologicheskie mehanizmy*, 33.
35 Ibid., 49.
36 Ibid., 147.
37 Michele Rivkin-Fish, *Women's Health in Post-Soviet Russia: The Politics of Intervention* (Bloomington: Indiana University Press, 2005); Nina L. Rusinova and Julie V. Brown, 'Curing and Crippling: Bio-medical and Alternative Healing in Post-Soviet Russia', *The Annals of the American Academy of Political and Social Science* 583 (2002): 160–72. DOI: 10.1177/000271620258300110.
38 Nikitin and Nikitina, *My, nashi deti i vnuki*, v. 1, 273.
39 Boris P. Nikitin, *Zdorovoe detstvo bez lekarstv i privivok*, 6th ed. (Moscow: List New, 2001).

40 Anna Nikitina, 'Ilia A. Arshavsky' in *Sem'ia Nikitinyh* (April–May, 2009) (http://nikitiny.ru/arshavskij?hc95b557dffd1c8279e209cf12e9b9ebe=0046a0bfd9a5daf51e4db533a474b48d&wrs4b390a4716ec4f18db62 cf7d8dd66e64=00fe2738e6eceaf776eb690501a88e9c).
41 Cit. in: Franzen, 'Kovarstvo komforta', 205.
42 Vladimir S. Skripalev, *Stadion v kvartire* (Moscow: Fizkul'tura i sport, 1981), 39.
43 Ibid., 94.
44 Arshavsky, *Fiziologicheskie mehanizmy*, 147.
45 Anna Ozhiganova, 'The Birth of a New Human Being: The Utopian Project of the Late Soviet Water Birth Movement and Its Inheritors', in Robbie Davis-Floyd (ed.), *Birthing Techno-Sapiens: Human-Technology Co-Evolution and the Future of Reproduction* (New York: Routledge, 2021), 193–207.
46 Steve Schenkman, 'Devochka-amfibiia', *Fizkul'tura i sport* 11 (1974): 36–7.
47 Erik Sidenbladh, *Water Babies* (New York: St. Martin's Press, 1982).
48 Anna A. Ozhiganova, 'Giving Birth to a Baby Dolphin: Esoteric Representations of Human-Dolphin Connections in the Late Soviet Waterbirth Movement', *Baltic Worlds* 4 (2021).
49 Daria Shevtsova, 'Dzhuna and Soviet (Para)Science Experiments', in *New Age in Russia*, 30 March 2021, https://newageru.hypotheses.org/5752.
50 Alexander G. Spirkin, 'Poznavaia psikhobiofizicheskuiu real'nost', *Tekhnika – molodiozhi* 3 (1980): 47–50.
51 Igor B. Charkovsky, 'K voprosu o vliianii vzveshennogo sostoianiia na prodolzhitel'nost' zhizni organizma', in *Materialy itogovoi konferentsii VNIIFK za 1973* (Moscow: VNIIFK, 1975), 123–4.
52 Igor B. Charkovsky, 'Vodnaia sreda kak faktor, raskryvaiushhii rezervnye vozmozhnosti cheloveka', in V.V. Kuznetsov (ed.), *Problemy rezervnyh vozmozhnostei cheloveka* (Moscow: VNIIFK, 1982), 156–61, quote on 159.
53 Ibid., 159.
54 Ibid., 161.
55 Gerard Yelensky and Peter Korop, 'Delo po obvineniiu', *Smena* 19 (1973): 21; Arshavsky, *Vash rebenok*.
56 Arshavsky, *Vash malysh mozhet ne bolet'*, 32.
57 Ibid., 36.
58 Porfiry Ivanov (1898–1983) was a Russian mystic and healer and the author of a cold strengthening and spiritual healing method called *Detka* ('Baby'). Ivanov's teachings prescribed bathing in ice holes, dousing oneself with cold water and walking barefoot in the snow to become closer to nature and become healed of all diseases. See: Boris Knorre, 'Sistema Porfirija Ivanova: kul't i dvizhenie', in M. Burdo and S.B. Filatov (eds.), *Sovremennaia religioznaia zhizn' Rossii: opyt sistematicheskogo opisaniia* (Moscow: Universitetskaia kniga, Logos, 2006), v. 4, 244–58.

59 Birgit Menzel, 'Occult and Esoteric Movements in Russia from the 1960s to the 1980s', in B. Menzel, M. Hagemeister, and B. Glatzer Rosenthal (eds.), *The New Age of Russia: Occult and Esoteric Dimensions* (München: Verlag Otto Sagner, 2012), 151–85.
60 See: Chaikovsky and Shenkman, *Iskusstvo byt' zdorovym,*
61 Arshavsky, *Vash rebenok*, 18.
62 Ivan M. Sarkizov-Serazini, *Osnovy zakalivaniia (s izbrannymi razdelami iz fizioterapii),* 4th ed. (Moscow: Fizkul'tura i sport, 1953), 26.
63 Ibid., 34.
64 Menzel, 'Occult and Esoteric Movements in Russia'; Nikolai Mitrokhin, 'Sovetskaia intelligentsiia v poiskah chuda: religioznost' i paranauka v SSSR v 1953–1985 godakh', *Novoe literaturnoe obozrenie*, no. 3 (163) (2020): 51–78.
65 Vladimir V. Komissarov, 'Funktsional'noe znachenie paranauki v zhizni sovetskoi intelligentsii 1960–80 gg', *Intelligentsiia i mir*, no. 3 (2012): 9–19.

Part Two

Care for older persons: Soviet geriatrics, spatial organization and social support

4

Ageing minds and bodies: Caring for older patients at a Soviet psychiatric hospital

Aleksandra Marta Brokman

After the Second World War the growing number of older people in the Soviet population led to increased societal interest in the processes of ageing, as well as the social and healthcare provisions aimed at addressing the specific needs of older citizens. The post-war period saw the significant development of gerontology and geriatrics, with researchers in those disciplines working to deepen understandings of health and illness in old age. This increased interest in ageing and conditions predominantly affecting older people was also visible in Soviet psychiatry, with researchers and practitioners turning their attention towards developing a better understanding of the mental health problems affecting older persons and improving the treatment of such patients.

This became particularly visible from the late 1950s and 1960s and was exemplified by the prominent place occupied by old-age psychiatry in the programme of the first congress organized by the newly created Russian Society of Neuropathologists and Psychiatrists, held in October 1962 in Moscow. Old age was among the most discussed topics at the congress, with papers covering a wide range of issues, from the factors that increased the risk of psychiatric disorders in old age, through their specific course and characteristics, to their incidence rate and prophylaxis. The final resolution of the congress emphasized that the ageing of the population necessitated the improvement of geropsychiatric services, more research into mental disorders affecting older persons and additional efforts aimed at their prevention.[1] Similar voices emphasizing the increased importance of old-age psychiatry could be heard throughout the following decades.[2] Although subsequent congresses of the Russian and all-Soviet associations of neuropathologists and psychiatrists did not feature these issues quite as prominently as in 1962, old-age psychiatry continued to grow as an important aspect of Soviet mental health research.

One popular argument in the Soviet field of geropsychiatry stated that old age did not have to be accompanied by any significant disorders. Soviet researchers rejected the idea that conditions such as dementia were a constituent and perhaps unavoidable part of the processes of ageing, although they admitted that present understandings of these processes were limited.[3] This strand of thinking was most visible in the writings of psychiatrists who focused their attention on preventing mental health disorders. Some went a step even further, suggesting that everyone could enjoy a healthy, fulfilling old age if only they made a conscious effort to work on themselves and adopt an appropriate lifestyle.[4]

The theme of working on oneself and self-improvement had long been present in Soviet ideology, permeating various aspects of life in the USSR. The belief in the plasticity of human beings was deeply ingrained in the ideology of the Soviet state, which from its early years set out to transform its people into the ideal of the New Soviet Persons: rational, disciplined citizens, committed to the ideals of the revolution and exercising perfect control over their minds and bodies.[5] The emphasis on self-improvement and perfecting one's body quickly became integrated into Soviet healthcare, particularly in the 1920s, when the People's Commissariat of Public Health headed by N. A. Semashko championed prophylactically oriented medicine.[6] Echoes of the conceptualization of individuals as capable of perfecting themselves through the conscious effort of their wills[7] could be found in post-war writing on mental health in old age, according to which old age could be overcome through individual effort: 'people who succeed at not getting old are the ones who do not want to get old'.[8]

Such arguments could often be found in texts written for the general public. While it is understandable that these ideas were put forward in order to motivate readers to take care of their health, they were a very visible part of discourse, implying that people who got old and suffered from serious age-related disorders must have failed in their self-improvement and struggle against old age. Just like twentieth-century Western health and wellness movements, which came under criticism for carrying exclusionary implications for society and not leaving much space for an '85-year-old man with a disabling respiratory ailment or the obese and severely arthritic elderly woman in a wheelchair',[9] the Soviet emphasis on healthy living and working on oneself in old age did not leave much space for a bedridden man suffering from acute old-age psychosis or for an older woman with severe dementia. Evaluating the discourse promulgated around old age in the early Soviet period, Stephen Lovell observed that 'old age, death and decrepitude represented a huge challenge for intellectuals propounding a faith in voluntarism and world transformation' – a challenge that was partially met when older persons were constructed as still potentially productive members of the Soviet workforce. This did not, however, leave much space for those who did not or could not work.[10] The issue clearly continued into the post-war decades, when significant emphasis was put on living an 'active' old age and pensioners were encouraged to engage in socially useful activity.[11]

This chapter focuses on the severely ill older persons who were left far outside this discourse, finding themselves unable to transform or even control their minds and bodies, and thus representing a stark case that demonstrates the limits to the plasticity of human material. Some older persons inevitably fell through the cracks of the narratives about self-improvement, active lifestyles and continued involvement in Soviet society. Older psychiatric patients presented a particularly stark example, as the progressing deterioration of their minds made them unable not only to be productive and socially useful, but in many cases also to express any desire, or lack thereof, to do so. What happened to these people? What care did they receive and how was their condition approached? Comprehensive answers to these questions would greatly exceed the scope of any single article; this chapter aims only to shed light on some particular examples, focusing on the care provided for older patients at one psychiatric hospital: Moscow's Clinical Psychiatric Hospital No. 4 named for P.B. Gannushkin.

The chapter's analysis is based on the hospital's archival files, chiefly the annual reports delineating the work of its wards. The available files cover the period from the early 1950s until the end of the 1970s, presenting a window into the hospital's activity across a sizable portion of the Soviet post-war era. The image of psychiatric care that emerges from them is a bleak one, in which patients whose bodies and minds deteriorated with no hope for recovery consequently disappear as people with social ties, needs relating to mental well-being or even distinct selves. They were instead cared for strictly as *bodies*, the physical and safety needs of which had to be managed. The wards caring for such patients, while still formally responsible for treatment, became liminal spaces between life and death, whose inhabitants, although still not dead, existed separately from social life, as their marks of personhood continued to diminish.

Elder care at the Gannushkin Hospital

Throughout the post-war decades, the Gannushkin Psychiatric Hospital had several different wards dedicated partially or primarily to caring for its older patients. In the early 1950s such patients were housed in Ward no. 4, which was formally dedicated to the care of women in infirm condition, as well as being scattered around several other wards.[12] While the profile of Ward no. 4 became significantly diversified towards the beginning of the 1960s,[13] several other wards dedicated entirely or largely to older patients began to emerge around that time. In 1957, the hospital opened Ward no. 17, located not in its main buildings, but in Liublino on the outskirts of Moscow. Dedicated to caring for particularly infirm patients of both genders, it focused primarily on those suffering from 'organic psychoses',[14] although it also housed people suffering from chronic alcoholism.[15] After it was transferred to the main hospital buildings in 1963, Ward no. 17 received a more clearly defined profile and became dedicated to caring for older men.[16] At the same time in the early 1960s, Ward no. 15 also began to predominantly house older patients and eventually became a ward for older women.[17] Both wards retained this old-age profile until the end of the period covered by the available files. In addition, Ward no. 22 also largely provided care for patients suffering from disorders common in old age from the late 1960s;[18] however, its yearly work is less well documented. Some older patients were also cared for in the wards with more general profiles.

Most of the older patients admitted to the Gannushkin Psychiatric Hospital suffered from old-age psychoses as well as neurological conditions that produced psychiatric symptoms such as cerebrovascular diseases and brain atrophies. Those patients constituted a majority in wards nos. 15 and 17. The prevalence of people with neurological conditions in psychiatric wards is not that surprising given the fact that neurology and psychiatry in the USSR were more intertwined than in the Western countries at the time.[19] The two disciplines shared professional associations, conferences, a journal and institutions, while old-age psychiatrists commonly researched and wrote on neurological conditions and accompanying mental health problems.[20] Patients with schizophrenia, who had often been living with this illness for fifteen or more years already, were also regularly listed in yearly ward reports.[21] From time to time, Ward no. 17 reported a small number of alcoholic patients, which increased in 1978, when ten beds were specifically designated for older and infirm alcoholics.[22]

Some patients improved enough to return home, but many needed help with basic activities, and had no chance for recovery. In some cases, they were admitted in a very serious state, which only worsened until their death. Their condition can be illustrated by the case of M., a woman sixty-four years of age, who was admitted to Ward no. 13 on 16 June 1961, and who died a week later of pathologies in the blood and lymph circulation in the brain. Her symptoms had begun to manifest a month prior to her admittance to the hospital, beginning with irregular behaviour: she put sugar on her sausages, placed a silk ribbon in the pot when cooking soup, became careless and stopped caring for her sick husband. She was examined by a neurologist, but her condition continued to deteriorate, necessitating hospitalization. At the hospital she was withdrawn and indifferent to her surroundings, did not know where she was and had a distorted sense of time. She repeated words and phrases during conversations, did not control her bowel movements and appeared neither to care about nor be aware of her condition. Due to her age, 'active intervention' (i.e. surgery) was impossible and she received only symptomatic treatment. Her speech deteriorated and she spent a lot of time lying on her back, with her legs bent towards her abdomen.[23]

In any given year, the wards dedicated to elder care housed a significant percentage of bedridden patients, patients with no chances for recovery, and those who, while able to walk, suffered too severe symptoms to take care of themselves. While not all reports give the number of such patients, some of the available data suggests that caring for them occupied a significant portion of the staff's time. For example, during 1960 in Ward no. 17, out of sixty-three patients who stayed at the ward, thirty were bedridden and forty-four suffered from urinary or bowel incontinence.[24] In 1969, the much larger Ward no. 22 reported having 75 patients who had no chance for recovery,[25] and a year later out of 263 patients who passed through this ward, 160 suffered from conditions accompanied by pronounced dementia and required prolonged hospitalization.[26] In 1973, out of the 215 patients who passed through Ward no. 15, only 53 were released home (which constituted an improvement on the 36 out of 220 patients released a year before). An almost equal number, fifty-two patients, died at the hospital in 1973.[27] Many patients were hospitalized for years, due to the severity of their conditions, problems with arranging transfers to a nursing home, and familial unwillingness to care for them at home.

The Gannushkin Psychiatric Hospital, like many Soviet medical institutions, struggled with overcrowding, shortages of staff and necessary equipment, as well as the poor conditions of the ward buildings themselves. The standard complaints in yearly reports included the lack of regular access to hot water and too low temperatures in the wards,[28] the insufficient amount of necessary furniture[29] and necessary renovation work not being done.[30] The insufficient provision of some medications and lack of access to certain medical equipment also remained an issue throughout the period documented in the available files. Among the most persistent of such problems were the difficulties with access to x-ray examinations, which plagued Ward no. 17 throughout the two decades covered by the files. The issue was reported already in 1958, a year after the ward was created. The Liublino branch of the hospital did not have its own roentgen (x-ray) equipment, and while the hospital had made an agreement to use the equipment at the relatively nearby Hospital No. 37, only patients who could be taken there by public bus were able to receive the examination. Since many patients in Ward no. 17 were in no condition to travel by bus, they could not be x-ray examined, causing the staff to report that in practice, they were 'unable to use the roentgen lab for diagnostic purposes'.[31]

This situation persisted until the ward was moved to the main hospital buildings in 1963. However, the move did not fully solve the problem of accessing roentgen equipment since the lack of a working lift in the building still made it impossible to transport many of the ward's older patients to the x-ray examination room.[32] The issue with the lift continued into the first half of the 1970s, with the ward's staff repeatedly reporting that as a result their severely ill patients could not receive the necessary examination.[33] The problem became even more complicated during the second half of the decade when the x-ray room closest to Ward no. 17 stopped functioning, necessitating the transport of patients to another building.[34] In 1979, the last year covered by the available files, Ward no. 17 reported that although three of its staff members had received lift-operator training, it still lacked a working lift.[35]

Management of bodies

Poor conditions in medical institutions and shortages of staff and equipment are of course not a new story in the history of Soviet healthcare.[36] Nevertheless, some of the issues faced at the Gannushkin Psychiatric Hospital deserve a closer look, as they intersected with the specific conditions and needs of older patients and shaped the nature and focus of care they received while suffering from severe mental health problems. Many of these patients needed chest x-rays to receive a proper diagnosis of lung diseases, which were dangerous in their age and led to many deaths among the older patients.[37] Their age and related weakened state were factors both making them more likely to suffer from these diseases and preventing them from accessing the necessary examination. The lack of x-ray equipment as such was not a problem: the equipment existed and was physically available. The issue arose from the hospital's inability to account for the specific needs of its older patients, who suffered not only from the psychiatric disorders that had led to their hospitalization, but also from multiple physical diseases, which also needed treatment and made transporting them to the examination room much more difficult.

Overcrowding and staff shortages also had particular outcomes in the context of psychiatric elder care. Both issues were reported year after year by all the wards dedicated to housing such patients and the situation remained dire throughout the evaluated period. One visible improvement occurred in terms of access to specialists, such as dentists, dermatologists or neurologists, with which Ward no. 17 struggled while it was located in Liublino.[38] The ward's move to the main hospital buildings improved the situation, and in later years such problems became much rarer.

Shortages of nurses and orderlies (*sanitarki*) were prevalent, which caused considerable difficulty in providing care to older patients, many of whom required help with eating, bathing and toilet visits, as well as a lot of basic supervision. For example, in 1959 Ward no. 17 reported that it was desperately in need of more personnel, having only one nurse and two orderlies available to tend to its fifty-five patients overnight between 5 pm and 7 am. The report openly stated that this staff was unable to adequately fulfil its task, since if they focused on caring for bedridden patients, they could not watch over more agitated ones, who easily fell and were prone to breaking bones.[39] The problem continued after the ward moved to main hospital buildings, with only sixteen to twenty nurses and orderlies working, while according to the ward's employment plan there should have been thirty-two.[40] Other wards experienced similar problems. In 1966, Ward no. 15 reported that while it was overcrowded, it was also at a risk of being left without orderlies. New staff could not be found to replace the current orderlies, who were already of retirement age and thus, because of their own ailments, less able to carry out their sometimes physically demanding work.[41] Nurses and orderlies were often older people themselves, which made it more difficult for them to supervise and manage severely mentally ill patients, who frequently became agitated or resisted feeding and bathing, physically attacking the staff and causing injuries.[42]

In the 1970s, the situation did not improve, but actually deteriorated. Ward no. 15 reported increasing overcrowding, with the average number of patients in the ward oscillating between ninety and ninety-three, instead of the planned sixty-three, while the number of its staff decreased.[43] In 1979, the situation continued to get worse, as some of the staff retired and were not replaced. Ward no. 15 was left with only fourteen orderlies, where there should have been twenty-one, and was able to allocate only one to two orderlies and one nurse to each shift, when the average number of patients in the ward was eighty-one.[44] Ward no. 17 had similarly small shifts, having been left with only fifteen orderlies, of which three more planned to retire the following year.[45]

Older patients in those wards not only often required help with basic hygiene but also suffered from conditions that severely affected their mental capacity, meaning that they needed greater supervision, which was difficult to provide with the insufficient number of staff. Alongside staff shortages, wards regularly reported fights between patients, often caused by their disorientation and arguments that broke out when somebody could not remember the way back to their bed and attempted to lie or sit on somebody else's.[46] The few nurses and orderlies left in charge of several dozen patients were unable to always prevent injuries and ensure the safety of severely ill older people. For example, in 1971 Ward no. 17 reported patients breaking their hips after falling in the toilet and in the corridor.[47] In 1969, in Ward no. 15, while the on-call orderly was in a bathroom washing garments soiled by one patient, another patient climbed onto a windowsill and fell out of the window.[48] Almost a decade later, in 1978, the limited staff of Ward no. 15 was notably struggling to provide basic care to its severely ill patients, while simultaneously maintaining order and cleanliness.[49] Together with requests for more personnel, reports of the difficulties related to simply keeping patients from injuring themselves show that preventing similar accidents was among the key activities in the geropsychiatric wards. These difficulties in meeting patients' needs in terms of basic care, as well as the problems with accessing x-ray examination described above, illustrate a notable trend emerging from the Gannushkin Hospital files: the fact that the bulk of its psychiatric elder care did not have much to do with patients' psyches, but instead focused largely on the management of their bodies.

Care for the bodies of patients features very prominently in the records of the work of psychiatric wards. This included both keeping them fed, clean and safe from injury and tending to other ailments from which they suffered. The difficulties with accessing x-ray examination became a significant problem for Ward no. 17 specifically because many of its patients suffered from lung and digestive system ailments. These and other conditions, such as heart diseases or cancer, were commonly found in the older patients at the Gannushkin Psychiatric Hospital. What is more, the older people often required not only treatment for psychiatric symptoms that warranted their hospitalization, but also needed a variety of other therapies aimed at strengthening their bodies, such as vitamin therapy,[50] heart medication[51] or healing baths.[52] An important activity of the staff in the wards housing such patients was preventing bed sores (by rotating bedridden patients),[53] as well as the previously mentioned tasks relating to basic care and supervision: feeding people who were unable to otherwise eat, changing and bathing those who suffered from incontinence, and preventing falls and bodily injuries. The care of patients' bodies constituted a significant portion of staff's activities, overshadowing their psyches and the human aspects of their suffering.

This is not to say that there was no care provided for patients' psychological well-being. Patients received psychotropic medication to stabilize their mood, improve sleep or combat psychotic symptoms and some improved enough to be released. In the mid-1970s cultural activities including daily television viewings and access to a library; lectures about upcoming elections to the Supreme Soviet were organized for 'the most lucid' patients in Ward no. 17.[54] Nevertheless, many cultural events present at other wards, such as concerts and meetings, were not organized, due to patients' condition: many were not well enough to participate in any sort of activities.[55] Similarly, work therapy was organized, but only about one fourth of patients were in a condition to take part.[56]

What is more, many of the patients were not expected to recover. Due to the progression of their diseases, some were not entirely aware of their condition and surroundings, nor could they take basic care of their weakened bodies. 'Significant degradation of personality' and severe dementia left them helpless. The staff at the Gannushkin Psychiatric Hospital admitted that not much could be done for such patients and that they should be transferred to nursing homes.[57] However, in practice they often stayed in the hospital wards, sometimes for years, as their condition deteriorated. While their minds were beyond recovery, their bodies still needed daily care and were managed by the hospital staff that worked to keep them fed and clean and prevent, or at least slow down, their further decline.

The lack of proper palliative care faced by clinicians at the Gannushkin hospital reflected broader issues related to the treatment of mentally weakened and dying patients across the world. Following an ethnographic study of hospitals in the UK, for example, Paula Boddington and Katie Featherstone highlighted a danger of dehumanization of older patients. They particularly focused on the issue of continence care – an issue that acts as a 'canary in the coal mine for the unravelling of dignity'. In their account, mental and bodily agency of dementia patients was often severely diminished, their remaining self-knowledge ignored and any remaining control eroded by ward routines.[58] The image of elder care at the Gannushkin Psychiatric Hospital that emerges from archival files reveals a similar 'crisis of dehumanisation', but also a significantly more acute one. While Boddington and Featherstone did write of the staff 'rescuing the moral dignity of patients',[59] the shortages of staff at Gannushkin Psychiatric Hospital created a situation in which nurses and orderlies struggled to take care of patients' basic bodily needs and were clearly unable to give each patient the careful care that might have protected their dignity. The overcrowding and short staffing of geropsychiatric wards led not just to difficulties in caring for older people, but also to their dehumanization. Cared for first of all as bodies, they disappeared as persons or human beings. Archival accounts of their care are dominated by tasks related to maintaining and managing their bodily functions. The people inhabiting those bodies are almost invisible, deprived of both voice and agency.

A particularly stark and grim example of this dominance of the body in the work of geropsychiatric wards comes from Ward no. 15 and concerns not the care given to the living patients but the practices of dealing with the bodies of the dead. The issue was first raised by the ward in 1966, when its annual report expressed concerns about difficulties related to transporting the bodies of its deceased patients to a newly opened hospital morgue. Since no transport was organized, the staff had to carry the bodies themselves, which was demanding on the orderlies, took about 45–50 minutes each time, and left the ward with only a single nurse available to tend to patients.[60] Ward no. 15 had the highest number of deceased patients at the Gannushkin Psychiatric Hospital, accounting for 34–54 per cent of all deaths; like other wards, it also struggled with overcrowding and understaffing.[61] The issue continued to be highlighted as one of the most pressing problems affecting the ward until the early 1970s and a few years later, in 1974, such problems also began to be reported by Ward no. 17.[62] Thus, for about a decade the bodies of deceased patients continued to take most of the staff away from caring for those still living, putting further pressure on staff already struggling to provide adequate supervision and care to older patients and thus contributing to their dehumanization.

Between life and death

Following an ethnographic study of an inpatient hospice in England conducted in the late 1990s, Julia Lawton concluded that such institutions functioned as places sequestering patients who through the deterioration brought on by disease lost control over their bodily functions or whose bodies began to rupture, causing the fluids and matter normally contained within the body to leak to the outside in an uncontrolled manner. Since the patients were sequestered in the hospice, the taboo of this 'unboundedness' of their bodies and consequent threat to their personhood remained hidden from society, allowing the symbolic maintenance of certain ideas about identities as persons.[63] The image of wards for older persons emerging from the files of Gannushkin Psychiatric Hospital reveals a similar place, hiding not only the taboo of bodily disintegration but primarily that of the disintegration of minds and wills, which together amounted to the disintegration of personhood. The patients at geropsychiatric wards became reduced to an existence akin to what Giorgio Agamben called 'bare life': a state in which only their bodies counted, but not the persons within the bodies. Those people became 'the living dead', inhabiting spaces between life and death, where their lives were stripped of rights, personhood and value.[64]

The tendency to conceptualize person and personhood through consciousness, rationality, awareness of self and others, as well as capacity for intentional action through the control over one's body had long been present in Western societies,[65] significantly influencing the perception of and language used to describe diseases that impaired cognitive functions in older age. Conditions such as dementia and Alzheimer's disease have been described as 'a living death' and 'a never ending funeral',[66] bringing about the death of the person and the dissolution of the self in stages as they progressed.[67] Since such conditions affect characteristics associated with personhood, they put the basic human status of their sufferers in question, leading to stigmatization and the perception of affected people as not quite human. By affecting reasoning and cognition, perceived as crucial aspects of a person's identity, dementia creates difference and otherness, which opens a way to stripping away people's full personhood and to marginalization.[68]

Old-age diseases affecting cognitive abilities posed the same kind of challenge to the conceptualization of a model Soviet person. The capacity for purposeful action, rationality, self-control and strong will were crucial characteristics of the ideal to which every Soviet individual was meant to aspire.[69] While by the post-war years old age had become somewhat integrated into that discourse and ageing Soviet citizens were assured that they could live productive and fulfilling lives by engaging in continued self-improvement and adopting an active, socially useful lifestyle,[70] this integration did not extend to severely ill older persons living out the rest of their lives in the wards of a psychiatric hospital. Unable to control their bodies, remember the way back to their bed and often unaware of their conditions, these people had no chance of exercising their will to perfect themselves or to engage in productive labour. They fell through the cracks of the Soviet discourse about self-improvement and were left outside it, present in physical bodies, but separated from the envisioned ideal of a person and society.

Robert Crawford observed that the body in illness and the dying body posed a threat to Enlightenment 'projects of control, transformation and perfection'. As health became a marker of personhood and the capability for self-enhancement (i.e., becoming a vehicle for progress), the sick were made different and othered.[71] The language around dementia, which often describes it as a gradual death and the dissolution of the self, amounts to making its sufferers less than full persons, showing that the diseased mind posed a similar threat and can be othered in the same way. It is not surprising, then, that diseased and deteriorating minds and bodies posed a challenge to the Soviet project, which, as historians such as Peter Holquist and David Hoffmann have shown, was a descendent of the Western Enlightenment in its drive to reshape and perfect society.[72] Severely ill older psychiatric patients did not and could not fit into a progressive narrative about remaking oneself and the world. Without a chance for recovery, they were beyond participating in progress or the struggle for a happy and fulfilling old age. They lived out what was often the last days, months or years of their lives hidden away in hospital wards, where staff tended to their bodies as their minds and selves deteriorated: a reality that fits into a broader tendency of exclusion and removal of disabled people from the public eye by the Soviet state.[73]

The geropsychiatric wards at the Gannushkin Psychiatric Hospital became liminal places between life and death, housing people whose bodies and minds were gradually decomposing and who, while physically still alive, were excluded from participating in social life in any meaningful sense. The older patients existed in a space with other similarly impaired people, many unable to engage in the few activities organized for them by the hospital staff or even to get out of bed at all. Their ties to people outside the hospital were often limited or non-existent. Many spent years at the hospital precisely because they lacked living relatives, or because their families did not want to take them home and did not come to see them. For example, one patient admitted to the hospital in 1961 was still in Ward no. 22 in the mid-1970s because her son categorically refused to take her home even for a short time.[74] Another patient, a certain Ms Ivanova, who spent over three years in the same ward, had only one relative, who was also sick and could not take care of her.[75] Patient Nakhodieva, hospitalized in Ward no. 15 from 1978, used to have a carer but after her death was left all alone, since her son never took any interest in her.[76]

Dehumanized and cared for primarily as bodies, these older patients existed in a state which rendered their previous lives and identities irrelevant, stripping them of who they were. This affected even such ingrained aspects of personal and social identity as gender. While patients were segregated into gendered wards, their gender did not shape their care. In both Ward nos. 15 and 17, older bodies were subject to the same routines and management, which in practice disregarded their gender. This fit into the phenomenon of older persons' de-gendering observed elsewhere, but while in other contexts it has had the freeing aspect of removing normative expectations,[77] here the diminishment of gender differences was tied to the reduction of identities and selves of patients who, while not yet dead, existed separately from any social life. Some patients at the Gannushkin Psychiatric Hospital did not even have a known identity, having been found in a condition in which they were unable to give their name or address. While such details were usually eventually established, it could take up to two months to clarify this information.[78] In the meantime, these older people existed even without these basic marks of identity, with their bodies tended to by the staff, but their selves and their history inaccessible and unknown.

Writing about patients with Alzheimer's disease, Annette Leibing has described the state in which they exist as one of biosocial death, which she understood as a specific form of social death occurring in some medical conditions 'in which a person's capability of participating in society diminishes to the point that the person is considered a nonperson or as not having full personhood'.[79] The term 'biosocial death' is also apt for describing the existence of the severely ill older patients at the Gannushkin Psychiatric Hospital, who in many cases were unable to live outside of an institution. Their cognitive abilities were diminished by illness to the point that they could not demonstrate an awareness of themselves and required help with the most basic activities. While not yet dead, they had no chance of escaping the state of biosocial death, since their condition offered no prospects for improvement or recovery. Thus, the psychiatric hospital wards became spaces in which older patients waited for a final and definite transition to death, secluded as their diseases eroded both their bodies and their minds.

Conclusion

Psychiatric hospitals, such as the Gannushkin Psychiatric Hospital in Moscow, were never intended to provide basic, everyday care to patients whose conditions progressed beyond any chance for recovery. The lack of readiness for that role is evident from regular complaints about this particular issue, as well as occasional suggestions on how to improve the situation and free up hospital beds for patients who required not basic care, but psychiatric treatment. Geropsychiatric wards had a noticeably lower patient turnover and took care to account for it in the reports. They explained that figures for patients released home will always be lower where older patients are concerned, due to the severe nature of their diseases, frequent loneliness and sometimes even lack of a home to which they could be released.[80] In 1965, Ward no. 15 began calling for the creation of special institutions for chronically mentally ill older people, to whence patients could be transferred instead of spending years at the psychiatric hospital.[81] Such specialized institutions, however, did not become available. Instead, the staff of the Gannushkin Psychiatric Hospital worked to transfer some of its patients to nursing homes, but the process was slow due to a shortage of places at those institutions and the fact that some patients did not have the necessary (or sometimes any) documents.[82]

Many patients spent years in the psychiatric wards before being transferred, while others never got a place at a nursing home. They died in the hospital, after days, months or years spent separated from social life, having their bodies managed by the staff as their minds continued to deteriorate. The geropsychiatric wards became spaces between life and death, occupied by older people who still lived but had lost their ability to fully participate in life as persons. While the hospital wards had not been intended to fulfil this role, it fell to them due to the reality of the psychiatric diseases affecting these older patients, as well as the lack of sufficient social and institutional support to provide such care elsewhere.

The wards at psychiatric hospitals such as the Gannushkin Psychiatric Hospital were obviously not the only places tending to older people with psychiatric conditions. Some such patients were cared for at nursing homes, some used outpatient services and some with less severe symptoms continued to live at home, without ever visiting a psychiatrist.[83] This chapter discusses only a very small fragment of the existence of mentally ill older people in the USSR. Nevertheless, even this fragment reveals something about the issues facing Soviet old-age mental healthcare, namely its lack of institutional support and plan for those older people who not only could no longer struggle against old age but were decisively defeated by it, to the point where their diseases threatened and diminished their personhood. While pathogenesis, diagnostics, treatment and prophylaxis of old-age mental disorders were said to be among the most pressing issues for psychiatry and healthcare,[84] caring for older people who had no chance for recovery was not stressed in a similar way.

Funding acknowledgement

This research was funded in whole by the Wellcome Trust [Grant No: 209842/Z/17/Z]. For the purpose of open access, the author has applied a CC BY public copyright licence to any Author Accepted Manuscript version arising from this submission.

Notes

1 *Trudy pervogo vesrossiiskogo s"ezda nevropatologov i psikhiatrov,* 2 vols (Moscow: Ministerstvo Zdravookhraneniia RSFSR, 1963).
2 See, for example: Gosudarstvennyi arkhiv Rossiiskoi Federatsii (GARF), f. a-482, op. 48, d. 3512; E.S. Averbukh, *Rasstroistva psikhicheskoi deiatel'nosti v pozdnem vozraste: psikhiatricheskii aspekt gerontologii i geriatrii* (Leningrad: Meditsina, 1969); D.F. Chebotarev, 'Sovremennye problemy gerontopsikhiatrii', *Zhurnal nevropatologii i psikhiatrii imieni S.S. Korsakova* 9 (1985): 1343–4.
3 Averbukh, *Rasstroistva*; GARF f. a-482, op. 48, d. 4577, ll. 107–14. Soviet authors attributed the view they argued against to unspecified 'Western authors', however, while early research on dementia indeed interpreted it as an extreme progression of normal age-related changes, by 1970s in the Western countries conditions such as dementia began to be seen as results of disease rather than ageing. J.F. Ballenger, 'Framing Confusion: Dementia, Society and History', *AMA Journal of Ethics* 19 (2017): 713–19.
4 For example: Iu. E. Rakhal'skii, *Psikhogigiena liudei pozhilogo vozrasta* (Kishinev: Kartia Moldoveniaske, 1959); I.B. Tarnavskii, *Chtoby osen' była zolotoi (kak sokhranit' psikhicheskoe zdorov'e v starosti),* 2nd ed. (Moscow: Meditsina, 1988).
5 David. L. Hoffman, *Stalinist Values: The Cultural Norms of Soviet Modernity, 1917– 1941* (Ithaca, NY: Cornell University Press, 2003); Catriona Kelly, 'The New Soviet Man and Woman', in S. Dixon (ed.), *The Oxford Handbook of Modern Russian History* (Oxford: Oxford University Press, 2013).
6 Tricia Starks, *The Body Soviet: Propaganda, Hygiene, and the Revolutionary State* (Madison: University of Wisconsin Press, 2009).
7 Raymond Bauer, *The New Man in Soviet Psychology* (Cambridge, MA: Harvard University Press, 1952).
8 Tarnavskii, *Chtoby osen'*, 10.
9 Meredith Minkler, 'Personal Responsibility for Health? A Review of the Arguments and the Evidence at the Century's End', *Health Education and Behaviour* 26 (1999): 126.
10 Stephen Lovell, 'Soviet Socialism and the Construction of Old Age', *Jahrbücher fur Geschichte Osteuropas*, Neue Folge, 51 (2003): 566.

11 Alissa Klots and Maria Romashova, 'Lenin's Cohort: The First Mass Generation of Soviet Pensioners and Public Acitivism in the Khrushchev Era', *Kritika: Explorations in Russian and Eurasian History* 19 (2018): 573–97.
12 Tsentral'nyi arkhiv goroda Moskvy (TsAGM) f. r-533, op. 1, d. 33.
13 TsAGM f. r-533, op. 1, d. 111.
14 'Organic psychoses' was a term used to describe psychiatric conditions believed to stem from physical defects or diseases of the brain, as opposed to changes occurring due to ageing.
15 TsAGM f. r-533, op. 1, d. 65. ll. 58–63.
16 TsAGM f. r-533, op. 1, d. 137, l. 109.
17 TsAGM f. r-533, op. 1, d. 125, l. 14.
18 TsAGM f. r-533, op. 1, d. 281, ll. 3–4.
19 Towards the end of the twentieth century the growing convergence of the two disciplines has also been observed in the Western countries. See: E.H. Reynolds, 'Structure and Function in Neurology and Psychiatry', *British Journal of Psychiatry* 157 (1990): 481–90. The fact that in the Soviet Union the dividing line between them became blurred sooner might be due to the Soviet psy-sciences' commitment to rejecting mind-body dualism and to providing physiological basis for their theories and methods. See: A.M. Brokman, 'The Healing Power of Words: Psychotherapy in the USSR, 1956–1985' (PhD thesis, University of East Anglia, Norwich, 2018).
20 For example: GARF f. a-482, op. 48, d. 2379;. E. Ia. Shternberg, *Gerontologicheskaia psikhiatriia* (Moscow: Meditsina, 1977).
21 TsAGM f. r-533, op. 1, d. 475, l. 61.
22 TsAGM f. r-533, op. 1, d. 595, l. 91.
23 TsAGM f. r-533, op. 1, d. 112, ll. 13–14.
24 TsAGM f. r-533, op. 1, d. 102, l. 118.
25 TsAGM f. r-533, op. 1, d. 281, l. 4 *oborot*.
26 TsAGM f. r-533, op. 1, d. 350, l. 4 *oborot*.
27 TsAGM f. r-533, op. 1, d. 444, ll. 58–9.
28 TsAGM f. r-533, op. 1, d. 112, ll. 86, 88.
29 TsAGM f. r-533, op. 1, d. 125, l. 48.
30 TsAGM f. r-533, op. 1, d. 626, l. 115.
31 TsAGM f. r-533, op. 1, d. 76, l. 133.
32 TsAGM f. r-533, op. 1, d. 166, l. 1.
33 TsAGM f. r-533, op. 1, d. 475, l. 160.
34 TsAGM f. r-533, op. 1, d. 567, l. 19.
35 TsAGM f. r-533, op. 1, d. 627, l. 45.
36 See for example: Mark G. Field, *Doctor and Patient in Soviet Russia* (Cambridge, MA: Harvard University Press, 1957); J.H. Bernstein, 'Emigrant Physicians Evaluate the Health Care System of the Former Soviet Union', *Medical Care* 32 (1994): 141–9.
37 TsAGM f. r-533, op. 1, d. 102, ll. 118, 123.

38　TsAGM f. r-533, op. 1, d. 112, l. 90.
39　TsAGM f. r-533, op. 1, d. 92, l. 111.
40　TsAGM f. r-533, op. 1, d. 137, l. 129 *oborot*.
41　TsAGM f. r-533, op. 1, d. 203, l. 9.
42　TsAGM, f. r-533, op. 1, d. 125, l. 10.
43　TsAGM f. r-533, op. 1, d. 379, l. 115.
44　TsAGM f. r-533, op. 1, d. 626, l. 116.
45　TsAGM f. r-533, op. 1, d. 627, l. 45.
46　TsAGM, f. r-533, op. 1, d. 125, l. 10.
47　TsAGM, f. r-533, op. 1, d. 379, l. 179.
48　TsAGM, f. r-533, op. 1, d. 311, l. 102.
49　TsAGM, f. r-533, op. 1, d. 595, l. 60.
50　TsAGM, f. r-533, op. 1, d. 507, l. 24.
51　TsAGM, f. r-533, op. 1, d. 125, l. 43.
52　TsAGM, f. r-533, op. 1, d. 112, l. 82.
53　TsAGM, f. r-533, op. 1, d. 444, l. 115.
54　TsAGM, f. r-533, op. 1, d. 475, l. 151.
55　Ibid., l. 151.
56　For example: TsAGM, f. r-533, op. 1, d. 379; f. r-533, op. 1, d. 626.
57　TsAGM, f. r-533, op. 1, d. 474, l. 1–2.
58　P. Boddington and K. Featherstone, 'The Canary in the Coal Mine: Continence Care for People with Dementia in Acute Hospital Wards as a Crisis of Dehumanization', *Bioethics* 32 (2018): 251–60.
59　Ibid.
60　TsAGM, f. r-533, op. 1, d. 203, l. 9.
61　TsAGM, f. r-533, op. 1, d. 279, l. 75.
62　TsAGM, f. r-533, op. 1, d. 475, l. 161.
63　J. Lawton, 'Contemporary Hospice Care: The Sequestration of the Unbounded Body and "Dirty Dying"', *Sociology of Health and Illness* 20 (1998): 121–43.
64　G. Agamben, *Homo Sacer: Sovereign Power and Bare Life* (Stanford: Stanford University Press, 1998).
65　A. Leibing, 'Divided Gazes: Alzheimer's Disease, the Person within and Death in Life', in A. Leibing and L. Cohen (eds.), *Thinking about Dementia: Culture, Loss and the Anthropology of Senility* (New Brunswick, NJ: Rutgers University Press, 2006); Boddington and Featherstone, 'The Canary'.
66　Pia C. Kontos, 'Embodied Selfhood: An Ethnographic Exploration of Alzheimer's Disease', in Leibing and Cohen, *Thinking about Dementia*, 195.
67　Sharon R. Kaufman, 'Dementia-Near-Death and "Life Itself"', in Leibing and Cohen, *Thinking about Dementia*.
68　U. Naue and T. Kroll, '"The Demented Other": Identity and Difference in Dementia', *Nursing Philosophy* 10 (2008): 26–33.

69 Bauer, *The New Man*; Kelly, 'The New Soviet Man.'
70 Klots and Romashova, 'Lenin's Cohort', Tarnavskii, *Chtoby osen'*.
71 Robert Crawford, 'The Boundaries of the Self and the Unhealthy Other: Reflections on Health, Culture and AIDS', *Social Science and Medicine* 38 (1994): 1347–65.
72 Hoffmann, *Stalinist Values*; P. Holquist, *Making War, Forging Revolution: Russia's Continuum of Crisis, 1914–1921* (Cambridge, MA: Harvard University Press, 2002).
73 Sarah D. Phillips, '"There Are No Invalids in the USSR!", A Missing Soviet Chapter in the New Disability History', *Disability Studies Quarterly* 29 (2009).
74 TsAGM, f. r-533, op. 1, d. 508, l. 145.
75 TsAGM, f. r-533, op. 1, d. 597, l. 57.
76 TsAGM, f. r-533, op. 1, d. 626, l. 108.
77 Catrinel Craciun, '(De)Gendering of Older Patients: Exploring Views on Aging and Older Patients in Romanian General Practitioners', *Actualidades en Psicologia* 30 (2016): 1–9; Catherine B. Silver, 'Gendered Identities in Old Age: Towards (De) Gendering?', *Journal of Aging Studies* 17 (2003): 379–97.
78 TsAGM, f. r-533, op. 1, d. 507, l. 1.
79 Leibing, 'Divided Gazes', 248.
80 TsAGM, f. r-533, op. 1, d. 125, ll. 40–3.
81 TsAGM, f. r-533, op. 1, d. 165, ll. 1177–8.
82 TsAGM, f. r-533, op. 1, d. 375, l. 61; f. r-533, op. 1, d. 566, ll. 42, 46.
83 V.N. Belousova, V.V. Listratenko, and G.I. Shestakova, 'Kliniko-statisticheskii analiz psikhicheskoi zabolevaemosti pozhilogo vozrasta v Amurskoi oblasti', in *Trudy pervogo vesrossiiskogo*.
84 GARF, f. a-482, op. 48, d. 3512.

5

A comfortable old age: Designing care homes for older Soviet persons

Susan Grant

The 2019–21 coronavirus pandemic drew attention to the precarious position of nursing homes and the vulnerability of older people living in them. It seemed all too easy for a deadly virus to spread and threaten lives in these closed or semi-closed institutions.[1] The pandemic restarted previous – and partially ongoing – arguments over how to organize such homes to both minimize epidemiological threats and maximize resident comfort.[2] The proper design of nursing or care homes for older people has been discussed and debated for decades – yet it seems unclear as to whether society has come any closer to creating a living space for older people that in fact does address their complex medical, social and cultural needs. Nor is this the first time that countries around the world have had to address the question of caring for ageing populations and older persons who can no longer live independently. Older people and their families must choose between options that include assisted living facilities, home help and nursing care homes, the latter often considered a last resort.

In this chapter, I focus on care homes. Although many older people continue to live at home,[3] with the demand for nursing homes in some countries in decline,[4] analysing care homes sheds light on current state and societal attitudes towards the old-age population. Even if fewer people are now living in nursing homes, the needs of those who must live in them should be assessed regularly. The Soviet Union, with its ageing population and interest in gerontology, can provide important insights for current conversations about nursing home design. The total number of beds in nursing homes rose continually in the Soviet period, jumping from 54,000 in 1950 to 101,000 in 1960 – and to 202,000 in 1980.[5] Contemporary discussions about nursing home design, moreover, show that Soviet architects knew what they were talking about when planning for older people's living needs. Having studied foreign models of planning and design, Soviet architects were on top of current trends and research in the field and their work can be read as part of a broader international story.[6] Today, moreover, the Soviet state might be gone – but the needs of older people have not changed so drastically over the last thirty (or even seventy) years as to render the Soviet experience irrelevant. Years of research on nursing homes, in both the Soviet Union and internationally, can help us to learn more about the needs of older people.

Homes for older people were not exactly a new phenomenon in the post-war Soviet Union, but in the 1950s these homes were singled out for development and construction. This was hardly surprising given the rising numbers of older people in the population: the percentage of the Soviet population aged sixty and over was 6.8 per cent in 1939; by 1961 it was 9.8 per cent.[7] The late socialist years saw much discussion about the role and function of homes for older people. Research focused on the construction, design and architecture of the homes, as well as ways of improving their living conditions and medical services.[8] In this chapter, I examine how architects and planners conceptualized and designed homes for older people from the 1950s to the 1980s. The timeframe spans the tenures of Nikita Khrushchev, Leonid Brezhnev and Mikhail Gorbachev, but care home design over these decades remained reasonably consistent. I examine the importance that architects, home directors and older people placed on the location of homes, their internal layout and amenities.

This chapter treats the physical space of homes for older people as a case study. Recent debates about the design and structure of care homes confirm that homes for older people have many shortcomings.[9] Some have looked to the past to shed light on current problems. In an article entitled 'The American Nursing Home Is a Design Failure', Justin Davidson writes: 'The nursing-home system is an obsolete mess that emerged out of a bureaucratic misconception.'[10] American and Soviet nursing home construction accelerated in the 1950s, and while the Russian and Soviet nursing-home system had their problems, the home system itself was not exactly ill-conceived. But as this chapter shows, the Soviet home system became increasingly like the US model that Davidson describes, that is, closer to a hospital environment. When initially conceived, the Soviet home system was supposed to allow older people to live and work in the care home, often tending to a plot of land, spending time in a labour therapy workshop and having leisure opportunities. This sometimes did not happen in practice because of a lack of resources or, as more often became the case, because homes ended up treating older people who were ill and required medical care. When that happened, the most cost-effective logistical solution seemed to lie in constructing homes that resembled hospitals. The preference was for older people to live at home and receive support from family, local volunteers, community nurses or Red Cross workers, but when none of these options were available or viable, an older person often ended up moving into a state-run care home.

When it came to older persons' health in the Soviet Union, the social and medical were inextricably entwined: how people lived, who they lived with and their place in society were never discursively separated from their health outcomes. In a country that placed much emphasis on prophylactic approaches to healthcare, design and orientation were to have an immediate bearing on the health and well-being of people living in care homes. The concepts behind the designs for care homes were also constantly evolving. Home design was an ongoing response to the needs of older people, the built environment and architectural developments. Hovering over all this was Cold War politics and the ideological battle between capitalism and socialism. Soviet architects were well-read on care home design abroad and frequently compared Soviet homes for older people to those in the West.[11] The fact that older people did not have to pay for their stay in a home was usually contrasted to the expensive care homes abroad, a narrative that architects used to show the superiority of socialism. Designing and building comfortable care homes, as well as funding them, was one of the ways in which the Soviet Union tried to show its commitment to welfare and public health.

Soviet nursing homes and their construction

For all the Soviet emphasis on care for older persons, ask a Russian today about Soviet homes for older people and they will likely tell you that they were deplorable. Much of this negativity is justified (and I examine the problems elsewhere), but that does not mean that the Soviet state or its bureaucracies set out to neglect older people. In principle, architects and social welfare administrators gave a great deal of thought to working out how best to serve the needs of older citizens. These plans fitted with broader design and planning projects to improve public health.[12] When it came to designing homes, architects, medical workers and social welfare representatives, as well as older people's opinions in the form of surveys, all shaped the approach to designing suitable spaces. The fundamental problem was that these spaces were not being built fast enough. Many Soviet older persons living in institutions of one sort or another continued to occupy pre-revolutionary buildings that were not designed for the physical needs of older people.[13] But private homes were hardly any better. Older people in the Soviet Union, especially in the Stalinist period, often lived in accommodation – apartments, communal spaces or houses – that might not have had hot water, sewerage or central heating.[14] In spite of these harsh realities, there was an understanding of what a good home should look like and there was an effort to design buildings that would cater to the greying generations, even if these homes were not being constructed in sufficient quantity.

There was also an understanding that older people had varied needs. Just one type of home could not cater to every 'old' person. Older people in the Soviet Union (just as anywhere else) were not a monolithic group, nor were they part of a truly unifying totalitarian society.[15] Class hierarchies and divergent levels of privileges were pervasive. Many benefited from the system and as many lost out. By the time the first Soviet generations reached old age, social divisions were already calcifying. Older Soviet citizens who had worked in the arts and sciences, or in industries with powerful trade unions, or who were old Bolsheviks or privileged pensioners (*pensionery soiuznogo znacheniia*), could avail themselves of special homes thanks to their profession or status. These homes were usually small in size, with cultural and social spaces tailored to their residents' needs. Another home with a comparatively privileged clientele was the fee-paying *pansionat* – a type of home that was partly state subsidized and partly funded by clients' fees. The focus of this chapter, however, is the general home for older and disabled people that was entirely state funded and under the remit of the Ministry of Social Welfare. In these homes older people dominated (in the 1970s, about 90 per cent were aged fifty and older) with 'young and middle-aged invalids aged 18–50' comprising only 10 per cent.[16] The gender balance changed over time as the male population shrank. The percentage of men in homes in 1958 was 35 per cent, in 1963 it was 28 per cent and in 1968 it was 25 per cent.[17] The overwhelming majority of homes were mixed (90 per cent) and just 10 per cent of homes were for women only.[18]

Soviet experts on ageing and architecture were familiar with foreign approaches to older people's accommodation. These included a variety of 'settlements', such as 'colonies' or 'satellite cities' for older people in France and Italy, villages for older people in Florida and Washington in the United States, Romania and Denmark, or living complexes for older people in Scandinavian countries.[19] But some Soviet experts felt that while this approach was tempting, 'segregating' older people was not beneficial.[20] Others also found these styles of living 'problematic' and more suited to capitalist countries but wanted to learn from foreign experience regardless (and some Austrian-style apartment homes were built in Cheliabinsk and outside of Moscow).[21] These foreign models did, in one form or another, influence the standard types of Soviet home which could be 'mixed' (including the practically healthy and disabled) or 'homogenous', i.e., exclusively for healthy older people. Designing these types of home was challenging for architects, whose designs needed to accommodate older people with different levels of mobility and medical requirements. The reality for many older persons was that, once they succeeded in getting into a home, the life that awaited them was often difficult and not the comfortable life foreseen by architects.[22]

One of the figures most frequently encountered in care home design in the Soviet Union is P. G. Rudakov. An architect, Rudakov wrote his dissertation and penned several publications on the subject. He worked in the Central Scientific Research and Design Institute of Standard and Experimental Accommodation Design (TsNIIEP zhilishcha), which continues to oversee architectural projects in modern Russia. This institute produced designs for Soviet care homes (as well as a wide range of other projects) in the post-war period. Established in 1949, its name changed a couple of times before reaching its final iteration in 1963, and was led by the academic Boris Rafailovich Rubanenko from 1959.[23] In 1960, the institute began to 'develop standard and experimental designs [for nursing homes] according to a scientifically grounded programme'.[24] Over the course of the 1960s it achieved an increase of 79,600 places and by the end of the 1970s there were about 1,200 homes in the USSR with 239,500 residents.[25] Despite such increases in the number of homes there were still long waitlists. In 1975 over 50,000 people were on a list to live in a home for older and disabled persons.[26] The growing population of older people placed additional demands on urban infrastructure and health services.[27]

The designs by Rudakov and others went to the Ministry of Construction and Architecture (hereafter, Gosstroi USSR) or one of its committees for assessment and approval. According to Rudakov, 'almost all' of the projects that Gasstroi recommended in the Ukrainian, Uzbek and Kazakh SSR's in 1961-2 were '*tipovoe*',[28] a style that was closely associated with the Khrushchev period (1953–64). After the All-Union Convention of Construction Workers in December 1954, architects began to follow a 'standard design construction from prefabricated parts' known as *tipovoe proektirovanie*.[29] This practice was supposed to save costs, but buildings ended up looking generic and architects raised questions about the quality of construction.[30] Statistics, however, confirmed the ubiquity of the '*tipovoe*' building model in the 1950s. In the RSFSR, more than 80 per cent of all new housing was of this type in 1959, compared to 1 per cent in 1951.[31]

Change came in the form of *tipizatsiia* – a new approach that 'allowed architects to achieve genuine diversity of form' without trampling on 'Khrushchev's stipulation that the construction components be pre-fabricated'. The materials were 'standardized', but the designs were individual.[32] *Tipizatsiia* was the subject of much discussion after Khrushchev's new party programme and the Twenty-Second Party Congress in 1961.[33] Architects sought 'a new type of architecture' for life under communism.[34] While the passage of years saw an increased focus on individual modifications, the underlying balance between standardized cost saving and localized change continued, and some general types of nursing home in the Brezhnev period (1964–82) continued to be in the *tipovoe* style.

Nursing home design depended on construction, and the Ministry for Social Welfare worked with other ministries and state agencies to turn ideas into reality. In the summer of 1976, G. N. Fomin, representative of the State Committee for Civil Construction and Architecture under Gosstroi USSR, which was answerable to the State Committee for Construction Affairs (Grazhdanstroi/Gosgrazhdanstroi), wrote that his committee had 'developed and approved sixteen projects, of which eleven are homes for elderly and disabled people, and one project is for a psychoneurological home with a technical training college'.[35] Projects included under the tenth Five-Year Plan (1976–80), he added, covered the further development of *tipovoe* designs for homes, as well as developing a 'home with apartments on the first floor for invalids using wheelchairs and a design for special apartments for single elderly people (with serviced accommodation at the first floor level)'.[36] As Fomin noted, Gosgrazhdanstroi had already 'approved and activated the design of homes for elderly and disabled people' in 1974. These designs satisfied 'all modern design and construction' demands.[37] Once designs were approved, the task then became that of financing and managing the building work to ensure that projects were completed. This is how the design and construction of homes was supposed to work. In practice, long delays were common.[38]

The built environment

Soviet architects and planners worked towards designing and building standard homes of different sizes in a range of locations. In a 1956 article about the design and construction of homes, S. Koriakov, the head of the Construction Department of the Ministry of Social Welfare, wrote that the ministry needed to build 'homes for invalids with 300 and 100 places' as part of the Sixth Five-Year-Plan (1956–60).[39] Homes for 300 places included a 'main building, bath-laundry, vegetable store, fuel depot, and garage in one block with a boiler, transformation substation, domestic store and workshop'. There were smaller out-buildings for heating, sewage, electricity and other needs. Rudakov seemed to respond to this demand for self-contained nursing homes and developed the idea further. He envisaged special complexes with a range of services and amenities in suburban or rural locations ('*poselki-kompleksy*') catering to those wanting to leave urban areas.[40] Complexes could include different styles of home in the form of apartment, *pansionat* and 'homes with constant medical care or small hospitals (*bol'nitsy-statsionary*)'. Older people could move between the different types of home according to their needs.[41] As well as having access to 'a good medical service and provisions' older people should also be able to undertake mass cultural work and have a garden for 'rest and work'.[42] Although much smaller in scale, the proposed homes resembled the resort complexes being built around the same time. These large complexes, set on the peripheries of urban centres, were also largely self-contained, with separate buildings for services and sleeping.[43] This pattern of separate service and sleeping buildings was common in Soviet designs for homes for older people.

Architects understood that older people's needs changed over time and that they required various amenities and services. They also realized that pensioners wanted to live in a familiar location, close to relatives and friends, and to be able to 'participate fully in public life'.[44] The opportunity for older people to participate in Soviet society was fundamental to the socialist conception of social life, and ideological thinking was deeply embedded in design philosophy. There was recognition of the important need for older people to be able to maintain social and cultural habits. One way of achieving this was to build care homes for older people close to urban areas. The 1950s and 1960s saw homes built to satisfy these requirements as architects continued their research into home location and design. In 1966 researchers in the Kiev Zonal Scientific-Research Institute for Standard and Experimental Design found that older people 'needed different types of homes', which included apartments and guest accommodation for the 'practically healthy' and more 'specialised' living for those in poorer health.[45] But the challenge in getting the design right lay in understanding the medical, social and cultural needs of older people.[46]

In 1973, Rudakov, now a senior researcher in TsNIIEP zhilishcha's Department of Typology (*otdel tipologii*), wrote about 'the new principles of designing a residential home for elderly people'.[47] The department had analysed 117 questionnaires that the directors and head doctors of standard homes had completed ('fifty surveys from the RSFSR and sixty-seven from other union republics'). Some 60 per cent of the homes had been 'specially built' and 40 per cent were 'adapted and reconstructed'. Rudakov's colleagues also visited twenty-five homes and conducted a survey of 744 older people living in thirteen state homes in the RSFSR. Rudakov noted that the environment and surroundings ranked high in importance for residents, with 71 per cent of older people preferring homes 'close to parks and green areas' in residential zones.[48] But he also acknowledged that care homes would need to accommodate the growing numbers of chronically ill and bedridden older persons as well as the healthy. In the coming years, he predicted, the number of places for the ill would increase to 60–70 per cent, with capacity for the 'practically healthy' falling to 30–40 per cent.[49] He emphasized the importance of cultural activities for mobile residents and 'round the clock medical service and care for the bedridden'.[50] Soviet designers realized that the broader built environment and the physical space of the home affected older people's health and well-being. Rudakov's claims about the change in the health condition of those needing to move to homes also showed that the USSR was moving closer to the United States in following a path towards medicalization.

Building in urban microdistricts, where larger construction plans came into play, presented architects with challenges of size and scale. This was particularly important in Moscow. Construction in Moscow had to adhere to the 'planned and harmonious development of the capital'. The city's general plan had eight zones, each with a population of 600,000 to one million people.[51] The vast majority (80 per cent) of general type homes for older persons in Moscow were to be in residential areas of the city, with 20 per cent 'close to green areas in the forest park protection zone (LPZP/*Lesoparkovyi zashchitnyi poyas*)'. The 'location criteria' recognized that older people often wanted to live in a familiar environment, close to home.[52] As well as endorsing proximity to neighbourhoods, architects also recognized that it was 'easier to organise cultural-domestic and medical service' in larger homes, which were more cost-effective to construct.[53] Even though 'national and foreign practice' showed that homes for 150–200 people were psychologically optimal for residents, planners, engineers and architects felt that 'the more economic expression in the short-term, and obviously in the long-term, is to construct home designs for 500–600 places in Moscow'.[54] Economics and wider planning concerns proved to be a powerful driving force in care home design. The original socialist plan to have care homes where older people could live and work was becoming more difficult to realize owing to the growing numbers of older people and their different healthcare needs.

In the early 1980s, surveys conducted by TsNIIEP zhilishcha of 'ministries, heads of regional and provincial departments of social welfare and home directors' still showed a preference for locating homes 'on the outskirts of towns, close to green areas' but a few also suggested locating homes 'far away from where [older people] lived' to help 'reduce the moral trauma of living in a home'. Distance from friends and relatives, went the argument, would lessen the likelihood of older people leaving the home to live with relatives. Unsurprisingly, older people strongly disagreed with the idea: 72 per cent of home residents wanted to 'live closer to their former place of residence or close to relatives'.[55] But the directors concerned about older people's trauma and longing to leave had a valid point. Older people did not want to leave their family home or community. Architects consequently had to design modern and comfortable care homes that older people would not want to leave.

Homes for life: Interior design and outdoor space

In the late 1950s, Rudakov acknowledged the 'complicated' nature of designing and planning homes for older people.[56] The task required 'the best architectural forces in the country'. In his opinion: 'The union of Soviet architects together with Gosstroi USSR and the Ministry for Social Welfare RSFSR needed to organise an open competition for the design of such homes, and the Academy of construction and architecture USSR – develop a basic position on their designs.'[57] Rudakov saw many issues with existing care homes.[58] Kitchens were too small to allow older people to make hot drinks or cook meals, laundry services were located far from their rooms and bathroom units were often shared and used for a variety of purposes.[59] Not only did he call on internal Soviet agencies to rise to the challenge of building better nursing homes, but he also looked abroad. For ideas on canteen and kitchen design, for example, he turned to the GDR and Czechoslovakia.[60] In the following years Rudakov's plea for improving nursing home design was heard as architects discussed increasing living and storage space and designed homes with common kitchens and lounge areas on each floor in multi-storey complexes.

Still, design challenges remained. One of the greatest difficulties lay in meeting older people's medical needs. Mobility was particularly important and architects included elevators in new multi-storey designs – a feature absent in many pre-existing homes that at times had left some older people with reduced mobility trapped on upper floors.[61] Some architects also recommended that homes be built with wide stairs with steps that were not too steep.[62] Designs for large homes, such as the 1960s MG-03-1 plan, included a room for an attending nurse on each floor.[63] In a TsNIIEP zhilishcha home for 200 people for which Rudakov acted as a scientific consultant in 1968, the home was 'a nine storey tower bloc' with a medical point and infirmary (*izoliator*) on the first floor. The 'practically healthy' older persons – divided into eight 'cells' of twenty-four people – lived on floors two through six, while the more infirm, in groups of twenty-six, lived on the upper floors. This design and structure differed from earlier iterations of homes but still considered the medical requirements of older residents.

One of the most advanced *tipovoe* designs of the 1960s was the MG-03-1.[64] It was used for a home in the Liublino District in southeast Moscow, the focus of a glowing *Sotsial'noe obespechenie* article in 1966. The author of this article directly connected the Liublino home to the Twenty-Third Party Congress and the Party's 'care' (*zabota*) for older people.[65] He introduced readers to an older woman who had been a party member since 1919 (and who was thus likely to have social privileges) but who recently struggled to live on her own. The Moscow city department of Social Welfare proposed she move to the home in Liublino and during her initial visit she found its rooms to be 'modern' and 'comfortable'.[66] It also impressed foreign visitors. A delegation from East Germany was effusive in their praise: 'We are delighted at everything we have seen. The good comfort and service speaks to the great care of elderly people and the desire to brighten the rest of their lives.'[67] Such fulsome reviews were perhaps supposed to reassure readers that the new homes were pleasant places to live. They also displayed socialist care for older people. The MG-03-1 design was used for a 580-bed home for older persons in Matveev, as well as one in Tushino.[68] The latter was a complex with two five-storey accommodation buildings and another, two-storey building with a 'vestibule, library, reading room, and auditorium for 400 people' that was linked to the other buildings via a passageway.[69] Soviet designs tried to accommodate the medical and social needs of Soviet citizens with a range of health issues.

Although later revised, another standard design, the P-03-2, was originally developed by the Giprogor[70] planning institute over the course of 1962–8. This design accommodated 300 people in a three-storey main building connected to a parallel building via passageway on each floor.[71] Rooms had a 'washbasin and built-in wardrobes' and a common-use bathroom, shower and bath. The home included social spaces for performances, club rooms, a library and reading-room, workshop for 'labour therapy' and administration offices.[72] But this design was also flawed. On the one-year anniversary of its opening, in 1970, the director of a P-03-2 home in Volgograd lamented that the design did 'not have enough storage for people's personal items, especially winter clothes in the summer'. He also claimed that 'grandmothers and grandfathers like to drink tea during the day but had no place to boil water' and so faced a 'long and uncomfortable walk to the canteen'.[73] Others noted that the halls leading to a summer veranda on each floor were empty and would benefit from some furniture.[74] The P-03-2 design had been the basis for various homes in the RSFSR, including in Tula and Leningrad provinces. But residents in these locations found the designs needed more work.[75] The director of the Lodeinopol'sk home in Leningrad province said the P-03-2 design had to satisfy the needs of 128 people aged 80–100 years, but the building 'did not have enough smoking rooms, toilets were unsuitable for older people who need support and space for wheelchairs, it had four bedrooms and fire regulations had not been followed'. The director felt that 'the overall design was good' but some modifications were needed.[76] Soviet care home design was still a work in progress.

By the late 1960s and 1970s Soviet care home design was largely defined by three or four styles. Some architects claimed there were only two: the three-to-five-storey 'pavilion style with accommodation buildings and services blocs connected by heated passages' and a nine-to-twelve-storey building with living and service zones 'on the first or upper floors'.[77] Others added centralized and bloc style homes alongside the pavilion style.[78] Lifts meant that architects could design 'short and bright' corridors. Newly built homes needed to have spaces for food storage and preparation, a dining hall, club, medical point with infirmary, pharmacy, rooms for dentistry, physiotherapy, exercise, doctors' and nurses' offices, a labour therapy workshop and general administration areas.[79] As the Brezhnev government, itself a gerontocracy, sought to establish 'developed socialism', architects and planners continued to push care home design forward. They also looked abroad and assessed care home designs in the United States, England, Sweden and Switzerland.[80]

Outdoor space was part of the design ethos. Architects realized the importance of landscaping and gardens.[81] As architects wrote in the 1970s:

> The zone for rest should flow from the home's main building and should have a garden with alleys for strolling and a courtyard for rest that is protected by the wind. The zone should have a shaded terrace, benches, fountain, pond and pool. It should also have a domestic area with garden and orchard tended to by residents.[82]

Conceptually, their position was not unlike today's understandings of the relationship between indoor and outdoor space, and the importance of the latter.

The British Regulation and Quality Improvement Authority's Care Standards for Nursing Homes, 2015, states:

> Garden space is safe and secure and easy to find from inside the home. Planting is used to soften hard features such as walls and fencing and to create points of interest for residents. Paths are wide enough to allow for two people to walk side by side. There are opportunities for resting and sitting throughout the garden and there is shelter available from the sun and wind. Consideration is given to using the garden to stimulate the senses through water features; planting and features that attract wildlife and birds; and fragrant plants and flowers.[83]

The role of outdoor space has been highlighted again recently. One UK-based architect observed: 'There is overwhelming evidence that access to quality, external space has a positive impact on physical and mental health, so an emphasis on providing quality outdoor space will be key to improving the quality of care home design in the UK.'[84] But the UK and other countries have, like the late Soviet Union, struggled to achieve better standards in home design due to lack of funding.[85] In the wake of the coronavirus pandemic, architects have highlighted that homes should have '[b]right, light spaces with plenty of windows for ventilation'.[86] Architects in the Soviet Union also valued the role of light. Most designs included open space such as a balcony with 'thorough ventilation mandatory in all premises'.[87] Designers and planners considered orientation important, with one noting that '80 per cent of wards in homes should be south facing'.[88] The physical environment was something that Soviet experts working in healthcare, design and architecture valued. The benefits of rest, leisure and resort stays for health and well-being were well-known in the USSR and the Russian Empire before it. Rudakov was critical of accommodation for older people that did not have insulated bedrooms and he noted that 'more than 16 per cent of old people needed to live in premises that did not get the sun'.[89] He argued that the 'infirmary and workshop should have north facing orientations'. In some homes people were spending 'fifteen to nineteen hours in a room' and the seriously infirm spent the entire day in their room.[90]

Researchers also paid attention to furniture and interior fittings, with some looking to American expertise for guidance on how firm or soft a mattress should be.[91] Interior design was important in creating a comfortable space. To that end, warm paint tones would cheer up north facing rooms and cooler tones would balance the brightness of south facing rooms.[92] Experts from the Kiev-based Institute of Gerontology of the Academy of Medical Sciences of the USSR also provided advice on geriatric institutions of different profiles and recommended colours from nature such as green and blue, as well as dark colours for big rooms and light colours for small rooms.[93] Indeed, TsNIIEP zhilishcha was developing a range of interior colours that could be used in care homes.[94] Floors in homes could also be covered in calm tones of linoleum, a practical material that was 'easy to clean'.[95]

TsNIIEP zhilishcha was active on several fronts in care home design. On 1 October 1975, the state construction body (Gosgrazhdanstroi) ratified a document titled 'Instructions for designing homes for elderly and disabled people'.[96] The main parties involved in the project were TsNIIEP zhilishcha, the Kiev zonal Institute of Gosgrazhdanstroi, the Russian Ministry of Social Welfare and the Institute of Gerontology in Kiev. This was hailed as the 'first normative document for designing homes of this type in our country' and was pitched as the culmination of 'many years of research'. The document included information on designs for two types of home: the general type that provided medical and cultural support; and a hospital type for the 'chronically ill, very old, and bedridden' who had the same needs as those living in general homes but with the additional requirement of constant medical care.[97] When it came to constructing new homes, the latter type of design was becoming increasingly common due to the growing number of people in need of constant medical attention.[98]

Soviet architects realized that designing care homes was an evolving process. The homes that were built in the 1970s had been the result of research conducted in the 1960s and so architects such as Rudakov considered them outmoded by 1982.[99] The 1974–5 instructions outlined by TsNIIEP zhilishcha in collaboration with Kiev-ZNIIP 'needed some corrections', primarily due to the number of seriously ill people who constituted '50–60 per cent of home residents' – figures that were on the rise.[100] The changing context – more numbers of older people with health concerns – led Soviet urban planners and architects to shift their original concepts for nursing home design to meet the higher numbers of older people requiring medical support. In the early 1980s the Russian Ministry of Social Welfare was planning for large increases in home places, construction of which was again associated with the government's 'great care' for its people. The eleventh Five-Year Plan (1981–5) would see some 32,000 places allocated in new builds.[101] According to the head of the administration for homes in the Russian Ministry of Social Welfare, A. Samarina, '62 per cent of residents are placed in standard designs (*tipovoe*) with all modern amenities; by the end of the Five-Year Plan this will be the case for the overwhelming majority'.[102] By 1982, the general style homes being built in Moscow were for 500–600 places, in Leningrad 900–1000 places, while the RSFSR average was about 200 places and increasing.[103]

The knowledge that smaller homes were better for older people's physical and mental health was proving less important than accommodating large numbers of older residents in more populous buildings. Aside from catering to the growing numbers of older people, architects also knew that building bigger complexes was less expensive. It was more economically efficient to cater to 500 people than 100, even if research showed – and still shows – that older people had a better quality of life in homes with fewer people. The demands of the Soviet planning system and need to economize, coupled with rising numbers of older people in the late 1970s and 1980s, shaped architects' response to home design.

Reforming eldercare continued under Mikhail Gorbachev and his government's *perestroika* or 'restructuring' programme. On 22 January 1987, the Party Central Committee, Soviet Council of Ministers and the Central Council of Trade Unions (VTsSPS) issued a decree on 'measures for further improving services to the elderly and disabled'.[104] This stipulated that territorial social welfare centres looking after the needs of pensioners be divided into three types with varying options for permanent and temporary stays and different cultural, social and medical services. All three types of centre also had to provide at-home care services to pensioners.[105] Architects might have put a good deal of thought into designing care homes, but the demand for places in these exceeded the pace of construction. Traditional homes for older people, often stretched to capacity, were no longer sufficient to cope with the needs of Soviet citizens who were living longer and experiencing a range of health problems.

In a 2007 article about changes in resident room design and long-term care facilities, Migette Kaup acknowledges that in the United States the objective has been 'achieving residential experiences within a setting that delivers medical services'.[106] But achieving the balance between the medical and home environment is difficult, as Soviet architects could attest. The intimate Green House home, first established in the United States in 2003, has recently come close to meeting this balance, offering a range of services to residents requiring little or considerable medical support.[107] The ethos of a small-scale care home where older people have the option to engage in social and cultural activities and have their medical needs met is something that Soviet architects understood to be important. But, as the Soviet experience shows, designing and building enough modern homes for significant numbers of older people with various medical and living needs is not easy. Nor is it always possible to construct enough homes. Societies around the world are ageing and it is imperative that we learn from past and present experiences to ensure that every one of us has the option to live out our lives in a dignified and comfortable environment.

Acknowledgement

My thanks to Isaac Scarborough and the anonymous reviewers for their comments and suggestions.

Funding acknowledgement

This research was funded in whole by the Wellcome Trust [Grant No: 209842/Z/17/Z]. For the purpose of open access, the author has applied a CC BY public copyright licence to any Author Accepted Manuscript version arising from this submission.

Notes

1. For an example of discussion of coronavirus spreading in the US care homes, see 'Nearly One-Third of U. S. Coronavirus Deaths Are Linked to Nursing Homes', *The New York Times*, 1 June 2021. Available online: https://www.nytimes.com/interactive/2020/us/coronavirus-nursing-homes.html, accessed 25 August 2021.
2. Research on nursing home care since the pandemic has raised questions about several issues, including nursing home size and the built environment. See Jennifer K. Burton, Gwen Bayne, Christine Evans, Frederike Garbe, Dermot Gorman, Naomi Honhold, Duncan McCormick, Richard Othieno, Janet E. Stevenson, Stefanie Swietlik, Kate E. Templeton, Mette Tranter, Lorna Willocks, Bruce Guthrie, 'Evolution and Effects of COVID-19 Outbreaks in Care Homes: A Population Analysis in 189 Care Homes in One Geographical Region of the UK', *The Lancet* 1, no. 1, E21–E31, October (2020): e 30. Available online: https://www.thelancet.com/retrieve/pii/S266675682030012X, accessed 25 August 2021. See also Diana C. Anderson, Thomas Grey, Sean Kennelly, Desmond O'Neill, 'Nursing Home Design and COVD-19: Balancing Infection Control, Quality of Life, and Resilience', *Journal of the American Medical Directors Associations* 21 (2020): 1519–24. For an interesting assessment of some of the ways in which care home design and architecture has changed since the middle of the twentieth century, see Sarah Nettleton, Christina Buse, and Daryl Martin, '"Essentially It's Just a Lot of Bedrooms": Architectural Design, Prescribed Personalisation and the Construction of Care Homes for Later Life', *Sociology of Health & Illness* 40, no. 7 (2018): 1156–71. Doi: 10.1111/1467-9566.127747.
3. A 2016 report showed that in the UK, 418,000 people or 4 per cent of the total population aged sixty-five years and older, were in care homes, rising to 15 per cent

for those over eighty-five years. See the Laing and Buisson 2016 survey, cited in Methodist Homes, Facts & Stats, available online: https://www.mha.org.uk/get-involved/policy-influencing/facts-stats/, accessed 25 August 2021.

4   U.S. Department of Health and Human Services statistics show that: 'From 1977 to 2014, the number of nursing home residents aged 65 and over per 1,000 population aged 65 and over fell by about one half'. National Centre for Health Statistics. Health, United States, 2016: With Chartbook on Long-term Trends in Health. Hyattsville, MD, 2017. Available at https://www.cdc.gov/nchs/data/hus/hus16.pdf#092, accessed 10 September 2021.

5   See table no. 8.29 'Beds in Stationary Social Service Organizations for Elderly and Disabled People', *Rossiiskii statisticheskii ezhegodnik/Russian Statistical Yearbook* (bilingual publication) (Rosstat, 2020), 231. Available at https://rosstat.gov.ru/storage/mediabank/KrPEshqr/year_2020.pdf, accessed 10 September 2021.

6   There is also an argument to be made for transnationalism in the field of ageing, but that is not my concern here. Other scholars provide strong arguments for considering late socialist transnationalism. In the GDR, see James Chappel, 'On the Border of Old Age: An Entangled History of Eldercare in East Germany', *Central European History* 53 (2020): 353–71. In relation to Black Sea resorts, see Johanna Conterio, '"Our Black Sea Coast": The Sovietization of the Black Sea Littoral under Khrushchev and the Problem of Overdevelopment', *Kritika: Explorations in Russian and Eurasian History* 19, no. 2 (2018): 327–61. Soviet architects looked to other socialist countries in Central and Eastern Europe, Switzerland, Austria, Scandinavia, as well as to the UK and United States. Rather than try to export their own style of home for older people, they primarily learned from home design in other countries.

7   N.N. Sachuk, 'Demograficheskaia i sotsial'naia kharakteristika naseleniia starshikh vozrastov', in *Osnovy Gerontologii* (Moscow: Meditsina, 1969), 493.

8   P.G. Rudakov, *Doma-Internaty dlia prestarelykh* (avtoreferat) (Moscow, ASiA USSR 1962), 4. See also the resolution from the Council of Ministers of the USSR 13/11/1967, No. 1031: 'Expanding the system of homes for the elderly and disabled and improving living conditions in them'.

9   'Calls for new minimum standards for UK care home design', Building Better Healthcare, 20 July 2020. Available at: https://www.buildingbetterhealthcare.com/news/article_page/Call_for_new_minimum_standards_for_UK_care_home_design/167833, accessed 20 April 2021.

10 Justin Davidson, 'The American Nursing-Home Is a Design Failure', *New York Magazine*, 25 June 2020. Available at: https://nymag.com/intelligencer/2020/06/the-american-nursing-home-is-a-design-failure.html, accessed 30 March 2021.

11 This applied to gerontology and geriatrics more generally. See Z.G. Revutskaia, 'Organizatsiia meditsinskogo obsluzhivaniia', in *Osnovy Gerontologii*, 601.

12 Conterio, 'Our Black Sea Coast', 329.
13 State Archive of the Russian Federation (hereafter GARF), f. 9527, op. 1, d. 1721, l. 150, 169.
14 Donald Filtzer, *The Hazards of Urban Life in Late Stalinist Russia: Health, Hygiene, and Living Standards, 1943–1953* (Cambridge: Cambridge University Press, 2010), chapter 1. The welfare reforms of Khrushchev and Brezhnev might have helped to improve the situation, but disparities still existed in the 1970s when some continued to live without basic amenities. For a comparison of pensioners living in different housing types and with access to amenities in three locations in the RSFSR, see Larisa Petrovna Tokareva, 'Kompleksnoe issledovanie ob'ema mediko-sotsial'noi pomoshchi i trudosposobnosti gorodskogo naseleniia pensionnogo vozrasta' (Vsesoiuznyi nauchno-issledovatel'skii institut sotsial'noi gigieny i organizatsii zdravookhraneniia imeni N. A. Semashko, Moscow, 1980), 68. Even by the 1980s some hospitals in rural areas of the Soviet Union and Eastern Europe lacked hot water, indoor toilet facilities and running water. Victoria Velkoff and Kevin Kinsella, *Aging in Eastern Europe and the Former Soviet Union* (US Department of Commerce, Bureau of the Census, Washington, DC, 1993), 63; information cited from 1987 Goskomstat publications.
15 For recent historiography on Stalinism, see James Ryan and Susan Grant, *Revisioning Stalin and Stalinism: Complexities, Contradictions, and Controversies* (London: Bloomsbury Academic, 2020), introduction.
16 *Perspektivnyi plan razvitiia i razmeshcheniia domov-internatov dlia prestarelykh i invalidov v g. Moskve* (Mosgorispolkom glavnoe arkhitekturno-planirovochnoe upravlenie Goroda Moskvy, Nauchno-issledovatel'skii i proektnyi institute general'nogo plana Goroda Moskvy) (Moscow, 1974), 13.
17 Rudakov, Antonova, *Doma-Internaty*, 5. There did not seem to be gender segregation within the living quarters. There are possible questions about venereal disease, but I currently do not have information about this. At least in the case of fee paying pansionats, wards with venereal disease, as well as infectious diseases, psychiatric illness or oncological diseases with a malignant tumour, alcoholics and drug addicts, would be removed from the home. GARF, f. A-259, op. 45, d. 8526, l. 1.
18 Rudakov, O.I. Antonova, *Doma-Internaty*, 5.
19 Sachuk, 'Demograficheskaia i sotsial'naia kharakteristika', 510. Revutskaia, 'Organizatsiia meditsinskogo obsluzhivaniia', 582–3. For similar, see P. Rudakov, 'O tipakh domov dlia prestarelykh', *Sotsial'noe obespechenie* 7 (1961): 46; O. Ia. Smirnova, 'K voprosu o tipakh zhilishcha dlia liudei pozhilogo vozrasta', *Obraz zhizn' i starenie cheloveka* (materialy simpoziuma) (Kiev, Zdorov'ia, 1966), 50–1.
20 Sachuk, 'Demograficheskaia i sotsial'naia kharakteristika', 510–11; Revutskaia, 'Organizatsiia meditsinskogo obsluzhivaniia', 583.

21 P.G. Rudakov, 'Doma dlia pensionerov', *Sotsial'noe obespechenie* 11 (1958): 43. Rudakov explored designing one-storey apartment style complexes, such as that in Cheliabinsk, and *pansionat* style homes. In particular, he drew on design ideas from Austria.
22 I deal with the harsh realities of life in a home for older people in a draft chapter from my book on older people in the Soviet Union.
23 A brief history of the institute can be found on its website. Available at: https://ingil.ru/about/, accessed 31 March 2021.
24 Goskomitet po grazhdanskomu stroitel'stvu i arkhitekturee pri gosstroe SSSR, *Doma-internaty dlia pozhilykh i starykh liudei v SSSR* (Moscow: Stroiizdat, 1972), 3; 1960 is also provided as the beginning of *tipovoe* design in Moscow in *Perspektivnyi plan*, 9.
25 *Doma-internaty dlia pozhilykh*, 3. In the United States at the time there were '25,000 homes for the elderly and disabled, alcoholics, drug addicts, and the mentally ill' with 450,000 beds; of these, some 7,000 were clinics or hospitals and the rest were *pansionats*. Revutskaia, 'Organizatsiia meditsinskogo obsluzhivaniia', 598.
26 GARF, f. 9527, op. 1, d. 4852, l. 2.
27 According to census data, the percentage of those age sixty and over in the USSR was: 6.8 per cent in 1926 and 1939; 9.4 per cent in 1959; and 11.8 per cent in 1970. In absolute numbers, those aged 60 and over in the USSR stood at 12,997,000 in 1939; 19,708,000 in 1959; and 28,514,000 in 1970. Iu. I. Alabovskii, *Sostoianie zdorov'ia i vnebol'nichnaia meditsinskaia pomoshch' litsam pozhilogo vozrasta (po materialom Stavropol'skogo kraia)* (Stavropol': Stavropol' Medical institute, 1970), 80. Some 20 per cent of the Moscow's population was of pension age in 1972. *Perspektivnyi plan*, 18.
28 Rudakov, *Doma-Internaty dlia prestarelykh (arkhitekturno-planirovochnoe reshenie)* (Avtoreferat dissertatsii na soiskanie uchenoi stepeni kandidata arkhitektury, Nauchno-issledovatel'skii institute teorii i istorii arkhitektury i stroitel'noi tekhniki, Moscow, 1962), 3. B. R. Rubanenko was Rudakov's scientific adviser.
29 Stephen V. Bittner, *The Many Lives of Khrushchev's Thaw: Experience and Memory in Moscow's Arbat* (Ithaca and London: Cornell University Press, 2008), 116. Conterio, 'Our Black Sea Coast', 335.
30 For discussion, see Bittner, *Many Lives of Khrushchev's Thaw*, 119.
31 Bittner, *Many Lives of Khrushchev's Thaw*, 116.
32 Conterio, 'Our Black Sea Coast', 346.
33 Bittner, *Many Lives of Khrushchev's Thaw*, 126.
34 Ibid., 127.
35 GARF, f. 5446, op. 111, d. 254, l. 7. 1976.
36 GARF, f. 5446, op. 111, d. 254, l. 7.
37 GARF, f. 5446, op. 111, d. 254, l. 7.

38 GARF, A-259, op. 46, d. 9168, ll. 77–9, l. 87. GARF, f. R-5446, op. 11, d. 254, l. 3. (1970s)
39 S. Koriakov, 'Tipovoi proekt doma invalidov', 3 (1956): 44. Giprogor had to fulfil this task, ratified in March 1956.
40 Rudakov, 'Doma dlia pensionerov', 43. These were meant to include shops, pharmacies, and polyclinics.
41 Rudakov, 'Doma dlia pensionerov', 44. Good transport links were also considered important: see Rudakov, 'Doma-internaty dlia prestarelykh', *Sotsial'noe obespechenie* 5 (1959): 34. For similar on location, see F. Babushkina and L. Shekhman, 'Novyi tipovoi proekt doma invalidov', *Sotsial'noe obespechenie* 11 (1959): 39. Rudeiko discussed Rudakov's 1960 work on apartment complexes, based on 'foreign experience', for older people and he and his colleagues in the Leningrad Sanitary-Hygiene Medical Institute also conducted research on hygiene in homes. V.A. Rudeiko, 'Gigienicheskie trebovaniia k zhilishchu dlia lits pozhilogovozrasta', in *Gerontologiia i geriatriia 1969–1970. Sotsial'naia sreda, obraz zhizni starenie* (Kiev, 1970), 206.
42 'Chitateli otvechaiut na anketu', *Sotsial'noe obespechenie* 3 (1966): 39.
43 Conterio, 'Our Black Sea Coast', 350.
44 Rudakov, 'Doma dlia pensionerov', 43, 45.
45 Smirnova, 'K voprosu o tipakh zhilishcha', 51. According to the architect Smirnova, apartment style living took two forms: 'distributed' (first floor accommodation in regular apartment blocks) and 'concentrated' (specifically constructed apartment blocks). Specialized living included general homes and the hospital type. Smirnova also discussed the logistics of locating these buildings in urban residential districts and referenced foreign experiences; see p. 52.
46 O. Ia. Smirnova, 'Osobennosti planirovochnoi struktury domov dlia preestarelykh', in Chebotarev (ed), *Gerontologiia i geriatriia 1969–1970*, 198. Smirnova had done field surveys on homes for older people in the Ukrainian SSR, Russian SSR, Estonia, Latvia, and Lithuania and found that 40.5 per cent of older people spent their time on recreation and 32.25 per cent of that time (especially in colder weather) was spent in the home. Smirnova, 'Osobennosti planirovaniia', 198–9.
47 P. Rudakov, 'Kakimi dolzhny byt' doma-internaty dlia prestarelykh?', *Sotsial'noe obespechenie* 9 (1973): 35.
48 Rudakov, 'Kakimi dolzhny byt', 35.
49 Ibid., 37.
50 Ibid.
51 *Perspektivnyi Plan*, 41.
52 Ibid., 29.
53 Ibid., 33.
54 Ibid., 33.

55 P. Rudakov and B. Kundryshev, 'Kakimi byt internatam?', *Sotsial'noe obespechenie* 9 (1982): 30.
56 Rudakov, 'Doma-internaty dlia prestarelykh', 35.
57 Ibid.
58 Ibid., 34.
59 Ibid.
60 Ibid., 35.
61 O. Ochkina, 'Nado vse predusmotret', *Sotsial'noe obespechenie* 5 (1959): 36.
62 Babushkina and Shekhman, 'Novyi tipovoi proekt doma invalidov', 40. For similar, see Koriakov, 'Tipovoi proekt doma invalidov', 43–5.
63 *Doma-internaty dlia pozhilykh*, 14.
64 Ibid. The design was also used in Kiev.
65 B. Sokolov, 'Starost' obespechena', *Sotsial'noe obespechenie* 7 (1966): 10.
66 Ibid., 12.
67 Ibid.
68 *Perspektivnyi plan*, 33.
69 *Doma-internaty dlia pozhilykh*, 14.
70 Giprogor (the Russian Institute for Urban Planning and Investment Development – *Rossiiskii institut gradostroitel'stva i investitsionnogo razvitiia*) was founded in 1929 and still exists today. On the history of Giprogor, see 'Iz istorii instituta', available at: http://www.giprogor.ru/about/history, accessed 13 September 2021.
71 *Perspektivnyi plan razvitiia*, 34.
72 Ibid.
73 P. Makaraov, 'Chto nuzhno uchest' na budushchee', *Sotsial'noe obespechenie* 3 (1970): 37.
74 N. Veselova, 'Proekt i zhizn': v poriadke obsuzhdeniia', *Sotsial'noe obespechenie* 11 (1969): 39.
75 P. Vanichev, 'Dorabotka proekta neobkhodima', *Sotsial'noe obespechenie* 3 (1970): 36. The 1970 articles were a response to Veselova's 1969 article.
76 Vanichev, 'Dorabotka proekta neobkhodima', 36.
77 *Perspektivnyi plan razvitiia*, 34.
78 Rudeiko lists three styles: pavilion, centralized and bloc. He describes the centralized style as exemplified by a 1956 Giprogor *tipovoe* design for 311 people that contained everything in one building, but only contained one or two storeys. He favoured the bloc style, which 'grouped related premises in blocs connected with heated passages'. It seems that it was less isolated than the pavilion style but less connected than the centralized style. Rudeiko, 'Gigienicheskie trebovaniia', 208–9.
79 *Perspektivnyi plan razvitiia*, 33.
80 Ibid., 99–105; *Rekomendatsii po ratsional'noi planirovke, zonirovaniiu i oborudovaniiu territorii domov-internatov dlia prestarelykh i invalidov i psikhonevrologicheskikh internatov* (Moscow: TsNIIEP zhilishcha, 1989), 27, 31.

81 For example, see Koriakov, 'Tipovoi proekt doma invalidov', 44.
82 *Perspektivnyi plan*, 39.
83 'Care Standards for Nursing Homes', Department of Health, Social Services and Public Safety, April 2015. Available at: https://www.rqia.org.uk/RQIA/media/RQIA/Resources/Standards/nursing_homes_standards_-_april_2015.pdf, accessed 20 April 2021.
84 'Calls for New Minimum Standards for UK Care Home Design', Building Better Healthcare, 20 July 2020. Available at: https://www.buildingbetterhealthcare.com/news/article_page/Call_for_new_minimum_standards_for_UK_care_home_design/167833, accessed 20 April 2021.
85 The funding challenge in the UK is noted here: 'Calls for New Minimum Standards for UK Care Home Design'.
86 'Calls for New Minimum Standards for UK Care Home Design'.
87 Revutskaia, 'Organizatsiia meditsinskogo obsluzhivaniia', 593.
88 Koriakov, 'Tipovoi proekt doma invalidov', 44.
89 Rudakov, 'Doma-internaty dlia prestarelykh', 35.
90 V. Strashnov, 'I tsvet, i forma (otdelka i okraska pomeshchenii v domakh-internatakh)', *Sotsial'noe obespechenie* 8 (1976): 32.
91 N.M. Ianko, 'Gigienicheskie trebovaniia k miagkoi mebeli dlia prodolzhitel'nogo otdykha lits raznykh vozrastnykh grupp', *Gerontologiia i geriatriia 1969-1970. Sotsial'naia sreda, obraz zhizni*, 223–224; 226–227.
92 Strashnov, 'I tsvet, i forma', 33. Ianko looked to I.I. Keegan (1962), E. Zink (1964) and J. Maxwell (1960).
93 Revutskaia, 'Organizatsiia meditsinskogo obsluzhivaniia', 593.
94 Strashnov, 'I tsvet, i forma', 34.
95 Ibid.
96 P. Rudakov, 'Liudiam budet udobno: Novyi normativnyi document dlia proektirovaniia domov-internatov', *Sotsial'noe obespechenie* 7 (1975): 26.
97 Ibid., 26–7; quotation page 27. I do not discuss the hospital type of home extensively here, but discussions on this to refer to an example in Leningrad. See for example, Rudeiko, 'Gigienicheskie trebovaniia', 207–8.
98 See A. Samarina, 'Vperedi – bol'shaia rabota', *Sotsial'noe obespechenie* 2 (1976): 33.
99 P. Rudakov and B. Kundryshev, 'Kakimi byt' internatam?', *Sotsial'noe obespechenie* 9 (1982): 29. For specific problems, see I. Khaliutkina, 'Dlia tekh, kto prikovan k posteli', *Sotsial'noe obespechenie* 3 (1982): 30.
100 Rudakov and Kundryshev, 'Kakimi byt' internatam?', 29.
101 A. Samarina, 'Vrach doma-internata', *Sotsial'noe obespechenie* 4 (1982): 25.
102 Ibid.
103 *Perspektivnyi plan*, 32.
104 *Programma-zadanie na razrabotku tipovykh i individual'nykh proektov territorial'nykh tsentrov sotsial'nogo obsluzhivaniia pensionerov* (Moscow, 1987), 3.

105 *Programma-zadanie na razrabotku tipovykh i individual'nykh proektov*, 3.
106 Migette Kaup, 'An Analysis of Resident Room Design in the Changing Culture of Long-term Care: Examining the Design of Spaces that Promote Resident Autonomy', in Interior Design Educators Council conference proceedings, *Design and Social Justice*, 44th Annual International Conference, University of Texas at Austin, 2007, 185.
107 Paula Span, 'The New Old Age: A Better Type of Nursing Home', *The New York Times*, 17 December 2017. Available at: https://www.nytimes.com/2017/12/22/health/green-houses-nursing-homes.html, accessed 26 April 2021. See the Green Hills example, available at: https://www.green-hill.com, accessed 28 April 2021. See also Davidson, 'The American Nursing-Home Is a Design Failure'.

6

Age and the city: Older persons in Soviet urban milieu and thought in the 1970s and 1980s

Botakoz Kassymbekova

This chapter analyses proposals made by Soviet urban designers to improve the conditions of older people in late Soviet cities, based on research about their lives in these cities.[1] I am interested in their visions of 'appropriate' urban environments for older age, and how they thought that cities should be adapted to the needs of older persons. There is no indication that these proposals were ever realized, but nevertheless they are important for our understanding about how older people's urban needs were conceived in the late Soviet Union.[2] The article focuses on the last two decades of the Soviet period (i.e., 1970s–80s) because discussions about old age and city environments emerged at this time.[3] These discussions were neither numerous, systematic nor encompassing of all Soviet cities and towns and were strongly influenced by Western architectural currents. Fragmentary research and planning ideas regarding accommodating old age in the city was published during this period and mainly addressed the issue in large central cities, including Moscow, Leningrad and Kiev, although some research on other cities also took place. This article draws on this literature to shed light on the urban dimensions of old age in the late Soviet Union and how these aspects were reflected in the contemporary understandings of 'good ageing' held by both planners and the ordinary Soviet citizens that they studied. It does not review all services that were discussed for older people, such as doctors' visits and various subsidies, but only those that were directly related to urban living and housing planning and design.

The post-Stalinist period was a time of rapid urban reconstruction: the administrations of Nikita Khrushchev (1953–64) and Leonid Brezhnev (1964–82) proclaimed housing policies and city development to be central components of their political agendas. This policy represented a considerable break with earlier housing policies in the immediate post-revolutionary and

Stalinist periods. Previously, mass housing provision in cities like Moscow, Leningrad and Kiev had been secured primarily through the nationalization of privately owned individual apartments and their reorganization into communal ones, along with the construction of limited individual apartment housing for Soviet political, artistic and technical elites. During the Khrushchev and Brezhnev periods, Stalinist architecture was criticized for its excessive lavishness and inaccessibility to most of the population: the vast majority of people in Soviet cities and towns up until the 1960s continued to live in communal apartments, barracks or dormitories with shared facilities such as bathrooms and kitchens.[4] In the post-Stalinist period, individual single-family apartments for each Soviet urban resident became a political promise: an amelioration of the tensions of shared living experienced in the Stalinist period. By offering Soviet citizens their most desired type of housing, the post-Stalinist leadership was appealing to citizens exhausted by decades of earlier deprivation.[5] Therefore, the Soviet government's highest priority since the late 1950s was the rapid mass construction of individual apartment buildings on the lowest budget possible to enable as many citizens as possible to move to individual apartments.[6]

At the same time, sociological research was permitted again, after sociology's ban during Stalinism as a bourgeois, unnecessary and dangerous science, and the distinct field of urban sociology was established in the 1960s.[7] Soviet scholars and planners paid special attention to Western urban planning and integrated it into their analysis and proposals.[8] Similar to their Western colleagues, Soviet urban sociologists began to stress human residents' needs and the interactions between the urban built environment and social worlds more generally. The idea of humanizing urban space that developed in post-war Western Europe became especially appealing to some Soviet urban scholars.[9] This differed from earlier Soviet approaches to housing as a 'machine for living' and 'functions of production processes', and creator of communes and collectives.[10] The new urban sociological thought stressed the importance of people's private lives, their life cycles and social relations for thinking about housing and urban planning.[11] This is how a group of architects explained what they saw as the new set of tasks for urban planning, which represented a body of thought embraced by Soviet urban designers:

> The human being needs a private place where he can separate himself from others, rest, sleep, and live his family life. Housing must respond to the need to restore the physical and moral forces that a man expends in his productive

and social life. The more intense the social interaction and the wider a person's relationships, the more he must be able to regenerate the energies socially expended, and the more profound and complete must be his physical and mental relaxation.[12]

This chapter draws on urban scholars' research and recommendations about older residents' urban needs and preferences in the Soviet Union during the 1970s and 1980s. As such, the chapter is less about how Soviet cities accommodated older persons in practice because most of these recommendations were not fulfilled. The focus of the chapter is instead on visions and proposals for improving urban residents' living. The urban scholarship adapted Western proposals to improve the built environment for older persons, but it also stressed family ties as key for older people's satisfaction of their needs and care in the cities. At the same time, older persons' desire for autonomy was stressed as important both for psychological and for social reasons. Urban scholars and housing designers proposed accommodating both the autonomy and familial connections of older persons in the city. At the same time, the post-Second World War demographic context and the Soviet state's priorities in terms of building micro-districts (*mikroraiony*, multi-storey housing districts outside of city centres) are key for understanding scholars' findings, concerns and proposals.

Older people in Moscow, Leningrad and Kiev

The Soviet Union's older population constituted 11.8 per cent (28.5 million people) of its total population in 1970.[13] Two million people over the age of fifty lived in Moscow (27 per cent of the city's total), one million (25 per cent) in Leningrad and 350,000 (20 per cent) in Kiev.[14] These individuals usually lived in central city areas in communal apartments, often with their adult children, whereas the newly built mass housing districts ('micro-districts') were populated largely by younger generations.[15] Even when younger persons moved to new micro-districts, the older people stayed in communal apartments that were located in city centres. The communal apartments offered less comfort than single-family apartments because their residents shared a single bathroom and kitchen with other residents; sometimes there were close to twenty neighbours sharing facilities. Moreover, communal apartments were often in poor physical condition. Urban pensioners' housing was less comfortable in comparison to new flats in micro-districts: only 69 per cent had a sewage system and gas, 57 per cent had central heating, 43 per cent had a bathroom or shower, 42 per cent had hot water and 13 per cent telephones.[16] This is how an older man in Leningrad described his communal apartment in the late 1980s:

> It's disgusting to enter our communal apartment. All of the residents consider themselves temporary – you know, there's not long left to live in it – and have turned it into a foul hovel. Each one keeps his or her room in some order, but the communal areas have turned into some sort of cesspit.[17]

And yet, some scholars reported, many older people still preferred to stay in communal apartments, rather than move to new single-family apartments in the new micro-districts as younger adults usually did.[18] This did not mean, however, that older persons preferred communal living to individualized living *per se*. On the contrary, the vast majority of older people, according to sociological research in Moscow, Kiev and Leningrad in the 1970s and 1980s, would have preferred to live in single-family apartments, a desire that can also be frequently found in the diary entries of Soviet pensioners.[19] Preference for single-family apartments, however, was not universal: individuals with disabilities or health conditions were more likely to prefer either staying in their communal apartments or moving to care homes.[20] Care homes, however, were generally the least preferred option.[21] Families preferred separate living not so much for economic reasons, but for 'social and psychological freedoms' and distance from 'intrusion' from adult relatives, even in the case of dependency.[22] The infrastructural development of the central city location was another crucial factor for the majority's preference to remain in communal apartments.[23] First, more than half of urban older persons, sociologists found out, were not satisfied with the quality of design and the sizes of new apartments in new micro-districts.[24] Importantly, central locations in cities offered access to parks, entertainment, medical services and other public facilities. Moreover, central communal apartments offered proximity to a better transportation network, which allowed travelling to visit family members and friends – but also to work, for those who continued working in old age.[25] Scholars found out that the most acceptable radius of movement (for grocery shopping, visits, etc.) for older people was 400 metres; moving to infrastructurally undeveloped regions increased daily distances and was thus avoided by older persons.[26] This is how one older person wrote to an acquaintance (also an older person) about his reluctance to move from a room in a communal apartment into a new individual apartment: 'We didn't want to endure inconveniences. A new apartment in a bad area, without greenery; and even with[out] a sick daughter it would be difficult.'[27]

Although proximity did lead to regular conflicts amongst neighbours in communal apartments, their co-residents did help each other in emergencies and also often socialized: they exchanged books, borrowed spices, money and medicine in case of illness, and simply talked.[28] Calling for medical help was an especially important positive factor in people's memories about Soviet communal living.[29] This is how the Soviet communal apartment experience was remembered: 'At least if worse comes to worst, even after peeing in your teapot they will still call an ambulance for you if you need it, or lend you a little bit of salt for your cooking.'[30] Retired older persons had particular cause to find communal living attractive since they did not hurry in the morning to work and could use common facilities during 'off-peak' hours.[31]

Older urban residents expressed a willingness to live autonomously, but family ties remained important.[32] Multigenerational families, i.e. families with older persons and adult children, constituted a quarter of all households in the Soviet Union.[33] Although most (72 per cent) Soviet older persons in 1970 lived with their adult children, in big cities like Kiev around half of these older people lived separately.[34] Hence, only around 10 per cent of urban families in Soviet cities lived with their older parents.[35] But even if older parents and adult children in big cities lived separately, close networks were maintained: around 70 per cent of respondents in Leningrad in 1972 and in Kiev in 1976 indicated that they wanted to live in proximity to older parents or adult children.[36] In Leningrad, for example, in the 1970s older parents visited adult children for communication (41 per cent), for common recreation (11 per cent) and offering household help (48 per cent). Two thirds of travel was done by the older parents to the homes of adult children.[37]

The post-war gender dimensions among older persons are important for understanding Soviet urban residents' preference to live near each other. The Second World War considerably decreased the male population, so that in the year 1970, for example, there were 2.8 times more women than men aged seventy or older. By 1979 there were 3.9 times more women over seventy, so that statistically single or widowed older women were more present in multigenerational households – also, because they were more likely to experience material difficulties.[38] Age was also an important factor: older and more dependent older persons lived with their adult children: in Ukraine, 90 per cent of single older persons and 50 per cent of couples over eighty years of age lived with adult relatives.[39]

Infrastructures for good ageing

Multigenerational apartments and age-specific apartment distribution

Urban scholars argued that familial networks and sociability should be integrated into city and housing planning to allow for connected, yet autonomous, ageing in the city. Immediate extended family (adult children and their families) were considered crucial for good ageing. Both official and academic conceptions of 'family' viewed this as an important factor of care for older persons. Family figured in academic texts as the 'social-economic cell of society', responsible for population reproduction and for the 'upbringing and socialization of children, organization of household and recreation of family members' and, importantly, care for older relatives [*popechenie prestarelykh*].[40] The 1969 Family Code legally obliged Soviet citizens to maintain and care for parents incapable of working or otherwise in need. Urban planners also argued that family would remain an important factor in delivering care, arguing that housing policies should assist older persons and their relatives in keeping ties and offering each other household help.[41]

Reacting to older individuals' desire to live separately but in proximity to their adult children, architects proposed constructing apartments specifically for multigenerational families. Dmitry Durmanov, for example, proposed five versions of such apartments. Depending on the needs and size of multigenerational families, he proposed designing apartments of various arrangements, such as with an additional bathroom, additional kitchen space, additional entrance and shared living room, or flexible room division, to accommodate the needs of different ages and family sizes. Durmanov offered several types of apartments: for those with one parent or a parental couple, which were supposed to be technically flexible in nature to allow the merger or removal of rooms or entire apartments in different configurations, depending on family dynamics.[42] This planning proposition was important because in the Soviet Union at the time most apartments (79 per cent) were one or two-room apartments, while 18 per cent were three-room apartments and only 3 per cent were four to five, or six-room apartments.[43] Since the dominant architectural policy concentrated on reducing the living area of single-family apartments to allow for the maximum provision of individual housing to families, flexible apartments for multigenerational families was a costly alternative. In practice, small and big families alike often received identically sized apartments.[44] As a consequence, providing apartments to older parents closer to their adult children was a more feasible option, a proposition popular among urban scholars.[45] Proponents of the familial approach to the distribution of apartments argued against settling older persons in compact settlements or in specialized homes. Instead, they argued that apartment distribution policies should be flexible and take family and personal situations into account. In the new micro-districts, for example, the argument was made that older persons should receive apartments on first floors. Those in need of intense care, moreover, could be settled in proximity with each other for more efficient organization of in-home care.[46]

Streets and services

One of the major difficulties faced by older persons in the city was their capacity to move around the city and neighbourhoods. Many could not physically leave their housing or use public transport because cities had been planned for healthy middle-aged adults.[47] Difficulties were not only to be found in the metro stations, which required a certain speed of movement (Soviet standards for walking movement in metro stations was calculated at more than one kilometre per hour) that was difficult for older persons, but also their built environment: metro hallways were calculated to allow 3,200 persons per hour, a standard considered inappropriate for older persons.[48] Another difficulty was access to buildings, since Soviet architectural standards dictated that buildings' entrances be higher than sidewalks: staircases were required to enter most buildings and access ramps were almost non-existent. Entering public transport such as buses and trolleybuses also involved climbing stairs, making it often impossible for older persons to access them.[49] The width of sidewalks did not allow space for slow walking for older persons (especially those with eyesight issues) – and the quality of roads themselves (e.g. slippery material or curbs between roads and sidewalks on the streets) also made movement for older persons a challenge.[50]

While physical movement in big cities was difficult due to the urban built environment, urban planners and sociologists criticized institutional services, such as geriatric cabinets[51] and health centres, which were important for older persons but were not available in many of the newly built micro-districts.[52] Some urbanists proposed organizing specialized care centres for older persons in the micro-districts to provide services such as grocery shopping, cleaning and so forth. Older persons who wished to continue to work, it was suggested, could work in such centres.[53]

The neighbourhood's built environment

Elena Pavlovskaia's 1985 dissertation, *Socio-cultural Aspects of the Formation of Material-spatial Leisure Environments and Older People's Interaction in Urban Near-house Territories*,[54] is probably one of the most detailed Soviet studies of older people's urban behaviour. It represents a unique depiction of Soviet urban micro-districts' challenges and the opportunities presented to accommodate older people. Pavlovskaia was the student of Selim Khan-Magomedov, a famous Soviet architectural historian of early Soviet constructivism; she was also inspired by the Tallinn school of urban sociology, which paid close attention to urban space as a communicative field and social space.[55] Citing research about older people in the Soviet Union and Western Europe, Pavlovskaia argued that it was by then a consensus that moving older people to nursing homes had negative effects on them, and since the 1970s new design methods developed in Western Europe had instead focused on adjusting older people's lives in the city as part of the humanization of urban space. Just as other urban critics at the time, Pavlovskaia argued that new housing micro-districts formed 'extremely weak neighbourhood contacts' and were 'psychologically uncomfortable', which negatively affected older persons as the spaces lacked cosiness, intimacy and 'humanness' (*chelovechnost'*). In comparison to central city districts, the contact between neighbours decreased and the 'majority of pensioners did not know their neighbours whatsoever'. Some types of neighbourhood leisure activities disappeared entirely in new micro-districts, since people used its public spaces only for necessities such as shopping or visits to the doctor.

Pavlovskaia's main concern was that micro-districts did not pay attention to the cultural dimensions of urban life. She observed that people dressed and behaved differently in old city-centres and micro-districts: they took more care in the centre, while more people vandalized physical surroundings, such as gardens, in the anonymous micro-districts.[56] The reason for this lay in the fact, according to Pavlovskaia, that micro-districts were products of functionalist planning and suffered from 'over-increased parameters, aesthetical poverty, empty spaces, absence of spaces for communication' and a lack of social infrastructure. As a result, many residents considered them less liveable and preferred staying in old city centres.

To evaluate older residents' needs, Pavlovskaia carried out 100 standardized surveys followed by open-ended interviews with residents in old-type housing and in new micro-districts in 1981. She also observed spatial usage and used photography to observe the space from within, i.e. 'see the space through the eyes of its inhabitants'. She determined that many older residents spent most of their time in the area surrounding their homes: 65 per cent of older people in the old yards, and 55 per cent in the communal spaces in the new micro-districts. Pavlovskaia concluded that in old-type yards communication and recreation were more intense – people used the yards to talk to their neighbours, do handicrafts, play chess, garden, walk with their grandchildren or read. In the new type of housing they almost never read or did handicrafts outside of their flats. As a result, in the old houses, 60 per cent of the older residents were satisfied with how they spent their free time, whereas in the new type buildings only 20 per cent expressed satisfaction.[57] At the same time, 75 per cent of residents of the city centre acknowledged having long-term relationships with neighbours, whereas in new micro-districts only a quarter knew their neighbours.[58] Pavlovskaia observed that spaces around houses and yards were gendered: there were, for example, benches that were used by male residents and those that were exclusively used by female residents. Women preferred protected and well-developed areas: they valued flowers and aesthetically pleasing and roofed areas. Female groups were larger in number and they usually gathered around a certain material structure or in an isolated place. Men were, on the other hand, more 'ascetic' and preferred public spaces to more intimate yards or areas immediately around houses.[59]

However, differences among older people's preferences were not only gendered. Age, personality and education also played a role. Pavlovskaia concluded that there were different preferences regarding the social and physical environment among older residents: (1) some wanted to influence their built environment, through gardening or cleaning, but also wished to have influence over the social atmosphere (keeping a certain microclimate by retaining relations with neighbours); (2) some preferred only certain kinds of communication and wanted to engage in certain kinds of activities; they also wanted to avoid excessive contact; (3) some wanted full isolation and prioritized personal safety; they were passive towards influencing surrounding territory; and (4) others did not want to use public space at all.[60] Urbanites tended to prefer anonymity and communicated with a small number of neighbours, whereas very old residents preferred isolation for health and safety reasons. Most older people did not express a desire to have contact with too many people – a characteristic of new micro-districts – because they could not remember them and as a result everyone seemed foreign.[61] At the same time, Pavlovskaia concluded, although old-type yards fostered more intense contact with neighbours, they were not a model for planning micro-district yards because they did not offer anonymity and privacy.

Good spaces for older residents were those that provided identification with space, the ability to influence it, but also the possibility of anonymity and choice of contacts.[62]

Based on her observations, Pavlovskaia proposed several small steps to improve older people's experience of outdoor spaces. First, she proposed organizing spaces that improved older people's agency. One of the steps was to allow the residents in the new micro-districts to fence off small garden plots in the communal areas around buildings. Since it was forbidden to fence them at the time, residents preferred to grow flowers on their balconies rather than on public plots, where the flowers were often destroyed. Older persons were less likely to enjoy out-of-town recreation, Pavlovskaia argued, and so allowing them to grow plants near their houses made sense not only as a way for them to get in contact with nature, but also, for all residents, as the greenery made the residential area cosier. So far, public spaces were 'nobody's spaces' and were seen by many older persons as 'foreign' (*chuzhaia*), as spaces without care and control.[63] In contrast, in old-type yard houses, older persons felt they had more ownership of their space.[64]

Secondly, Pavlovskaia proposed organizing comfortable spaces for older residents that would protect them from the sun, rain, noise, older children and noisy sport facilities. But these places, she proposed, should not be isolated, since older people also wanted to see what was happening in other, adjacent places.[65] Such areas could be organized, for example, near the entrances to buildings. Pavlovskaia determined that in bigger micro-districts, 70 per cent of older people socialized in the immediate entrance areas or on children's playgrounds. In the spring and summer those entrance areas were often overfilled, i.e. benches were so busy that pensioners often brought their own chairs out. In old-type yards older people socialized in central squares, but in new micro-districts the older residents rarely left the area near their house entrances. Twenty per cent said that they met and socialized at entrances to their buildings due to health and mobility issues, but it was also psychologically comforting to remain close to their houses for the feeling of protection. Pavlovskaia suggested organizing squares specifically made for older persons near the entrances, which would also improve the situation for other groups who often had to push through the crowds of older women near the entrances, which caused psychological discomfort for everyone involved.

For those older persons who looked after grandchildren or great-grandchildren, Pavlovskaia proposed improving child-focused infrastructure. Since it was not only grandparents, but often great-grandparents who took care of children, and on average spent three to five hours each day with their grandchildren outside, Pavlovskaia argued that playgrounds were in practice also places for older persons. Pointing to the falling prestige of grandchild-rearing and siding with the general Soviet discourse about usefulness of grandparents in terms of unburdening their children who were 'young workers', Pavlovskaia suggested improving the quality of playgrounds, for example, through more comfortable benches, for raising prestige not only of grandchild-rearing but also of the older people.

Finally, Pavlovskaia noticed that older people walked differently in microdistricts than in other parts of the city. In central city districts, the old-type of architecture invited 'attention to details and nuances of the environment', inspiring slow recreational walking. The strolling allowed meeting and communicating with other people 'spontaneously' and involved a cultural and 'emotional component'.[66] Older people, Pavlovskaia observed, prepared for strolls in such areas by dressing specially for the occasion and behaved in a mannered way, thereby increasing the special atmosphere of these places. This contrasted starkly to new micro-district behaviour: walking there was more functional, i.e. to the grocery or drug store, and did not foster recreational walking. Since there were few roads in the new micro-districts suitable for strolling, Pavlovskaia argued for constructing a non-linear pathway system in green zones, installing benches for occasional rest and lanterns to allow for recreational walking.

Conclusion

This chapter provided a survey of Soviet scholarship on older people's urban condition and their proposals for improving it. The research was not all-encompassing and mostly concentrated on major cities such as Moscow, Leningrad and Kiev, yet it sheds light on several aspects of ageing in urban environments across the USSR. First, Soviet scholars were inspired by and agreed with their Western colleagues on the necessity to adapt cities' built environment for older persons' physical experience of the city: to improve sidewalks, transportation, apartment building's yards, etc. Accommodating the city to meet the older persons' needs allowed them not only continuous mobility, but a feeling of belonging to the city. This latter point was important because Soviet scholars generally agreed (also with Western colleagues) that allowing older people to stay in their usual home environments was more preferential than moving them to care homes. At the same time, Soviet urban designers stressed that family connections and autonomy were crucial for older persons' good ageing. From one side they emphasized that older people wanted to live independent lives, while also noting that keeping family ties were important for both older people and their families. These considerations were rooted in the Soviet state's family policies and its dual – and sometimes contradictory – promotion of both welfare and care support and individual actualization within the Soviet project. Older person's experience of city environments, late Soviet urbanist scholars suggested, was one place where this actualization could have been improved and *humanized* to a much greater degree.

Funding acknowledgement

This research was funded in whole by the Wellcome Trust [Grant No: 209842/Z/17/Z]. For the purpose of open access, the author has applied a CC BY public copyright licence to any Author Accepted Manuscript version arising from this submission.

Notes

1. Soviet urbanists usually adopted the age threshold of sixty years of age when speaking of older persons. Sometimes, however, official pension age was taken to refer to elderhood: fifty-five years of age for women and sixty for men.
2. Olga Smirnova and Ludmila Barmashina, *Zhilye doma kvartirnogo tipa dlia prestarelykh* (Moscow: TsNTI, 1977), 7; V.I. Vilenchik et al. (eds.), *Zhilishcha dlia prestarelykh: Potrebnosti i puti ikh udovletvoreniia* (Minsk: Belorusskii nauchno-issledovatel'skii institut nauchno-tekhnicheskoi informatsii i tekhniko-ekonomicheskikh issledovanii Gosplana BSSR, 1989), 7–8.
3. Oleg Ianitskii, 'Sotsiologiia goroda', in V. Iadov (ed.), *Sotsiologiia v Rossii* (Moskva: Institut sotsiologii RAN, 1998), online: https://socioline.ru/pages/v-yadov-sotsiologiya-v-rossii; accessed 1 August 2021.
4. M.N. Fedchenko, *Povsednevnaia zhizn' sovetskogo cheloveka (1945–1991)* (Kurgan: Izdatel'stvo Kurganskogo gosudarstvennogo universiteta, 2009), 64.
5. Susan Reid, 'Happy Housewarming! Moving into Khrushchev-Era Apartments', in Marina Balina and Evgeny Dobrenko (eds.), *Petrified Utopia: Happiness Soviet Style* (London: Anthem Press, 2009), 137; Steven E. Harris, *Communism on Tomorrow Street. Mass Housing and Everyday Life after Stalin* (Baltimore: Johns Hopkins University Press. Washington, DC: Woodrow Wilson Center, 2013), 111–12.

6   Ol'ga Iakushenko, 'Sovetskaia arkhitektura i zapad: otkrytie i assimiliatsiia zapadnogo opyta v sovetskoi arkhitekture kontsa 1950-kh – 1960-kh godov', *Laboratorium* 8, no. 2 (2016): 81.
7   Oleg Ianitskii, 'Istoriia gorodskoi sotsiologii v Rossii: evolutsiia idei', *Sotsiologicheskie issledovaniia* 8 (2016): 123; Andres Kurg, 'Free communication: from Soviet future cities to kitchen conversations', *The Journal of Architecture* 24, no. 5 (2019): 680.
8   Iakushenko 'Sovetskaia arkhitektura i zapad', 76–81; Ianitskii, 'Istoriia gorodskoi sotsiologii', 122. Overviews of Western urbanist thought could frequently be found in Soviet publications on urban architecture and planning. See, for example, publications specifically about accommodating older people: Kalervo Leikho, 'Zhilishche dlia liudei s ogranichennoi podvizhnost'iu' and A.V. Sigaev, 'Peshekhodnye puti i transport dlia invalidov i prestarelykh', in V.K. Stepanova (ed.), *Arkhitekturnaia sreda obitaniia invalidov i prestarelykh* (Moskva: Stroizdat, 1989); *Zhilye doma dlia pozhilykh za rubezhom* (Moscow: Gosudarsvennyi komitet po grazhdanskomu sroitel'stvu i arkhitekture pri Gossstroe SSSR, 1975).
9   Ákos Moravánsky and Karl R. Kegler, *Re-scaling the Environment: New Landscapes of Design, 1960–1980* (Basel: Birkhäuser, 2017).
10 Ianitskii, 'Istoriia gorodskoi sotsiologii'; A.V. Baranov, 'Sotsiologicheskie problemy zhilishcha', in A.G. Kharchev (ed.), *Sotsial'nye problemy zhilishcha* (Leningrad: Gosudarstvennyi komitet po grazhdanskomu stroitel'stvu i arkhitekture pri Gosstroe, 1969), 17.
11 G.D. Platonov, *Demografiia i problemy zhilishcha* (Leningrad: Stroitel'stvo i arkhitektura Leningrada, 1967), 4; see also Alexei Gutnov et al. (eds.), *The Ideal Communist City* (New York: George Braziller, 1971).
12 Andrei Baburov et al., *Novyi element rasseleniia. Na puti k novomu gorodu* (Moscow: Stroiizdat, 1966), 47.
13 D. Valentei, 'Liudi "Tret'ego Vozrasta"', in D. Valentei (ed.), *Pozhilye liudi v nashei strane* (Moscow: Statistika, 1977), 3.
14 N.N. Sachuk and N.N. Lakiza-Sachuk, *Pozhiloi chelovek v urbanizirovannom obshchestve* (Moscow: Akademiia Nauk SSSR, 1977), 6.
15 Ludmila Barmashina, *Printsipy rasseleniia i tipy zhilykh iacheek dlia pozhilykh v sisteme gorodskoi zastroiki* (Ph.D. diss., State Committee on civil building and architecture of the State Building Commission of the USSR, Kiev, 1979), 19–24; Ruben Bagirian, *Sotsial'noe razvitie mikroraiona bol'shogo goroda* (Moscow: Akademiia Nauk SSSR: 1984), 11.
16 Vilenchik et al., *Zhilishcha dlia prestarelykh*, 11.
17 Kokotov, 'Dnevniki', as collected by the Prozhito Archive, St. Petersburg.
18 V. Kogan, 'Odinokie prestarelye – problema i puti ikh sotsializatsii', in Dmitry Valentei (ed.), *Naselenie tret'ego vozrasta* (Moscow: Narodonaselenie, 1986), 113; Sachuk and Lakiza-Sachuk, *Pozhiloi chelovek*, 9.

19 Bagirian, *Sotsial'noe razvitie mikroraiona*, 22; Barmashina, *Printsipy rasseleniia*, 22.
20 Barmashina, *Printsipy rasseleniia*, 33.
21 Ibid., 90.
22 Baranov, 'Sotsiologicheskie problemy zhilishcha', 12–13.
23 Barmashina, *Printsipy rasseleniia*, 104.
24 Vilenchik et al., *Zhilishcha dlia prestarelykh*, 9; Elena Pavlovskaia, 'Sotsial'no-kul'turnyi aspekt formirovaniia Predmetno-prostranstvennoi sredy otdykha i obshcheniia liudei pozhilogo vozrasta na gorodskikh pridomovykh territoriiakh' (PhD diss., Moscow, 1985), 5.
25 Ol'ga Smirnova, 'K voprosu o tipakh zhilishcha dlia liudei pozhilogo vozrasta', in Ol'ga Smirnova and Ludmila Barmashina (eds.), *Zhilye doma kvartirnogo tipa dlia prestarelykh* (Moscow: Gosudarstvennyi komitet po grazhdanskomu stroitel'stvu, 1977), 5.
26 Vilenchik et al., *Zhilishcha dlia prestarelykh*, 24.
27 Kokotov, 'Dnevniki'.
28 Smirnova and Barmashina, *Zhilishcha dlia prestarelykh*, 5; Philipp Pott, *Moskauer Kommunalwohnungen 1917 bis 1997. Materielle Kultur, Erfahrung, Erinnerung* (Zürich: Pano, 2009), 206–12; Vilenchik et al., *Zhilishcha dlia prestarelykh*, 26.
29 Pott, *Moskauer Kommunalwohnungen*, 208.
30 Svetlana Boym, *Common Places: Mythologies of Everyday Life in Russia* (Cambridge, MA: Harvard University Press, 1994), 150.
31 Deborah A. Friedman, 'Everyday Life and the Problem of Conceptualizing Public and Private during the Khrushchev Era', in Choi Chatterjee (ed.), *Everyday Life in Russia Past and Present* (Indiana: Indiana University Press, 2015), 174.
32 V.D. Shapiro, 'Vzaimootnosheniia starshego i srednego pokolenii sem'i', *Sotsiologicheskie Issledovaniia* 1 (1981): 127; Barmashina, *Printsipy rasseleniia*, 55; Baranov, 'Sotsiologicheskie problemy zhilishcha', 13.
33 I.A. Gerasimova, *Struktura sem'i* (Moskva: Statistika, 1976), 58; T.N. Roganova, 'Chislo i sostav semei v SSSR', in *Vsesoiuznaia perepis' naseleniia 1970 goda. Sbornik statei* (Moskva: Statistika, 1970), 262.
34 Barmashina, *Printsipy rasseleniia*, 31.
35 V.Iu. Durmanov, *Tipologiia kvartir dlia semei s pozhilymi roditeliami* (PhD diss., Moscow, 1978), 8.
36 Barmashina, *Printsipy rasseleniia*, 22; Vilenchik et al., *Zhilishcha dlia prestarelykh*, 17.
37 Durmanov, *Tipologiia kvartir*, 28.
38 Kogan, 'Odinokie prestarelye', 107; Barmashina, *Printsipy rasseleniia*, 70; Roganova, 'Chislo i sostav semei', 262; I.V. Kaliniuk and A.Ia. Kvasha, 'Starenie naselenia: problemy i perpsektivy', in Dmitry Valentei (ed.), *Naselenie tret'ego vozrasta* (Moscow: Mysl', 1986), 17.
39 Durmanov, *Tipologiia kvartir*, 8.

40 Gerasimova, *Struktura sem'i*, 3.
41 Durmanov, *Tipologiia kvartir*, 24–6.
42 Durmanov, *Tipologiia kvartir*.
43 E.P. Fedorov, 'Formirovanie gorodskogo fonda v zavisimosti ot semeinoi struktury naselenia', in K.K. Kartashova (ed.), *Sem'ia i zhilaia iacheika* (Moscow: Gosudarstvennyi komitet po grazhdanskomu stroitel'stvu i arkhitekture pri Gosstroe SSSR, 1974), 107–8; see also B.L. Krundyshev, 'Naselenie starshei vozrastnoi gruppy i zhilishche', in V.K. Stepanova (ed.), *Arkhitekturnaia sreda obitaniia invalidov i prestarelykh* (Moscow: Stroizdat, 1989), 288.
44 A.D. Vasserdam, 'Zaselenie kvartir i demografiia', in K.K. Kartashova (ed.), *Sem'ia i zhilaia iacheika* (Moscow: Gosudarstvennyi komitet po grazhdanskomu stroitel'stvu i arkhitekture pri Gosstroe SSSR, 1974), 43.
45 Smirnova and Barmashin, *Zhilye doma kvartirnogo tipa*, 5–8.
46 Smirnova, 'K voprosu o tipakh zhilishcha dlia liudei pozhilogo vozrasta', 50; Vilenchik et al., *Zhilishcha dlia prestarelykh*, 26.
47 Sigaev, 'Peshekhodnye puti', 600.
48 Ibid., 555–9.
49 Ibid., 555–601.
50 Ibid., 590–600.
51 Geriatric cabinets (*geriatricheskie kabinety*) were a type of drop-in consultation office that provided medical treatment to older people and undertook 'sanitary enlightenment' work. They were attached to polyclinics or hospitals.
52 Barmashina, *Printsipy rasseleniia*, 91–2.
53 Vilenchik et al., *Zhilishcha dlia prestarelykh*, 25.
54 Pavlovskaia, 'Sotsial'no-kul'turnyi aspekt formirovaniia'.
55 Interview with Elena Pavlovskaia, Setptember 2021.
56 Pavlovskaia, 'Sotsial'no-kul'turnyi aspekt formirovaniia', 55–7.
57 Ibid., 66.
58 Ibid., 73–4.
59 Ibid., 67–8.
60 Ibid., 67–8.
61 Ibid., 121.
62 Ibid., 180.
63 Ibid., 78–81.
64 Ibid., 105–6.
65 Ibid., 77.
66 Ibid., 88.

Part Three

Narratives of ageing, public and private

7

The modern babushka: Rethinking older women in late socialism

Danielle Leavitt-Quist

In 1979, the popular weekly newspaper *Nedelia* published a series of 'family portraits' – exposes in instalments about members of the classic Soviet family: mother, father, daughter, son and grandmother, or in Russian, *babushka*.[1] As an institution, the babushka often conjured pre-revolutionary, even biblical associations. She was wise and frail, pious and superstitious, tethered to the earth and its crops. The classic babushka waxed almost mythological in historical memory, often resembling Alexander Solzhenitsyn's iconic protagonist in *Matryona's Home*.[2] But, by *Nedelia*'s 1979 account, that kind of grandmother, 'quiet and tireless, like a mouse, scurrying around the house, pleasing everyone and demanding nothing in return', was almost entirely limited to historical memory and had been replaced by a new type. The 'modern babushka', sociologists and journalists called her, went on dates and socialized, exercised, wore fashionable clothing and makeup, and exhibited great emotional and professional strength. Most controversially, she did not attend to the daily care of her grandchildren. The modern babushka had 'destroyed firmly-held beliefs about who she was and her role in the home', *Nedelia* alleged, and everyone could feel it.

Modern babushkas represented a new generation of Soviet working women who, as they grew older and became grandmothers, forged new paths in their ideological approach to grandmother-hood. Their choice to opt out of customary grandchild care in favour of other activities unearthed generational tensions that spurred discussions on what was considered valuable, socially useful labour and who in society had obligations to perform that labour. The heart of the issue was rather pedestrian: who will take care of the kids? While pedestrian, this question fundamentally mattered in socialism's algorithm, as it determined who could and could not work outside the home. Although modern babushkas did not represent all older women, they gained significant attention from the state, sociologists and journalists, spurring conversations about older women's role in society and the family, older people's right to free time and leisure, and what really constituted socially useful work.

The discussions surrounding the modern babushka, which spanned most of the 1970s and 1980s, reveal Soviet perspectives on gender, old age and labour – and where those intersect. This chapter explores these discussions as they took place in Soviet periodicals, academic research, film and written correspondences, which was, we might assume, an extension of private, interpersonal conversations on the issue throughout the late socialist space. How old women were perceived and discussed in late socialism highlights not only how integral the labour of the babushka was in the functioning of Soviet society, but how old men and old women were often understood as very different social actors, with distinct and separate roles to play. Discourse on modern babushkas highlights how older women's relationship to labour, consumerism and leisure in late socialism influenced multiple spheres of Soviet society, spurring debate and conflict over what was and was not appropriate for older women.

Literature on generational conflict in the USSR often focuses on how the behaviours and tendencies of youth concerned and affected older generations.[3] This often gives the impression that the changing behaviours of older persons had little impact on Soviet youth.[4] Sources on modern babushkas, however, demonstrate that how older people behaved and thought also dramatically affected younger generations: in their case, older women's changing approach to domestic duties posed significant problems for young and middle-aged parents who relied on grandmotherly help to keep all their proverbial balls in the air. Additionally, discussion about modern babushkas helps to reframe late socialist stereotypes about consumerism and individualism, which often centre on youth culture. As this chapter shows, older women were not exclusively critical of consumerism and individualism. In fact, many looked forward to their old age as a time when they would be afforded the space, time and resources needed to live leisurely. How to balance the Soviet emphasis on work with 'deserved rest' was unclear to many, and the ageing and retiring population dredged up questions and concerns in terms of what the state's responsibilities were to support older and more infirm members of the population – and which responsibilities were society's and which the family's.

This chapter highlights how power and authority in the Soviet family had to be renegotiated as a generation of skilled working women grew old and as older generations lived longer in general. One journalist wrote in 1980: 'The number of old people in families grows more rapidly than the number of children. Each one of them has the chance to live to seventy. Every third to eighty. What will await us then?'⁵ His comment suggests how dramatically the increasing lifespans of older people affected the status quo of Soviet families, requiring consistent negotiations on how resources, labour, time and space in the home were used.⁶ Discussions about the modern babushka struck at the core of communist morality, bringing into question what really constituted socially useful work and whether the young and the old – given their respective positions in life – were entitled to certain care from the other.⁷

The modern babushka, gender and the Soviet family

Until mid-century, grandmothers in the Soviet Union were often considered symbols of pre-revolutionary life: most were unskilled, many illiterate, and they possessed vague memories of the 'old world'. By and large, these women cared for children, enabling the transformation of Soviet territory into a socialist space by freeing millions of young, able-bodied women from the duties of household work to build communism. Historically, the babushka was logistically vital to the functioning of the Soviet project at the most prosaic levels. By the 1970s and 1980s, a vocal portion of the women becoming grandmothers emerged with different ideas about their roles in the home and in society. Their upbringing in the 1920s and 1930s had instilled in them the importance of socially useful work outside of the home, and an old age spent caring for children often seemed unattractive. Frequently referred to as a 'modern babushka' (*sovremmenaia babushka*), some of these women even asked that they not be called babushka at all, as the term carried with it undesirable connotations.⁸

Although the social and cultural changes that Soviet society underwent in the 1950s and 1960s were significant – especially related to ideas about retirement, private life and leisure time – the realities of Soviet life and labour still relied on traditional grandmothering norms to provide care for children and households while younger mothers tended to their careers.⁹ The impact of modern babushkas, whether actual or simply anticipated, was significant. Although modern babushkas likely did not represent the majority of women in their age cohort, they nonetheless gained the attention of the state, sociologists and journalists throughout the 1970s and 1980s; these actors took increasing interest in modern babushkas and their 'mysterious personality' (*zagadochnaia lichnost'*), which prioritized self-fulfilment outside the home.

Self-fulfilment often took two forms: continuing to work past retirement age and involvement in leisure and activism. Two operative issues motivated modern babushkas' transition away from traditional norms. First, that they did not consider childcare (or household work generally) as socially useful as the skilled professional or industrial labour which many of them performed daily in their jobs. The second issue, often contrasting with the first, had to do with their right to a deserved rest in their old age. These modern babushkas assumed what sociologists called a 'second youth', meaning a period of life meant for leisure, socializing, exploration and entertainment.[10]

Survey data from a study conducted in 1984 can help make sense of how prevalent these broader ideas were. The study revealed that only 15 per cent of people working at retirement age (fifty-five years old for women and sixty years old for men) thought it better for a pensioner to raise grandchildren instead of remaining in the workforce.[11] Of those surveyed, 47 per cent felt strongly that a pensioner should not help with childcare, suggesting that pensioners believed they could offer more socially useful labour in their places of work, or that they deserved a rest in their old age.[12] Meanwhile, a large portion of these older people lived in three-generation households: of the 59 million households recorded in the 1970 All-Union Population Census, 11 million were families including three or more generations.[13] Typically, women became grandmothers between the ages of fifty to sixty, which was considered by many to be the prime of life, although on the cusp of Soviet pension age.

Although modern babushkas represented a new generation of older women with Sovietized ideas about the value of certain kinds of work, societal demand for childcare had not significantly changed since the 1920s. Children still needed care to enable adult women (and men) to fill the workforce, and state day cares and nurseries simply could not meet the demand on their own. For example, in 1974 *Krasnaia Zvezda* reported that pre-school day care centres could accommodate only about ten million children, or one third of the country's children in the under-seven age group – statistics that were likely optimistic. Big cities such as Moscow tended to be favoured, and people in the countryside and in medium-sized factory towns were often left to fend for themselves. They relied extensively on the help of a nearby or live-in babushka or on private, semi-legal day care and childcare co-ops.[14] Discussions about modern babushkas generally observed that modern grandmothers were ready to share with young parents the pleasure that children brought, but, in many cases, resolutely dissociated themselves from daily care for grandchidren.[15]

The volume of discourse suggests that this phenomenon seemed to many to potentially threaten the existing Soviet order and had the potential to be disruptive. Ideas surrounding grandmotherhood and the roles of older women in late Soviet society proved to be particularly charged subjects for families, which were deeply invested in maintaining the tradition of grandmothers' help at home. Natalya Baranskaya's novella *A Week Like Any Other*, for example, describes in exhausting detail the routine of a family navigating work/life balance without a babushka in late socialism.[16] Her story leaves little room for doubt that having a babushka's assistance at home significantly advantaged family life and alleviated some of the weight of the gruelling 'double burden' that Soviet women infamously bore: the burden of working full time and serving at the same time as the sole manager of a household.[17]

Early discussions about the modern babushka dating from the late 1970s and early 1980s can be characterized by their tones of frustration and indignance. Some suggested that babushkas choosing to forego childcare led to a decline in birth rates because Soviet women simply could not manage the double burdens of work and domestic responsibilities on their own and were therefore unwilling to have additional children.[18] In letter responses to the 1979 *Nedelia* article on the babushka in Soviet families, several readers argued that older women who chose to forgo childcare were selfish, unpatriotic and unwilling to dedicate themselves to the well-being of the family. One woman from Saratov, L. Doronina, wrote: 'Before, the grandmother considered it her DUTY to raise her grandchildren. Now if she does it, then only as a FAVOR.' She lamented that 'My children, at our mention of grandmothers, can hardly remember them although both grandmothers are in full health'.[19]

Although some families likely supported modern babushkas in their deserved rest, many families publicly bemoaned them. Doronina's letter to *Nedelia* suggested that grandmothers who consciously chose to be absent in their grandchildren's lives had no reason to lament not being taken care of themselves in their very old age.[20] This was a common sentiment: many argued that modern babushkas' behaviour would only hurt them in the long run, and that a 'second youth' would lead to loneliness as deeper old age set in. One journalist, Valery Kadzhaia, wrote that loneliness in old age is retribution for the kind of egoism that modern babushkas exhibited. 'For today's grandchildren their grandmothers and grandfathers are more often kind acquaintances as, for instance, are the friends of their parents. In the same way, those who break the threads that tie the three generations together doom themselves to loneliness in their old age. And it will come for sure.'[21]

Some considered continued household labour in old age an issue of fairness, since the decades after Stalin's death had seen a significant scientific and technological revolution. This meant, some argued, that younger generations' 'first half of life' was marked by a heavy workload burden, as individuals amassed new levels of education and qualifications to meet the demands of the technological revolution. Under these conditions, shifting a significant part of household chores onto the shoulders of the older generation was only fair, since it meant a kind of equalization of the overall load.[22] One additional justification was that by the 1970s and 1980s household labour had fundamentally changed, becoming easier and more attractive than it had been in the 1920s, 1930s or 1940s. New luxuries – such as hot water, gas stoves, indoor plumbing, sewage systems, garbage removal, as well as new technologies, such as refrigerators, vacuum cleaners, washing machines, etc. – all made household work less burdensome.[23]

This approach – to shift more household labour onto the shoulders of older persons in the name of equality – was laughable to many older people, especially the women who would bear the brunt of domestic work. One woman, L. Ermakova, wrote to *Nedelia* in response to their 1979 article on babushkas: 'Do not forget what the current grandmothers have gone through and suffered. We survived a terrible war and a difficult post-war period. We worked (during the war, day and night), and many fought. We lived in barracks, in communal apartments without amenities. We didn't have nice, good furniture (sometimes there weren't even baby carriages), didn't visit cafes and restaurants, didn't go to the sea, couldn't dress nicely, didn't wear fashionable things like sheepskin coats, boots, or jeans. Our clothes were altered from our parents' clothes. Some of us have learned to open taxi doors only in old age.'

Comparing the burdens of the 'first half of life' of older persons with youth in late socialism was bound to ignite fires, and older people rebuffed that there was nothing *fair* in terms of their generational experiences, highlighting the loss, sacrifice and poverty the older generation experienced in youth. As Ermakova continued in her letter to *Nedelia:* 'So, is it worth reproaching us that, at least a little, albeit belatedly, we want to make up for what we did not have in our young years? ... Let the grandmothers travel, if they are interested and healthy, let them dress beautifully and enjoy all the joys of life. Yes, the idea of what is allowed for grandmothers has to be changed. When the young themselves are grandmothers, they will agree with this.'[24] Ermakova's letter highlights that although consumerism and individualism were issues that older persons often identified and criticized in young people, they were not the exclusive preoccupation of younger generations in late socialism.[25] Many older people were interested in enjoying the finer things of life and had highly nuanced feelings about collectivism in general.

Discussions related to the idea of the modern babushka reveal a clear attempt to reframe the issue of socially useful work, eschewing notions that childcare and housework were inherently inferior labour. Articles proliferated characterizing the noble, gruelling, vital work of the babushka.[26] 'How wonderful when there is a babushka in the family – and how difficult without her!' one article began, before regaling readers with all of babushkas' immutable virtues – economy, strength and experience.[27] Articles suggested how useful it was for older women to quit their jobs to engage in household labour and childcare, putting their great experience to work raising the younger generation. Indicatively, these same publications often celebrated older men who continued formal work in some capacity, suggestive of conflicting societal interests: as the Soviet Union faced a shrinking labour force in its major cities, industries often petitioned for permissions to employ retirees while allowing them to receive pensions. Men were less likely to be conscripted into household work even if they weren't formally working, so their continued employment at a workplace seemed their comparative advantage. Household labour, in contrast, was in desperately short supply and considered – by the state and much of society – more appropriately within older women's wheelhouse.

The 1977 Soviet film, *For Family Reasons* (*Po semeinym obstoiatel'stvam*), follows a modern babushka, Galina, as she makes the decision – at a high cost to family harmony – not to be the primary caretaker of her new grandchild. Despite her daughter's desire for Galina to stay home with the child and provide care, Galina was a working woman who had sacrificed to become a tough boss at her workplace. Galina bemoans: 'After raising a daughter without a husband you think you'll get some help in old age, but just the opposite happens.'[28] The film follows Galina and her daughter in their acrobatic search for a suitable childcare alternative. At one point they employ another babushka who quits promptly upon gauging the heavy weight of the infant grandchild. Later they hire an older man with a higher technical education who was avoiding taking care of his own grandchild. He offered his own childcare service to help his adult daughter pay for her nanny. (It is worth noting, however, that he was available only three times a week because of a new hobby, artistic whistling, which claimed some of his new free time.) When Galina asks why he chose not to just care for his own grandson, he replies: 'It's not good for me', to which Galina responds: 'How can you be so cold to the child? Are you not ashamed? You should be'. The man responds: 'At least I quit my job when the baby was born', suggesting that Galina was making the more selfish choice by remaining at her workplace.

As Sarah Ashwin has written, men and women were meant to play distinctive roles in the building of communism – roles not limited to youth or middle age.[29] Even in old age and retirement, men and women continued to be urged and conscripted into those clear roles. Women's prescriptive role as 'worker mother' and manager of the household remained almost unchanged from youth to middle age to old age. Men's role as the manager and builder of communism either remained intact or shifted slightly in old age away from actively building communism to instead inspiring and advising younger workers based on their own extensive experience.[30] Modern babushkas disrupted this model by claiming that their responsibilities as working mothers had been fulfilled in youth and middle age – that they could now seek and achieve their own goals.

The state and labour in the household

Wrapped up in conversations about the modern babushka was the issue of labour – what was considered truly socially useful work and how maintaining a household fit within that. There was a clear attempt over the 1960s to 1980s to reframe household labour not just as useful and valuable, but as *optimal* at certain stages of life. One example of this reframing can found in the USSR's main ideological journal, *Kommunist,* which often provided clarification on issues of ideology and communist morality. In the late 1960s, the editors of *Kommunist* took it upon themselves to discuss the idea of 'adult dependents' (*izhdiventsy*). Often, dependents had been labelled with the unsavoury stereotype of feeding off other people's work, and modern babushkas strove to avoid this characterization. Modern babushkas' decision to remain at work instead of assisting in childcare was, many sociologists argued, the result of a desire to avoid becoming financially dependent, notwithstanding their modest pensions. The editors of *Kommunist* were aware of the struggle faced by modern babushkas and others who engaged household labour. One letter to the editors of *Kommunist* asked about the moral standing of dependents who engaged exclusively in household labour. In response, the editor fervently decried discriminatory attitudes towards such workers, writing that 'their work (yes *work* and not insignificant) is socially useful, socially imperative work. There's no getting around this reality. And the current reality is that society cannot entirely take upon itself the care and rearing of children and the everyday service of the population. And that which society cannot do is accomplished by these "dependents"'.[31]

Another late-1960s letter to *Kommunist* enquired whether, if given the choice, older people ought to remain at their places of employment or help with household and domestic duties, including getting involved with collective housing administration and maintenance. *Kommunist* responded that it was better for a pensioner to register their party membership with their local housing office and deregister from their former place of employment, which could often mean retirement from work. 'The fact is that party organizations and institutions are strong, powerful organizations', the editor wrote, 'They can continue their full-blooded activities even if several communist pensioners are removed from their register', a statement perhaps meant to console pensioners who were worried about how their workplaces would fare without them.[32] Meanwhile, the editor continued, thousands of Soviet citizens were living in housing complexes surrounded by 'remnants (*perezhitki*) of the past, [and] who need the experienced, guiding hand of an elderly communist'. The idea was that at their stage of life the most useful work older people offered society was in making a home environment (broadly speaking) conducive to communist ideals, not in continuing labour at a place of employment. Older people's role, fundamentally, was in rearing the masses. For older women, this typically meant working in Housing Maintenance Offices (*ZhEK*), where they could organize and assist their local communities (keeping order and protecting against 'hooligans', maintaining the cleanliness of courtyards, etc.), as well as taking care of individual households and children. For older men, this often involved speaking at schools, summer camps, institutes, universities and serving as consultants for younger workers at their places of work.

One late Soviet compromise between the state's needs for older women at home and older women's desire to remain independent was found in private plot gardening. Older women who wanted both to retire from work and to assist their children and grandchildren – but with clear boundaries – often split their time between the city and private garden plots and dachas. The garden plot was a place of relaxation and leisure, but also considered productive, as it yielded food and other goods. Importantly, it was usually only a short train ride away from children and grandchildren, so the grandmother could leave for an entire weekend or longer holiday.[33] 'For older people, the recognition of the importance and social usefulness of their activities on their personal subsidiary plots is of primary importance', a pair of sociologists wrote in the mid-1980s. 'The widespread dissemination of this sentiment will contribute to older people's enthusiasm for working on personal subsidiary plots, which can be considered one of the important tasks of today.'[34] The usefulness of private plots was not just limited to production: private plot gardening improved the aesthetic, moral *and* economic conditions of the USSR. Of course, care for grandchildren was never far away in discussions about older people's social contributions. In the same book that encouraged older people's private plot gardening, the authors made a further push for childcare: 'In addition, they [older people] help to introduce their grandchildren to work and solve the problem of summer vacations. In this we see older people's socially useful work.'[35]

How to provide the babushka the independence she desired while still maintaining her value for the family was a complex problem in late socialism, which private plot gardening could solve only in part. Entire teams of demographers, psychologists, sociologists and architects studied the problem: what should be done so that older persons and the young could live together and yet maintain the space they clearly desired? As early as the late 1960s, specialists proposed a new type of household dwelling: a configuration of living space and community that would allow grandparents, adult parents and their children to have their own spaces and still live together – in practice, separate flats conjoined as pairs.[36] The developers of the plans described the arrangement as consisting of two flats with one large common room, two kitchens and two bathrooms. 'With such planning', they said, 'close association and privacy could be combined'.[37]

Soviet leaders and demographers feared that the separation of the babushka from the rest of the family threatened the moral undergirding of Soviet society because Soviet society relied on three generation households to transmit moral strength from generation to generation.[38] Sociologists criticized some modern babushkas' practice of only providing financially or materially for grandchildren – i.e. buying toys and gifts, paying for special outings, etc. Although they suggested that it was sometimes healthy for all parties to live separately and maintain boundaries, they recommended that older people be closely involved in the moral and ethical rearing of the younger generation. Trying to slough off the responsibility for children's moral education by instead buying them gifts was condemned as behaviour inherently out-of-line with communist values.[39] One prominent sociologist, V.D. Shapiro, suggested that if grandparents (primarily grandmothers) dedicated themselves to rearing grandchildren they would experience a level of satisfaction that would compensate for their loss of their social status and important social roles.[40]

Although the proposed Soviet 'mother-in-law' apartments were never built, the fact that workers and thinkers from a variety of disciplines coalesced to work on solving this specific conflict speaks to its salience in the minds of many Soviet citizens. It also indicates that modern babushkas took their new lifestyles seriously, and that they – as a cohort – were often treated seriously in return. Debates about the modern babushka demonstrate that for Soviet society to function smoothly, older people and youth relied on each other's reciprocity in caretaking and household labour. Modern babushkas went head-to-head with the state and younger generations alike over the issue of childcare and care for a household, revealing that this question – who took care of whom – fundamentally mattered in communism's algorithm.

Soviet sociologies of grandmotherhood

In addition to families and the state, Soviet sociology was a further site of increasing interest in the modern babushka.[41] Sociologists took interest in how the changing role of the babushka complicated Soviet family and work life, writing about them in books on Soviet family life, the role of older people in Soviet society and pension policy. Although some sociologists perpetuated the stereotype that modern babushkas' selfishness – and the generational conflict it caused – contributed to a decline in birth rate and housing and childcare crises, many sociologists took a more nuanced approach to the older Soviet population. As research on old age showed increasing interest in the psycho-social worlds of older people, Soviet sociologists demonstrated a strong focus on making sense of older citizens' social, psychological and spiritual needs, often with the implicit intent to understand what motivated people like modern babushkas to disrupt the traditional model. Sociologists perceived the 'very way of life of the older population' to be fundamentally changing – becoming more and more dynamic.[42] They encouraged families to work to create hospitable environments for retired members of the family. 'The attitude of the family towards an older person who has become a pensioner', Shapiro urged, 'is an indicator of its cohesion and stability'.[43] Of the three main populations weighing in on modern babushkas' behaviour – families, the state and sociologists – the latter had the least to lose, and their responses were generally less emotive and more sympathetic to modern babushkas in many cases.

According to sociologists, an older woman's desire to keep boundaries between herself and children or grandchildren was driven by two primary factors. The first was maintaining financial independence. Leaving the workplace to help with childcare was often a financial strain on older skilled and professional workers. A pair of sociologists identified that an older person leaving the workplace to assist in domestic work constituted a fundamental shift in the power dynamics of a Soviet family. They described a process in which one ages from youth to middle age, developing increasing importance and power in the family as he or she becomes established in a career, earns more money and serves as the family's financial provider. 'However, as one approaches old age', they wrote, 'this process stops and even reverses. The role of the older person in the family becomes different due to the loss of economic independence. In the family, he no longer performs active functions and becomes a consumer of both various kinds of services and material resources, while earlier he could be one of the main persons providing the family materially. The increasing dependence of older persons on family members is not seen by them as favorable'.[44] One sociological survey of pension-aged people living in Moscow asked why they felt disincentivized from retiring. Many cited issues related to family (an increase in household labour, becoming financially dependent on relatives and a decrease in familial authority).[45] Of course, by retiring to engage in childcare, an older person in the late 1970s or 1980s would have received a pension, albeit often much smaller than their salary, and, as noted above, many pension-aged people were permitted to receive both a pension and a limited salary if they continued working.

The second main factor that sociologists cited was characterized by the term 'second youth' – a time focused on career advancement, leisure, travel, socializing and developing new skills and hobbies. In practice, for most grandmothers in late socialism their 'second youth' was more than just a repetition of youth, since their actual youth had been spent in the turbulent first half of the century when, as Seth Bernstein has written, they were forced to grow up very quickly.[46] For many older women, this was likely the first time in their adult lives when they were afforded some social and professional space from the grinding 'double burden' of work and household duties.[47]

The active and leisurely lifestyles of modern babushkas were attractive demonstrations of older people's standard of living in the USSR, and they received positive attention in internationally directed periodicals, such as *Soviet Woman*. For example, babushkas who did not remain at work often joined a variety of clubs – not just activism-focused, as Klots and Romashova have shown in this volume and elsewhere – but purely for leisure and entertainment.[48] Amongst the sample of retired older women featured in *Soviet Woman* in 1979, there were those who spent their free time at the Women's Club of Anglers at the Moscow Angler-Sportsman Society, at the Leningrad Club of Service Dogs or in writing a book on how to continue looking attractive in old age.[49] Articles such as this proliferated in *Soviet Woman*, which crafted a feminine ideal meant to advance Soviet interests at home and abroad, as Alexis Peri has shown.[50] In newspapers and forums aimed at a domestic audience, however, such as in *Nedelia*, the active and leisurely lifestyles of modern babushkas were often the subject of controversy and debate.[51] An active old age spent developing hobbies and interests was an ideal the USSR supported in theory, but, like many of the images proliferating on *Soviet Woman*'s pages, fell short of reality.

Sociologists and gerontologists, however, consistently argued that a 'second youth' was good for the physical and emotional health of older women. One study conducted by researchers at the Institute of Gerontology in Kiev in the mid-1980s collected survey data in the Ukrainian SSR and the Georgian SSR and found that older women who cared for young children in families with multiple children had on average worse health and hygiene norms than those who did not.[52] The health of the babushka became a popular concern as more grandmothers lived into older age (75+ years) in the 1970s and 1980s. Even grandmothers who chose to stay home with children were often encouraged to take time off, and one 1986 *Nedelia* article suggested that without deliberate breaks, too much involvement from the babushka was detrimental for the family all-around. 'The trouble is that the grandmother completely removes her daughter from parental concerns, with the best intentions, of course. But as a result, the babushka is overworked, tired, and the daughter is not able to realize herself as a mother and is therefore dissatisfied, although she does not understand what is the reason for her nervousness.'[53] The solution, according to the author, was for the babushka to leave the house recreationally 'twice a week or at least twice a month', in order to meet with people, relax, visit a museum or see a movie. This was absolutely necessary, the author insisted, 'precisely because the whole family relies on her.'[54] The *Nedelia* article suggests a softer popular approach to babushkas – and the older population more generally – in the mid-1980s, which highlighted that the family and individuals had an obligation to support older persons in addition to receiving support from them.[55]

The operative issue became clear as babushkas asserted their right to leisure time: free time, just like every other Soviet commodity, was not impervious to scarcity; as one generation took more, another generation inherently had less. There was a struggle for free time between different age groups, and the babushka was the figure most often relied upon to relinquish access to such free time.[56] Conversations often centred around obligations that one generation had to another. For example, as retired grandparents took on a significant load of their children's (the middle generation's) child-rearing responsibilities, the question of the younger generation's obligation to their grandparents arose. Should the grandchildren be obligated to give back to them in some capacity? The middle generation was already employed full time, but the younger generation – teenagers, especially – were considered prime candidates to help balance things out. Adolescents and teenagers were consistently reprimanded for exploiting the older generation, as suggested in the *Krokodil* cartoon below (Figure 7.1), which ran with the following admonition: 'Some young people forget that care for the elderly is not only their moral duty, but an obligation which is emphasized in our constitution.' The cartoon's authors depict the 'obnoxious' nature of a young woman immersed in materialism and leisure, while her grandmother attends to the physical care of their apartment. The cartoon emphasizes the young

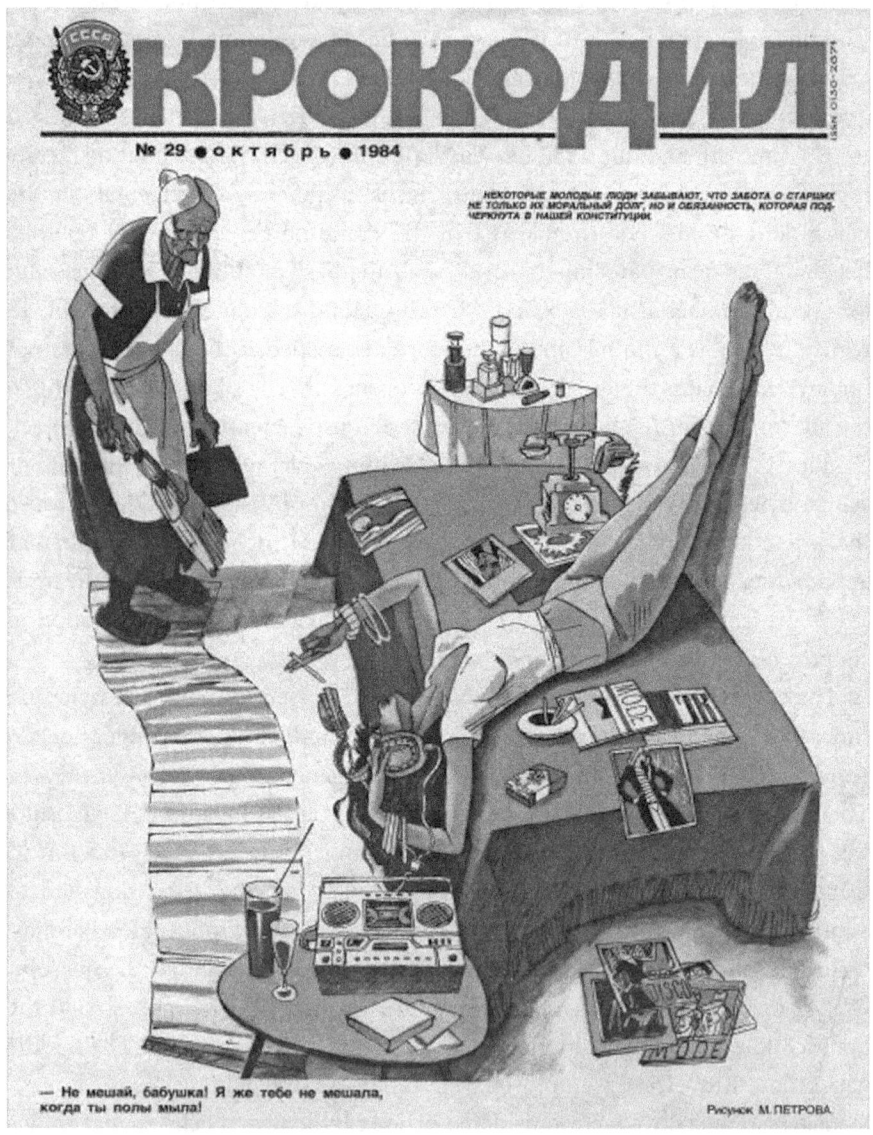

Figure 7.1 Cover of the satirical magazine *Krokodil*: 'Don't bother me, babushka!'

woman's lack of self-awareness about her relationship with her grandmother and implicitly calls for young peoples' reorientation away from vain and self-centred lifestyles towards conscious care for older people.

Conclusion

Who takes care of whom? Whose work matters more? Who has the right to leisure and when? The modern babushka debate, although seemingly mundane, unearthed questions at the core of communist ideology and morality, revealing late socialist tensions about age, gender and labour. The emergence of the modern babushka was representative of the late Soviet move towards individualism and consumerism and away from a single-minded focus on the collective. Debates and discussion about the modern babushka reveal how the behaviours and ideas about older persons impacted younger generations and show that the lifestyles of a relatively marginalized Soviet population – older women – had profound effects on how society functioned generally. It forced discussion on what constituted useful labour, and whether older persons deserved breaks from labour altogether. Debates surrounding modern babushkas demonstrated that men and women were often expected and urged to play specific roles in their old age – even once they retired, they were often conscripted into roles similar to those they had occupied in youth and middle age. While leisure and free time were often ideals that the Soviet state wanted to support in old age, the practical needs of family life were often too pressing to fully release older people, and older women in particular, from their family responsibilities. Despite the social provisions that the USSR promised women and families, the babushka was often Soviet families' most vital and reliable safety net. The lifestyles of older women, the debates reveal, proved to be fundamentally determinative in how Soviet families and workplaces functioned.

Notes

1   Tamara Afanas'eva, 'Babushka', *Nedelia*, no. 42 (1979): 18–19.
2   Alexander Solzhenitsyn, 'Matryona's Home', *Encounter* 20, no. 5 (1963): 28.
3   See, for example, Juliane Fürst, *Stalin's Last Generation: Soviet Post-War Youth and the Emergence of Mature Socialism* (Oxford: Oxford University Press, 2010); Juliane Fürst, *Flowers through Concrete: Explorations in Soviet Hippieland* (Oxford: Oxford

University Press, 2021); and S.L. Zhuk, *Rock and Roll in the Rocket City: The West, Identity, and Ideology in Soviet Dniepropetrovsk, 1960–1985* (Washington, DC: Johns Hopkins University Press, 2010).

4   For more on generational divergence in the USSR, see (particularly the last chapter): Stephen Lovell, *Generations in Twentieth-century Europe* (New York: Palgrave Macmillan, 2007).

5   Valery Kadzhaia, 'Elders Are Always Dear', *Soviet Woman*, no. 11 (1980): 6–7.

6   Between the 1930s and the 1960s, the average Soviet lifespan increased by about twenty years. For more on ageing demographics, see N.N. Sachuk, 'Sotsial'no-demograficheskaia kharakteristika starshykh vozrastnikh grupp naseleniia SSSR', in *Obraz zhizni i starenie cheloveka* (Kiev: Zdorov'ia, 1966), 8–19; A.N. Rubakin, 'Osnovnye problemy starosti v nastoiashchee vremia', in *Obraz zhizni i starenie cheloveka* (Kiev: Zdorov'ia, 1966), 45–50; also: Michael Ryan, 'Life Expectancy and Mortality Data from the Soviet Union', *British Medical Journal* 296 (1988): 1513.

7   Alissa Klots and Maria Romashova have shown that older women were often driven to activism in their pension years as a way of keeping busy and continuing to contribute after they formally left the workforce; see Alissa Klots and Maria Romashova, 'Lenin's Cohort: The First Mass Generation of Soviet Pensioners and Public Activism in the Khrushchev Era', *Kritika: Explorations in Russian and Eurasian History* 19, no. 3 (2018): 573–97. I add to this narrative by exploring the deliberate turn away from caretaking as the type of socially useful work older women chose to engage in. It's important to note, as Donald Raleigh has documented in his oral history work, that modern babushkas did not represent all older women, and that grandparents, particularly grandmothers, continued to play important roles in shaping younger generations' attitudes, particularly in the decades after Stalin. See, Donald J. Raleigh, *Soviet Baby Boomers: An Oral History of Russia's Cold War Generation* (New York: Oxford University Press, 2011). On communist morality, see Deborah A. Field, *Private Life and Communist Morality in Khrushchev's Russia* (New York: Peter Lang, 2007).

8   Afanas'eva, 'Babushka', 18–19.

9   For discussions about leisure time, see chapter six in, Stephen Lovell, *Summerfolk: A History of the Dacha, 1710–2000* (Ithaca: Cornell University Press, 2016). On Soviet pensions, see Lukas Mücke, *Die allgemeine Altersrentenversorgung in der UdSSR, 1956–1972* (Stuttgart: Franz Steiner Verlag, 2013).

10 Kadzhaia, 'Elders', 6–7.

11 Per the 1956 pension reforms, Soviet pension ages were fifty-five years for women, sixty years for men. For more detail, see Mücke, *Die allgemeine Altersrentenversorgung*.

12 M.Ia. Sonin and A.A. Dyskin, *Pozhiloi chelovek v sem'ie i obschestve* (Moskva: Finansy i statistika, 1984).

13 V.D. Shapiro, *Chelovek na pensii* (Moskva: Mysl, 1980), 127.

14 Hedrick Smith, 'In Soviet Union, Day Care Is the Norm', *The New York Times*, 17 December 1974.
15 Kadzhaia, 'Elders'.
16 Natalya Baranskaya, *A Week Like Any Other: Novellas and Short Stories* (Seattle, WA: Seal Press, 1989).
17 For more on the double burden, see Francine Du Plessix Gray, *Soviet Women: Walking the Tightrope* (New York: Doubleday, 1990); Sarah Ashwin, *Gender, State, and Society in Soviet and Post-Soviet Russia* (London and New York: Routledge, 2000).
18 L. Doronina, 'Chtoby vnuki tsenili vas', *Nedelia*, no. 46 (1979): 9.
19 Ibid.
20 Ibid.
21 Kadzhaia, 'Elders'.
22 Sonin and Dyskin, *Pozhiloi chelovek*, 149.
23 Ibid., 152.
24 L. Ermakova, 'Ne v ushcherb sebe', *Nedelia*, no. 46 (1979): 9.
25 For more on materialism and generational conflict, see Natalya Chernyshova, *Soviet Consumer Culture in the Brezhnev Era* (London: Routledge, 2013), ch. 4.
26 See, for example, A. Strel'tsova, 'V sem'ie, gde est' babushka', *Sovietskaia kul'tura*, 13 August 1982, 6.
27 Ibid.
28 Aleksei Korenev (dir.), *Po semeinym obstoiatel'stvam*, directed by (Moscow: Mosfil'm, 1977).
29 Ashwin, *Gender, State, and Society*.
30 Male pensioners and veterans were mobilized to share their experiences and inspire young audiences at workplaces, factories, summer camps and schools. See: Tsentral'nii derzhavnii arkhiv vishchikh organiv vladi ta upravlinnia ukraini (TsDAVO), f. P-2605, op. 8, dd. 3883, 4662.
31 Rossiskii gosudarstvennyi arkhiv sotsial'no-polititicheskoi istorii (RGASPI), f. 599, op. 1, d. 187, ll. 18–20.
32 Ibid.
33 Sonin and Dyskin, *Pozhiloi chelovek*, 161.
34 Ibid. In Soviet Ukraine, a television program also featured interviews with pensioners who worked on their own plots. These included a pensioner who raised 400 chickens, one who raised roses, and one who kept bees in an apiary while working on his personal memoirs. See: Tsentral'nyi derzhavnyi kinofotofonoarkhiv Ukrainy (TsDKFFA), *Radianskaia Ukraina*. Ukrkinokhronika Newsreel, August 1972. № 33. Arch. № 5071. 1599, III.
35 Sonin and Dyskin, *Pozhiloi chelovek*, 162.
36 For more on generational conflict related to housing, see Lynne Attwood, *Gender and Housing in Soviet Russia: Private Life in a Public Space* (Manchester: Manchester University Press, 2010), 187–8.

37 Ibid. For more on early discussions of older persons' living spaces, also see O. Ia. Smirnova, 'K voprosu o tipakh zhilischa dlia liudei pozhilogo vozrasta', in *Obraz zhizni i starenie cheloveka* (Izdatelstvo 'Zdorov'ia', Kyiv, 1966), 50–2.
38 Kadzhaia, 'Elders'.
39 Sonin and Dyskin, *Pozhiloi chelovek,* 143–62.
40 Shapiro, *Chelovek na pensii,* 113.
41 For more on how sociology developed as a social science in the post-Stalin USSR, see Vladimir Shlapentokh, *The Politics of Sociology in the Soviet Union* (Boulder: Westview Press, 1987).
42 Sonin and Dyskin, *Pozhiloi chelovek,* 161.
43 Shapiro, *Chelovek na pensii,* 117.
44 Sonin and Dyskin, *Pozhiloi chelovek,* 143–62.
45 V.D. Shapiro, *Sotsial'naia aktivnost' pozhilykh liudei v SSSR* (Moskva: Nauka, 1983), 59.
46 Seth Bernstein, *Raised under Stalin: Young Communists and the Defense of Socialism* (Ithaca: Cornell University Press, 2017).
47 Gray, *Soviet Women.*
48 'How Do You Live, Grandmother?' *Soviet Woman,* 1979, no. 11, 22–3.
49 In fact, fashion and beauty increasingly became a subject of interest to many older women, who by the 1960s and later began wearing makeup, fashionable clothing and fixing modern hairstyles. For more, see V. Vasil'ev, '... i vsegda neotrazima', *Nedelia,* no. 42 (1985): 15.
50 Alexis Peri, 'New Soviet Woman: The Post-World War II Feminine Ideal at Home and Abroad', *The Russian Review* 77, no. 4 (2018): 621–44.
51 For more on pensioners' social activism, see Shapiro, *Sotsial'naia aktivnost'.*
52 N.N. Lakiza-Sachuk and N.N. Sachuk, 'Pozhilye zhenshchiny v mnogopokoleniiakh sem'iakh', in *Mekhanizmi stareniia i dolgoletiia – materialy konferentsiia. Sukhumi, September 29–30, 1986* (Institute of Gerontology: Kiev, 1986).
53 Anna Spivakovskaia, 'Pozdravtye, Ia—babushka!' *Nedelia,* no. 17 (1986): 17.
54 Ibid.
55 On this, see 'Teper' my ne odinoki', *Nedelia,* 1988; Aleksander Savvin, 'Pomoshch' nashim starikam', *Nedelia,* no. 31 (1989): 9; N. Bazhanov, D. Venediktov, V. Menshikov, and V. Pokrovsky, 'Kto pomozhet starym liudiam?' *Nedelia,* no. 19 (1990): 15.
56 Sonin and Dyskin, *Pozhiloi chelovek,* 143–62.

8

The right to a permanent collection: Archiving the lives of Soviet pensioners

Alissa Klots and Maria Romashova

'You and I think of ourselves as too ordinary to have a permanent collection in an archive', wrote the sixty-eight-year-old retiree and member of the Perm city women's soviet Valentina Grigor'evna Sokolova in her diary in 1975, recollecting a conversation with another older activist.[1] Indeed, Sokolova could not claim a model biography, high posts or outstanding achievements – and until recently could not have hoped to have her personal documents preserved in the local archive. Yet now Sokolova was preparing her diaries, letters, memoirs, autobiographies, photographs, lectures and autographed books to be deposited at the State Archive of the Perm Oblast. Moreover, she was recruiting other older activists to follow suit and also donate their personal papers to the archive.

This chapter uses Sokolova's quest to create an archival collection for older activists like herself in order to preserve her own memory and that of her generation as an entry point into the study of memory and old age in the late Soviet period. Historians have noted that during the later decades of its existence, Soviet society experienced an increased interest in its past.[2] Scholarship on this 'historical turn' in Soviet culture has focused on two interconnected developments. The first one included the state's campaigns to bolster the regime's legitimacy through memory politics. The Soviet state encouraged the publications of memoirs by participants in revolutionary events, as well as fictionalized biographies of historical figures; they also supported local initiatives to bring back forgotten revolutionary names and invested into commemorative projects that celebrated the Great Patriotic War as a victory for the entire Soviet system.[3] The second key component of the 'historical turn' was an explosion of grassroots initiatives

---

Some material from this chapter has previously appeared in Alissa Klots and Maria Romashova, '"Tak vy zhivaia istoria?": sovetskii chekovek na fone tikhoi arkhivnoi revolutsii pozdnego sotsializma', *Antropologicheskii Forum/Forum for Anthropology and Culture* 50 (2021): 131–61.

dedicated to studying and preserving local history, including pre-revolutionary heritage.[4] What has remained unrecognized, however, is the role that older Soviet citizens themselves played in late Soviet commemorative practices of the times through which they had lived.

Post-Stalinist Soviet discourse marked the 'older generation' as carriers of revolutionary memory and emphasized their duty to pass their legacy down to the 'youth'.[5] Increased life expectancy and well-being among older Soviet citizens thanks to improvements in living standards, developments in healthcare and the introduction of universal old-age pensions allowed a small but vocal group of Soviet retirees to heed this call and actively engage in memory politics. Older members of the Soviet intelligentsia, who had dedicated their lives to building the first socialist state, saw participation in local history initiatives as a way to commemorate themselves and the contributions of their generation – the generation of builders of socialism. These older activists sought to make sense of their lives as historical actors by writing themselves into 'big history'.[6] While framing themselves as 'ordinary' Soviet citizens, they emphasized the extraordinariness of their generation and the world-historic task that had befallen them.

A close look at senior citizens' commemorative practices reveals the central role that archives played in late Soviet memory culture, a phenomenon we have dubbed the 'quiet archival revolution'.[7] The post-Stalin decades saw an attempt to rethink how state archives should select materials for preservation, as well as what kinds of individuals deserved to have their documents deposited. Throughout the 1950s–70s, professional archivists, historians and literary scholars, as well as lay members of the intelligentsia, debated how to best document the lives of 'ordinary' builders of socialism. As a result, 'ordinary' citizens like Valentina Sokolova were not only inspired to organize their papers into 'personal archives' in their homes but were able to donate these collections to local archives, museums and libraries. For these active older Soviet citizens, archiving their legacy became their last contribution to the communist project.

The campaign against the 'cult of personality' that followed the death of Joseph Stalin also reignited discussions about the role of individuals in history. On the one hand, denunciations of Stalinism sparked new interest in the revolutionary heroes that had been excluded from the official pantheon.[8] Moreover, the period saw a growing interest in personality (*lichnost'*) as a psychological phenomenon and the complexities of an historical figure's inner world.[9] On the other hand, historians had become weary of 'great personalities' and were eager to explore the creative role of the 'masses'.[10] In order to create such new narratives, the professional communities of historians and archivists had to address the issue of primary sources.

The first to respond to the challenge were local history museums (*kraievedcheskie muzei*). From the mid-1950s on, they started building coalitions with members of the local public to replenish museum collections with personal artefacts and testimonies. Returning to early Soviet commemorative practices, which had relied on the voices of participants in historical events, was a way public-facing historians sought to destalinize their discipline. New opportunities also opened up for state archives, which were transferred in 1960 from the Ministry of Internal Affairs, the infamous organization responsible for mass arrests, incarceration and executions under Stalin, to the direct control of Council of Ministers. No longer part of the state security system, archivists could claim professional autonomy and re-evaluate archiving practices. Following the example set by local museums, some archives began collecting diaries, letters, photographs and memoirs that spanned the pre-revolutionary times to the most recent Soviet achievements, such as the Virgin Land campaign in Northern Kazakhstan.

Museums and archives sought to engage broad sections of the public, from the Komsomol to labour unions, but their efforts particularly attracted volunteers from among older cohorts of Soviet citizens. Across the country, party veterans and participants in the revolution and the Civil War came together under the auspices of local museums. Their tasks included recovering the names of forgotten revolutionaries, reviewing memoirs and evaluating exhibit items, meeting with the local youth and creating 'people's' museums.[11] Sessions of collective reminiscing produced 'new material' meant to paint a 'truthful' picture of historical events.[12] In Orsha, Belarus, the city archive received multiple submissions from retirees – 'old communists' and 'first Komsomol members'. Pensioners were happy to share their memories of meetings with Lenin or even the storming of the Winter Palace.[13] In Tselinograd, Kazakhstan, a city pensioners' soviet delegated a group of 'archival inspectors' – retirees who assisted professional archivists in auditing archives at institutions. The pensioners' soviet also sent its representative to the city archival commission.[14]

The mobilization of older citizens was a unique feature of late Soviet memory politics. During the first post-revolutionary decade personal testimonies from 'ordinary people' became an important component of commemorative campaigns aimed at preserving evidence of early Soviet achievements.[15] Numerous commissions charged with the writing of party, union and Komsomol histories, as well as societies of former political prisoners and 'Old Bolsheviks', regularly held so-called evenings of reminiscence and collected retrospective accounts that helped bring to life pre-1917 revolutionary history.[16] However, early Soviet commemorative campaigns focused on very recent historical events and did not rely on a specific age cohort. In fact, even members of the All-Union Society of Old Bolsheviks, which brought together individuals who had joined the party before the revolution, were on average between forty-five to fifty-five years old at the time of these earlier recollections.[17]

The situation looked very different forty years after the revolution. Most participants of the revolutionary events were now of advanced age. Moreover, the visibility of older citizens in Soviet society had greatly increased since the early revolutionary years due to the rapid decline of the birth rate and modest increases in life expectancy.[18] In particular, women's life expectancy had risen, outpacing men's, and making older women a particularly visible social category, much in contrast to earlier periods.[19] As the individuals in this article show, it was often *women* who were most active and activist in their older years, further complicating the field of state-individual negotiation in memory politics. Finally, the reform of 1956 that introduced universal old-age pensions for urban residents created a distinct social category of pensioners: men and women who had left gainful employment not because of disability but because of reaching a certain age, sixty for men and fifty-five for women.[20] The pension reform was officially hailed as another great achievement of the socialist regime: its older citizens could now enjoy their 'well-deserved rest'. At the same time, the new law created a mass category of relatively healthy citizens that no longer worked in a society where labour was central to an individual's life. Shortly after the introduction of universal pensions for urban residents, the state began promoting volunteerism among its retirees, framing it as a way for pensioners to continue contributing to society. While many older Soviet citizens were happy to shed their societal obligations and enjoy quiet time with their families, a small but vocal group of pensioners sought to remain active.[21] For them, participation in commemorative initiatives was a way to continue contributing to the project of building communism.

A collection of letters published in 1976–7 by the major cultural newspaper *Literary Gazette* (*Literaturnaia gazeta*) in response to a series of publications on archiving personal documents offers a window into older citizens' conflicting understanding of their role in the late Soviet commemorative project. The newspaper publications had been staged as a debate between two groups of archivists. Those in the first group argued that state depositories had to be very selective in terms of which documents to preserve and therefore should not accept personal papers submitted by the public. Representatives of the other fraction, however, supported the democratization of the archives in order to preserve the voices of the 'ordinary people'. Publications from the latter group noticeably outnumbered those by their opponents.²² As a result, the discussion was read as an appeal to the public, as well as the professional community, to join their efforts to preserve the personal documents of 'ordinary people' in state archives. These publications encouraged older readers to speak up in support of broadening the scope of archival collections and to argue that their documents were indeed worth preserving. While their letters revealed the multiple tensions in the older cohort's understanding of their value as carriers of memory, there was shared commitment to preserving historical evidence for the collective benefit of Soviet society.

'I am seventy-two years old', wrote the retired economist Elena Vladimirovna Shumeiko. 'My peers are also at the end of their life journey. [...] We, the disappearing witnesses of the past, had a chance to see life in its development, participate in it and evaluate it from the position of historicism, that is often lacking in judgements made by youth.' To make sure that the state's 'grandchildren' would not destroy the older generation's legacy, Shumeiko asked the newspaper to create an 'Archive for Private Persons'. She was hoping that this sort of archive could prevent the disappearance of documents as she had witnessed when 'a big archive of an old person with an interesting life' was burnt in 'a bout of hopelessness' or when her own ninety-one-year-old mother destroyed her notes on her encounters with composer Mily Balakirev and translator and literary figure Fyodor Fidler. Shumeiko herself had memoirs about the early decades of Soviet power. These memoirs, however, were 'strictly autobiographical' and Shumeiko was unsure if they had any historical value.²³

Shumeiko's letter demonstrated contradictory ideas about the value of older people's testimonies and the responsibility for preserving them. The letter began by setting up a dichotomy between the 'old' and the 'young'. The older generation had not only participated in the creation of the first socialist state, but also had a much better understanding of Marx's historicism than did the youth. Therefore, the younger generations could not be trusted with making sound decisions when it came to preserving historical documents. Yet, the two examples Shumeiko provided about the destruction of valuable historical evidence showed that it was in fact representatives of the *older* generation who selfishly burnt their papers on their death beds. Thus, older people were at once the carriers of historical memory – and its potential destroyers. They were both to be celebrated and disciplined. The value of older citizens' documents was also ambiguous. Were their papers only worth saving if they contained information about famous cultural figures or historical events – or did the personal lives of unremarkable 'private persons' also deserve to be preserved?

Readers' responses to the newspaper debate, published by *Literary Gazette*, showed that older members of the Soviet intelligentsia who were evaluating their personal legacy had competing ideas about what made it worthy of preservation. Some older citizens saw themselves only as tools for preserving the memory of others, especially those who had heroically fought for their country in wars and revolutions. A former teacher from Kurgan, for example, had spent her retirement collecting war-time letters from her region.[24] A 'veteran of two wars' from Voronezh had been trying to find an institutional home for his notebooks that 'reflected daily life in the trenches and accounts of military activities of many people on the way from Volga to Berlin'. Others felt the need to preserve the memory of their ancestors for their children and grandchildren, like the retired lieutenant colonel who wrote a family history that spanned a hundred years. Whether or not the younger generation would appreciate those efforts, though, remained a source of anxiety. A sixty-six-year-old reader worried about her seven notebooks of memoirs and five notebooks of a family chronicle compiled by her deceased mother. Her thirty-year-old son and daughter-in-law appeared to have no interest in the documents, and, she believed, would probably destroy them once their mother passed away. Creating an archive for personal use by family members, moreover, was not just a private affair but also a tool for raising the younger generation's historical awareness through an intimate connection with the country's foundational events. As the head of the newspaper's literary department and the editor of the series on personal documents, A. Latynina, argued, it was the duty of Soviet society to combat young people's 'indifference to the lives of their fathers and grandfathers' and urged the readers to foster their children's 'historical consciousness'.[25] By emphasizing the need to preserve the memory of 'fathers and grandfathers', Latynina's comments revealed the tension between the official revolutionary narratives, which privileged men, and the personal narratives and file of the increasingly female cohort of older Soviet citizens involved in late-Soviet archiving.

While some readers saw themselves only as carriers of the memory of others, either heroic contemporaries or familial predecessors, others believed themselves to be worthy of commemoration. A seventy-seven-year-old researcher from Kiev believed that her diaries had to be preserved because she was one of those, who 'never ignores what she sees, hears, and feels'. While seeing and hearing emphasized an ability to capture events and people around her, the reference to feeling implied that the woman's inner world was also of historical significance. The value of these people's lives, moreover, was defined by their belonging to the unique generation of the builders of socialism. 'We participated to their best of our abilities in the October revolution, in the struggle to bring our party's decisions to life, in the building of socialism, [and] in the creation of the scientific and technological base of communism', wrote a party veteran from Leningrad. This feeling of generational distinction, fostered by official state rhetoric, made some older Soviet citizens re-evaluate their personal contribution to history and take steps towards preserving their own legacy.

Letters from readers published in the *Literary Gazette* present only static snapshots of older citizens' understanding of their historical role. They were selected, excerpted and edited by the newspaper staff who used the letters to make a point about the value of personal documents. Yet similar belief in the societal value of historical evidence, together with feelings of ambiguity about the place of an older individual's legacy in the state commemorative project, is also evident in the unpublished personal documents of the retired propagandist Valentina Sokolova. Moreover, her diaries and correspondence paint a dynamic picture of an older woman's developing interest in history – and her gradual realization of her personal role in history through conversations with professional historians and archivists, as well as family members and fellow pensioners. Sokolova's story demonstrates the complex interaction between the official rhetoric that encouraged historical enquiry and glorified the 'older generation' as carriers of revolutionary traditions, professional archivists who validated 'ordinary' retirees as historical actors, and pensioner's own individual biographies and senses of self.

Valentina Grigori'evna Sokolova was born in 1907 in the town of Orenburg into a family of underground revolutionaries. After her parents' divorce, she moved to Perm with her mother and brother and in 1930 graduated from Perm State University with a degree in education. As a newly minted teacher, Sokolova took part in the contemporaneous Bolshevik campaign against illiteracy, the late 1920s and early 1930s collectivization drive, and continuous promotion of atheist propaganda. She eventually became a professional propagandist: a lecturer on scientific atheism. After the lecture bureau that had employed her was reorganized in 1956, Sokolova took a library job in Sverdlovsk (Ekaterinburg) and then in Perm, where she worked until her retirement in 1962. Having failed to join the party four times, Sokolova reinvented herself as a 'non-party Bolshevik', actively participating in various state campaigns.[26] Her work and activism left little time for her daughter Galina, who was born in a short-lived marriage and was mostly raised by her grandmother. Galina eventually moved to Kuibyshev (Samara), leaving her mother free to pursue her professional interests without having to take care of grandchildren, a burden held by many older women in the Soviet Union.[27]

In the late 1950s, against the background of the fortieth anniversary of the October Revolution, Sokolova developed an interest in local revolutionary history and started collecting materials about Lenin's relatives in the Urals, thereby joining the ranks of amateur local historians. She also reconnected with her estranged father, the Old Bolshevik Grigorii Sokolov, who had met Lenin in Paris. Now a pensioner, he gave lectures to the youth and wrote articles about party history for children's magazines *Murzilka* and *Pioner*.[28] Sokolova eventually offered her father help with the memoirs that he intended to write for young audiences. In regular correspondence, father and daughter discussed Grigorii Sokolov's texts, exchanged opinions about new publications on party history and shared family documents and published articles. It was through this communication with her father that Sokolova began to reflect on the place of her family in history: 'Hello, papa! I am reading the history of the Communist Party in Kuibyshev and for the first time learning about your biography. You write that it mentions you five times. I only found four [references]: on pages 38, 43 and 136 and in the autobiography'.[29] The inclusion of her father's name in the party account meant that her family was now part of the state's official history, thus creating a direct connection between Sokolova and the foundational events of the Soviet state.

Grigorii Sokolov did not live to see his memoir published: he died in 1966, two years before 'An Old Communist's Story' was released by the main Soviet publishing house for children, Children's Literature (*Detskaia literatura*).[30] For Valentina Sokolova, her father's death was a final tragedy in a series of personal losses: in 1959 she had lost her maternal aunt, in 1964 her uncle died, and in 1966, just a few months before her father passed away, so did her mother. The deaths of her closest family members made Sokolova engage with the question of historical memory on a very personal level. Not only did she have to come to term with her loss, but she also faced decisions about her family's legacy. While her father's memory was secure, with his memoirs published and a street in Kuibyshev named after him, the fate of her mother's legacy remained unclear. Moreover, Valentina Sokolova was now the owner of her family's house, which was filled with old documents and family heirlooms. Unable to simply throw away things that until recently had belonged to her closest family, Sokolova started offering parts of her inheritance to local museums, libraries and schools as historical artefacts. However, her donations at this stage were limited to pre-revolutionary items. While aware of the historical value of personal items, Sokolova still only recognized this in dealing with material objects from the 'previous era'. Whether collecting information about Lenin's relatives in the Urals, helping her father write his story of underground revolutionary activity or donating her family's heirlooms to museums, Sokolova still saw 'history' as something that preceded her own time.

This vision of history as external to Sokolova's own life, however, was about to change. After her retirement in 1962, Valentina Sokolova had become an active member of the newly organized Perm City Women's Soviet, one of the many volunteer organizations of the Thaw era that actively recruited pensioners.[31] To her dismay, in the late 1960s, members of the Women's Soviet began to hear rumours about the impeding disbandment of the organization.[32] The feeling that the 'end of an era' was upon them only intensified with the serious illness of the Soviet's long-time chairwoman, the pensioner Tatiana Ivanova. Realizing that a decade of their hard work on behalf of the women of Perm would soon fall into oblivion, a group of activists decided to create an archive for the organization. As the soviet's secretary, Sokolova was responsible for preparing the documents. In 1969 she compiled several albums with materials on past and present activists in the city Soviet and organized the documents of several district Women's Soviets. She then spent the following eighteen months working with Tatiana Ivanova's sister to create a personal collection for Ivanova's personal documents at the State Archive of Perm Oblast. Luckily for the activists, the archive had just moved to a new building and its staff, staunch believers in the power of personal documents to democratize history, had begun accepting donations. While conceived as an initiative to preserve the memory of an organization, the Women's Soviet's archival project was to a great degree structured around individual women: first and foremost, its late chairwoman Tatiana Ivanova, but also 'ordinary' activists who were profiled in the albums. Tatiana Ivanova clearly deserved a permanent collection in the archive, as she qualified as an 'outstanding' individual: she had been the leader of a city-wide mass organization.[33] Yet, the initiative also raised questions about the historical significance of the lives of 'ordinary' members, including women like Valentina Sokolova.

It is in this context that Sokolova received a letter from a local archivist that changed her understanding about her own personal documents' importance. In the mid-1950s the State Archive of Perm Oblast received a collection of letters from the Perm region's early Soviet Komsomol leaders. Sent from the Main Political Education Committee (*Glavpolitprosvet*), these documents were meant to serve as primary sources for a series of publications about the village Komsomol and the campaign against illiteracy of the 1920s. The main protagonist of this local revolutionary story was the Komsomol activist Vasilii Rakitin, who had died of pneumonia in 1927.³⁴ His papers contained letters from a certain Valya Sokolova, who worked in the village reading room after Rakitin had left for mandatory military service. The correspondence offered unique evidence of young people's emotional engagement in the anti-illiteracy campaign. The young woman's identity remained a mystery, until one of the archivists recognized the older amateur local historian Valentina Grigorievna Sokolova as Valya from Rakitin's letters. The archivists immediately reached out to the newly discovered witness of the revolutionary changes in the countryside.

In 1971 Valentina Sokolova wrote to her daughter Galina:

> I recently found out that my name has been circulating in newspaper and journal articles and mentioned in TV programmes on the history of the Komsomol in the Perm region and will soon appear in such a serious publication as an edited volume published by Perm State University. I would love to put on airs, but unfortunately have no ground [to do it]. I was neither an organizer, nor a leader in the Komsomol. [I was a] rank-and-file Komsomol member of the Lenin levy.³⁵ I joined in 1924. My name is mentioned next to the name of the Komsomol-chekist Vasia Rakitin. [...] This is how I made history. This discovery got me so agitated that I couldn't work in the GAPO [archive]. [...] I walked all the way to Sverdlov Park and could not collect myself for a long time.³⁶

In the letter, Sokolova emphasized her status as a 'rank-and-file' participant in historical events, as opposed to 'leaders' and 'organizers', whose place in history was clear. However, despite her 'ordinary' status, Sokolova ultimately decided to offer the archivist the personal documents that captured her own life. As a response to the archivists' request, she wrote:

> I am sending you a copy of my notes about Vasya Rakitin from my diary. I haven't had time to copy the pages about [poet Vladimir] Maiakovskii and [People's Commissar of Enlightenment Anatoly] Lunacharskii's visits to Perm. I am unwell, my hands are shaky after the bout. You found me as Vasya's addressee. Maybe you will be interested in how I lived my life.³⁷

In this text, Sokolova acknowledged for the first time her value not only as a witness to the lives of 'great' others, such as Maiakovskii, Lunacharskii or Rakitin, but also as a historical actor in her own right. This transition is key to understanding Sokolova's and many of her peers' involvement in the late Soviet commemorative campaign. Sokolova's case demonstrates how an 'ordinary' Soviet pensioner came to recognize herself as a historical subject: one whose documents were worthy of a permanent collection in a state archive.

Sokolova's initiative to create a collection of her own personal documents, which would capture the life of an 'ordinary' Soviet person, received immediate support from the local archivists. As she wrote in her diary: the 'employees of the archive made clear that they value people. And [archivist Leon] Kashikhin even called me "our gem" for my detailed accounts of the past'.[38] This support encouraged Sokolova to organize her papers and develop a plan for the gradual deposit of her documents in the archive.

Working through her documents, Sokolova began constructing a new biography for herself: that of a member of the 'older generation'. The importance of *generation* as a framework through which Sokolova started to see her past came through especially in her correspondence with her daughter Galina. Although mother and daughter had a complicated relationship, Galina was interested in her mother's life story, and Sokolova used the correspondence to essentially write her autobiography in letters. When Galina criticized Valentina for being too reliant on class analysis, the older Sokolova responded with an appeal to the values of her generation:

> I need to comment on your remark about the class nature of my memoirs[;] it was not the official line, it was life itself. Our youth coincided with the greatest revolution: the exploited overthrew the exploiters. That had never happened in a class society before. And the class approach permeated everything. [...] Observe other party and Komsomol veterans. The habit of evaluating everything from the position of class is 'in their blood,' from their youth to their old age.[39]

Sokolova juxtaposed her and her daughter's generations, emphasizing the former's unique role in history, which had enabled them to truly understand the class approach. Sokolova's positioning herself as a member of the 'older generation' also justified her efforts to preserve her legacy. While she had not been a 'leader' of the Komsomol or not even a party member, the fact that she belonged to the *generation* of the builders of socialism made her life story and her interpretation of it historically significant. Therefore, even though she was happy that her daughter was interested in her past, Sokolova chose not to send her any original personal or family documents. Those were valuable historical sources, and it was her duty to have them securely stored in an archive so that future generations could learn about the exceptional achievements of her generation.[40]

While working on her own collection, Sokolova also began actively recruiting her fellow retirees – volunteers at the Women's Soviet – to donate their materials to the archive and eagerly helped her friends create their own personal collections. For Sokolova, these women's documents had historical value because they were history themselves. Although in line with the Soviet State's broader push to institutionalize the history of the builders of socialism, Sokolova's initiative shows how she and women like her were able to reframe the state's heroic and often male-dominated public narrative to include a variety of female voices that represented life not just fought and won but lived as well. As she noted in her diary when one of her colleagues finally donated her personal papers to the local party archive, 'Our descendants will study how we lived and worked, what made us happy and what made us sad, and read and reread her diaries.'[41] While preserving the memory of her generations' contributions to the building of the Soviet state, Sokolova equally did not shy away from documenting their suffering during Stalin's terror. She assisted the former Gulag prisoner Mikhail Al'perovich, a party veteran and an active member of the Revolution and Civil War Veteran's Soviet of Perm Region under the auspices of Perm Local History Museum, in creating a catalogue of 'individuals wrongfully accused under Stalin'.[42] For Sokolova, this catalogue was another way of preserving the memory of her generation.

Gradually, working on her personal archival collection took up all of Sokolova's time. By the early 1980s, preparing her papers for deposition into the archive remained the only thing on the to-do lists the ageing Sokolova wrote at the beginning of each year.[43] Her diary, which she had kept since she was a teenager, was now filled with retrospective accounts of her own life and those of her friends and peers. These diaries, Sokolova knew, would also be part of her personal file: they too would serve to preserve her and her generation's legacy. A few years before Valentina Sokolova's death in 1990, her daughter Galina received an urgent request to visit the retirement home where her mother had been residing since she had gone blind. Afraid that her mother's health had turned for the worst, Galina got on the first train to Perm. It turned out that there had been no changes in Valentina Sokolova's health, but she needed her daughter's help: the last part of her personal collection was finally ready for deposit into the archive.[44]

In the article that concluded the discussion about the documents of 'ordinary people' in the *Literary Gazette*, the head of its literary department, A. Latynina, remarked that she hoped the publications about archiving personal documents had been interesting for all of the readers and not just 'specialists, historians and older people, who had amassed lots of papers during their lives'.[45] Latynina's words were a recognition of the fact that professional historians and retirees were indeed the two groups most invested in preserving the personal documents of 'ordinary' Soviet citizens. The selection of readers' letters published by the newspaper supported this observation. At the same time, these two groups were not enough for Latynina, as they appeared to be natural carriers of memory. It was their responsibility to awaken the historical awareness of the 'younger generation'. Yet, as this chapter has demonstrated, it was in fact older members of the Soviet intelligentsia that experienced a historical awakening in the 1960s–70s. Pensioners who responded to the newspaper discussion included a former economist, a retired lieutenant colonel and a party veteran. Up to that point, they had not been engaged in the state's commemorative projects and were only beginning to recognize their own role in history. The case of Valentina Sokolova shows that this was a gradual process that unfolded in conversation with professional archivists, other retirees and family members – and ultimately allowed a wide variety of individuals, from 'ordinary' older women to professional activists (or those who were one and the same) to reframe the state's push to commemorate public narratives of socialism into personal histories of life as socialism was built. Thus, the late Soviet historical turn did not only encourage Soviet citizens to look more closely into their country's past to make sense of themselves in the present. For older members of Soviet intelligentsia, the historical turn meant reimagining themselves as members of a distinct generation that laid the foundations of the first socialist state. It was now their duty to preserve their legacy.

Notes

1 *Gosudarstvennyi arkhiv Permskogo Kraia* (GAPK) f. R-1610, op. 1, d. 196, l. 3. *Dnevniki*.
2 Denis Kozlov, 'The Historical Turn in Late Soviet Culture: Retrospectivism, Factography, Doubt, 1953–91', *Kritika: Explorations in Russian and Eurasian History* 2, no. 3 (2001): 577–600.
3 On autobiographies, see Marianne Liljeström, 'Monitored Selves: Soviet Women's Autobiographical Texts in the Khrushchev Era', in Melanie Ilic and Jeremy Smith (eds.), *Soviet State and Society under Nikita Khrushchev* (Basingstoke: Palgrave Macmillan, 2004): 131–48; on biographies, see Polly Jones, *Revolution Rekindled: The Writers and Readers of Late Soviet Biography* (Oxford: Oxford University Press, 2019); on local history, see Victoria Donovan, *Chronicles in Stone: Preservation,*

Patriotism, and Identity in Northwest Russia (DeKalb: Northern Illinois University Press, 2019); on World War II memory, see Lisa A. Kirshenbaum, *The Legacy of the Siege of Leningrad, 1941–1945: Myth, Memories, and Monuments* (Cambridge: Cambridge University Press, 2006); Vicky Davis, *Myth Making in the Soviet Union and Modern Russia: Remembering World War II in Brezhnev's Hero City* (London: I.B. Tauris, 2018).

4   Donovan, *Chronicles in Stone*; Ekaterina Melnikova, 'Rukami naroda: sledopytsloe dvizhenie 1960–1980-kh gg. v SSSR', *Antropologisheskii Forum* 37 (2018): 20–53; Catriona Kelly, '"Ispravliat" li istoriu? Spory ob okhrane pam'atnikov v Leningrade 1960-1970-kh godov', *Neprikosnovennyi zapas* 2, no. 64 (2009), online: https://magazines.gorky.media/nz/2009/2/ispravlyat-li-istoriyu.html, accessed 1 September 2021.

5   Alissa Klots and Maria Romashova, 'Lenin's Cohort: The First Mass Generation of Soviet Pensioners and Public Activism in the Khrushchev Era', *Kritika: Explorations in Russian and Eurasian History* 19, no. 3 (2018): 582.

6   In her analysis of the autobiographical boom in the 1980s and 1990s, Irina Paperno argues that the explosion in autobiographical publications was a manifestation of the need to rethink individual lives as the Soviet system was collapsing. Yet, as this chapter will demonstrate, long before the Soviet regime began showing signs of strain, during the relatively stable 1960s and 1970s, individual life-stories became the site on which 'big history' was written. Irina Paperno, *Stories of Soviet Experience: Memoirs, Diaries, Dreams* (Ithaca: Cornell University Press, 2009).

7   For more on the 'quiet archival revolution', see Klots and Romashova, '"Tak vy zhivaia istoria?"'

8   Polly Jones, '"Life as Big as The Ocean": Bolshevik Biography and the Problem of Personality from Late Stalinism to Late Socialism', *The Slavonic and East European Review* 96, no. 1 (2018): 157–8.

9   Ibid., 166–9.

10 I.F. Petrovskaia, *Khranilishcha chelovecheskogo znania i opyta* (Moskva: GAU SSSR, 1959), 30.

11 V.I. Zlatoustova, 'Gosudarstvennaia politika v oblasti muzeinogo dela (1945-1985 gg.)', in *Muzei i vlast'. Gosudarstvennaia politika v oblasti muzeinogo dela (XVIII-XX vv.)* (Moskva: NII Kul'tury, 1991), 251–4; R.S. Likhacheva, 'Vstrecha uchastnikov octabr'skih boev v muzee revolutsii SSR', *Vorposy istorii* 6 (1957): 196–8; V.A. Korolev, 'Veterany – v strou', in *Na Zapadon Urale* (Perm: Permskii Oblastnoi Kraevedcheskii Muzei, 1969), 257–8; I. Punin, 'Sekzia veteranov Oktabr'skoi revolutsii i grazhdanskoi voiny pri muzee', in *Materialy po istorii Evropeiskogo severa SSSR* (Vologda: Vologodskii pedagogicheskii institut, 1973), 435–6.

12 Likhacheva, 'Vstrecha uchastnikov octabr'skih boev v muzee revolutsii SSR', 196.

13 Z.A. Zhuravlev, 'Sobiranie dokumentov lichnogo proiskhozhdenia – zadacha kazhdogo arkhiva', *Voprosy arkhivovedenia* 2 (1963): 48.

14 G.I. Gabdul'manov, 'Uchastie obshestvennosti v rabote arkhivnykh uchrezhdenii', *Voprosy arkhivovedenia* 1 (1963): 69.
15 Elizabeth Papazian, *Manufacturing Truth: The Documentary Moment in Early Soviet Culture* (DeKalb: Northern Illinois University Press, 2008); Katerina Clark, '"The History of the Factories" as a Factory of History: A Case Study on the Role of Soviet Literature in Subject Formation', in Jochen Hellbeck and Klaus Heller (eds.), *Autobiographical Practices in Russia* (Göttingen: Vandenhoeck und Ruprecht, 2004), 251–77; Sergei Zhuravlev, *Fenomen 'Istorii fabrik i zavodov': Gor'kovskoe nachinanie v kontekste epokhi 1930-kh godov* (Moscow: IRI RAN, 1997).
16 On party history, see Frederick C. Corney, *Telling October: Memory and the Making of the Bolshevik Revolution* (Ithaca: Cornell University Press, 2004); on Komsomol history, see Sean Guillory, 'The Shattered Self of Komsomol Civil War Memoirs', *Slavic Review* 71, no. 3 (2012): 546–65; on Istprof, see Roman Gil'mintinov, *Istprof i osobennosti profsoiuznogo istoriopisania v SSSR v 1920-e gg.* (Ph.D. dissertation, Tomsk State National Research University, 2019).
17 It is telling that some of those eligible to join the organization refused to do so because they perceived it as an organization of 'invalids'. See: Aleksandra Trofimova, 'Obschestvo starykh Bol'shevikov: put' ot leninskoi gvardii k stalinskoi lektorskoi gruppe', *Vestnik KGU. Istoricheskie nauki i arkheologia* 1 (2018): 170.
18 Stephen Lovell, 'Soviet Russia's Older Generations', in Stephen Lovell (ed.), *Generations in Twentieth Century Europe* (Basingstoke: Palgrave, 2007), 209.
19 On the causes and consequences of women's increase in life expectancy in the USSR, see Botakoz Kassymbekova's and Danielle Leavitt-Quist's chapters in this volume.
20 On the 1956 pension reform, see Lukas Mücke, *Die allgemeine Altersrentenversorgung in der UdSSR, 1956–1972* (Stuttgart: Franz Steiner Verlag, 2013).
21 Klots and Romashova, 'Lenin's Cohort'.
22 For more on the discussion on *Literaturnaia Gazeta* and the broader context of the debate, see Klots and Romashova, '*Tak vy zhivaia istoria?*'.
23 '*Chitatel' predlagaet temy*', *Literaturnaia Gazeta*, 3 September 1976, 6.
24 Ibid.
25 A. Latynina, '*Istoria i kazhdyi iz nas*', *Literaturnaia Gazeta*, 22 June 1977, 6.
26 The reasons for Sokolova's repeated failure to be accepted into the party are not clear. One possible reason was that her stepsister from her father's second marriage had been arrested as an 'enemy of the people'. When Sokolova applied for party membership for the last and fourth time, already after her retirement, her application was rejected as she was deemed to be 'futureless'. GAPK. F. R-1610, op.1, d.509, l.202.
27 Maria Romashova, '"Defitsitnaia Babushka": Sovetskii diskurs starosti i tsenarii starenia', *Novoe Literaturnoe Obozrenie* 3 (2015): 55–65.

28 GAPK. f. R-1610, op. 1, dd. 237, 238, 239, 830, 831.
29 GAPK. f. R-1610, op. 1, d. 237, l. 8.
30 Grigorii Sokolov, *V dom starogo Tomasa prishol khozian. Rasskaz starogo kommunista* (Moscow: Detsakaia literatura, 1968).
31 Klots and Romashova, 'Lenin's Cohort'; Melanie Ilic, 'What Did Women Want? Khrushchev and the Revival of *Zhensovety*', in Melanie Ilic and Jeremy Smith (eds.), *Soviet State and Society under Nikita Khrushchev* (London: Routledge, 2011), 104–21.
32 GAPK f. R-1610, op. 1, d. 196, Dnevniki t. 3, ll. 12-15.
33 According to the 1941 State Archival Regulations, only government leaders, eminent scientists, artists, labour heroes and other distinguished citizens were entitled to have their personal collections permanently preserved in a state archive. See: E.M. Miagkova, 'Fondy lichnogo proiskhozhdenia: etapy istorii, opyt raboty, kratkaia istoriografiia voprosa', *Vestnik VNIIDAD* 4 (2020): 16–26.
34 GAPK f. R-1610, op. 1, dd. 503–4.
35 Those who joined the party or the Komsomol as a response to the death of Vladimir Lenin became known as 'Lenin levy' (*leninskii prizyv*).
36 GAPK. f. R-1610, op. 1, d. 929, l. 8
37 GAPK. f. R-1610, op. 1, d. 196, l. 107
38 GAPK, f. R-1610, op. 1, d. 824, t. 10, l. 72.
39 GAPK. f. R-1610, op. 1, d. 929, t. 1, l. 54.
40 GAPK f. R-1610, op. 1, d. 821, t. 7, l. 22.
41 GAPK f. R-1610, op. 1, d. 822, t. 8, l. 6.
42 GAPK f. R-1610, op. 1, d. 258, l. 63; d. 822, t. 8, l. 60.
43 GAPK f. R-1610, op. 1, d. 816, t. 3, ll. 29-33.
44 Interview with Galina Efimovna Gol'dbukht, 3 May 2018, conducted by Alissa Klots.
45 Latynina, '*Istoria i kazhdyi iz nas*'.

9

Soviet life cycle and ageing: Through the lens of museums of medicine

Katarzyna Jarosz

Over the course of the twentieth century, museums of medicine started to appear throughout the republics of the Soviet Union, both in provincial towns and in large cities. They played a dual function: firstly, thanks to their exhibitions of modern educational charts, wax models of human bodies and pictures presenting venereal diseases, among other things, they served to promote and educate on matters of health and hygiene. Secondly, thanks to the passion and determination of many of the retired medical practitioners who made up their staffs and built up collections of medical artefacts, they helped understand the medical past as a significant part of human travail. Most of these museums' collections had been developed to save 'old material' from being lost or destroyed, preserving them for future generations. The museums tend to have been established in buildings with a pharmaceutical, medical or scientific history, such as hospitals or universities, and were also often built on the premises of former or still operating anatomical theatres, pharmacies and hospitals. Their layout, design and appliances were all once used, or are even, in some cases, still in use. The collections in these museums were often made up of personal objects belonging to doctors, medical institutions and hospitals, as well as a range of original documents. Such museums began to play a significant role in Soviet republics' medical institutions in the late 1940s, when the history of medicine became a compulsory subject at Soviet medical universities and, with few exceptions, was taught (and in many cases still is taught) as a separate course in faculties of social medicine.

Museums of medicine, like other museums, are not simply a collection of objects but rather a powerful visual medium. Museums can be described as 'memory machines', through which curators and directors create stories through their specific choice of exhibits, labels and captions. Heritage tourist sites and museums streamline memory, history, events and emotions into a powerful and unified vision imparted to posterity. For the sake of this chapter, the notion of 'narrative' will be built on the work of the psychologist Jerzy Trzebiński,[1] who observed that the idea of the world and human life existing in culture always takes the form of a story. Stories are a means of understanding the world. People see stories as a stream of events and problems. The universality of this narrative way of understanding the world is demonstrated by the fact that stories are a common element in religion, mythology, legends and fairy tales, as they are in literature, opera and cinema. The past is also often retold in this narrative way. Museums, as machines meant to streamline and spread information about the past, also tell stories: important ones, in fact, with wide audiences.

This paper aims to analyse what sort of stories were being told by Soviet museums of medicine, and what stories continued to be told today in the post-Soviet world. In particular, it investigates whether and to what extent museums of medicine in the post-Soviet bloc dealt with questions of the human life cycle (ontogenesis), including birth, development, ageing and death. It seeks to understand if and how these museums contributed to Soviet and post-Soviet citizens' awareness and perception of ontogenesis. Is it possible to explore a realm of Soviet culture and practice regarding the attitude to life through the lens of museums' exhibitions? When, according to the museums' narratives, does life begin, and when does it end? What are its boundaries? Does it begin with insemination, pregnancy or birth? What illnesses do people have in their lives, and how are they cured to keep people healthy? When and how does their life end? When and how did a Soviet citizen die? What were the causes of his or her death? In this chapter I analyse four stories, as seen through the lens of museum exhibitions. These are the beginning of life: reproduction, pregnancy, birth and birth control; development from a newborn child to a grown-up person; older people; and death.

Methodology and literature

The analysis of Soviet and post-Soviet medical museums in this chapter is based on both secondary literature and fieldwork. Academic works were analysed that referred directly or indirectly to issues related to the history of medicine, museums of pharmacology and museums of medicine. Based on this, nine medical museums were selected for fieldwork.[2] Fieldwork consisted of visits to all the selected museums and the collection of photographic documentation. Three key resources or features distinguished the museums as best able to provide information on the history of medicine. The first was their visual materials, that is, the museums' archives and photographs related to the history of medicine. Second was the museums' premises, which consisted of reconstructed chambers from the turn of the nineteenth and twentieth century and thematic halls. The third resource was the museums' exhibits, including antique furniture, vessels, tools and medicines. I also analyse the museum buildings, exhibitions and exhibits, the way in which they are displayed at these museums and the spaces of the museums themselves. By choosing such an approach, and by looking at museums across an array of vastly different countries, I hope to consider and compare the multitude of narratives regarding human development and ontogenesis in the researched countries.

Markedly little has been written about medical museums in the post-Soviet landscape, or about their place in the history of science. Other aspects of Soviet medicine have been analysed to a larger extent. Tricia Starks has written about the role of hygiene in the Soviet Union,[3] while Nikolai Krementsov devoted many of his works to Soviet medical experiments.[4] Loren Graham wrote about the history of Soviet medicine, pointing out that the history of medicine and public health during the Soviet period of history is a 'fascinating subject, crying out for careful, empirical research'.[5] Susan Grant has written about the Russian and Soviet healthcare system,[6] and Alexander Grando, the founder of the Ukrainian National Museum of Medicine, wrote several works on the history of Ukrainian medicine.[7] Velma Gudiene has shown the significance of prescription books as a historic source, using prescription books from the Museum of the History of Lithuanian Medicine and Pharmacology in Kaunas.[8] Anatoliiu Kostukijukievicus and Taurus Mekas[9] have also researched the history of this particular museum as well. While the broad contours of the Soviet medical system are receiving increased attention, and some individual works have begun to analyse the holdings and importance of post-Soviet medical museums, little work has been done to compare or consider in wider context the place of Soviet and post-Soviet medical museums. This chapter builds on the existing literature to synthetically evaluate medical museums in the post-Soviet landscape and suggest their place in the current writing of medical history in the region: the story not only on individuals' Soviet ontogenesis, but the ontogenesis of the Soviet medical system itself.

Reproduction

In the Soviet Union, sexual life, reproductive capacity and maternity were all considered to be social and political issues: questions of ideology rather than personal or phenomenological concerns. Fertilization, pregnancy, birth and motherhood went far beyond the problems of future parents. Bringing up healthy citizens, helping single mothers and providing proper medical care, both for pregnant women and for infants, were the subjects of both public discussion and propaganda, the aim of which was to promote birth-rates and maternity. State officials, politicians, health experts, intellectuals and women's organizations were active in resolving problems connected with bearing and raising children. Already at the very beginning of the new Bolshevik regime, a decree issued on 19 December 1917 stated:

> All the establishments, large and small, of the People's Commissariat of Public Assistance that serve the needs of children, from the foundling homes in the capitals to modest villages crèches, are being amalgamated in a single State organisation, under the charge of the Department of Maternal and Child Health, in order to form a single integrated system with the goal of serving pregnant women and mothers, a system which will strive to achieve the purpose to which the efforts of the State are directed: the production of citizens of a high mental and physical calibre.[10]

In the great majority of post-Soviet medical museums, human life is described as beginning at birth. In the Soviet Union, after a short 'daring and progressive'[11] period in the early 1920s, sexuality was unmentionable in social discourse and love was ideologically limited to married, monogamous, heterosexual couples. This attitude is reflected in the significant lack of exhibitions in medical museums that might present sexual life. Visitors can learn hardly anything about the history of birth control, contraception or abortion in the Soviet Union.[12] There are references to sexual activities, though they mainly inform visitors about the dangerous consequences of improper sexual behaviour.

An example of this can be found at the Museum of Healthcare in Tashkent, Uzbekistan (uz: *Toshkent Sog'liqni Saqlash Muzeyi*), which was founded in 1973. Along with a section dedicated to the medieval Central Asian medic Ibn Sina, Tashkent's museum focuses heavily on rules of hygiene, including sexual hygiene. One of the exhibits is a detailed chart describing how it is possible to catch venereal diseases and what the consequences can be. There is a picture of a woman affected by syphilis, with charts setting out precise explanations about the ways of catching this disease, its symptoms and its consequences. The only post-Soviet museum that refers directly to sexual life and birth control is the 'Medical exhibition with an exposition of birth control items', organized in 2019 in Daugavpils, Latvia (lat. *Medicīnas izstāde ar kontracepcijas ekspozīciju*). This exhibition was created by the Latvian Society for the Promotion of Health and Education. The aim of the exhibition is to show visitors the history of medicine in Daugavpils, but with a special focus on contraception. One entire hall is completely dedicated to contraception, and various contraceptives and birth control artefacts can be seen here.

With the exception of the Latvian exhibition, the issue of birth control is omitted from the narrative told in post-Soviet medical museums, even though it used to be a topic of interest and discussion for both politicians and medical staff. Already in 1923, the People's Commissariat of Public Health (Narkomzdrav) recommended that women should be informed about contraception in gynaecological clinics' consultation rooms. In an article in the medical journal *Feldsher and Midwife* (*Fel'dsher i akusherka*), Shibaeva states: 'Every year, the number of contraceptive devices grows and becomes more varied. Contraceptive devices allow one to carry out a successful fight against abortion, which is extremely harmful to women's health.'[13] At the same time, however, the Soviet Union, except for a short break between 1936 and 1955, had a very liberal attitude to induced abortion and, more than 251 million induced abortions were conducted in the Soviet Union.[14]

In the Soviet Union, reproduction was government-regulated, with the state showing a keen interest in controlling the health of future generations. Unlike the silenced narrative of birth control, in the majority of post-Soviet medical museums the issue of maternity and child-rearing is well documented. Visitors can see propaganda materials aimed at raising awareness about how to bring up healthy children, as well as numerous exhibits documenting the state's policy regarding the proper methods of raising children to be healthy citizens. To give just one example, a poster from the National Museum of Medicine of Ukraine (ukr.: *національний музей медицини україни*) in Kyiv, which was published by the Red Cross Infant Nursery, presents a mother, baby and a doctor. In the background, one can read the words '*Zdorova zmina*' (a healthy new generation). This is in keeping with the general character of the collections at the National Museum of Medicine of Ukraine, which was opened in 1982 and which presents the development of medicine in Ukraine. From the interior of a bathhouse dated to the time of Kievan Rus, to Soviet medical practices, the museum contextualizes posters like that of the Red Cross Infant Nursery in the longer history of Ukrainian and Soviet medicine.

It is clear from this and other museums' narratives, moreover, that the focus was firmly on a healthy child, rather than its mother. Mothers' bodies were generally considered as vessels: first used to carry a child inside them, and then to provide food for that child. The Soviet government intervened to regulate reproduction and began to provide material support for mothers, such as payment of allowances for single mothers and for mothers raising many children. They also received full paid maternity leave and an allowance of 400 roubles after giving birth to a child.[15] Women who bore and raised ten or more children were awarded the honorary title of 'Mother Heroine' and received a medal of maternal glory. The first step in this regulation was the process of childbirth: women were supposed to give birth in maternity houses (rus.: *rodil'nye doma*), under the supervision of qualified staff. At both the Latvian Medical Exhibition and the Pauls Stradins Museum of the History of Medicine (lat.: *Paula Stradiņa medicīnas vēstures muzejs*) in the Latvian capital of Riga there are reconstructions of such birthing facilities (Figure 9.1). In keeping with its status as one of the world's leading medical museums, the Pauls Stradins Museum has an extended exhibit and large-scale reconstructed birthing house. This includes a clean and spacious reception room, consultation room, labour preparation ward, labour ward, neonatal babies ward and operating theatres. This may have been somewhat unusual in practice: a WHO report from 1962

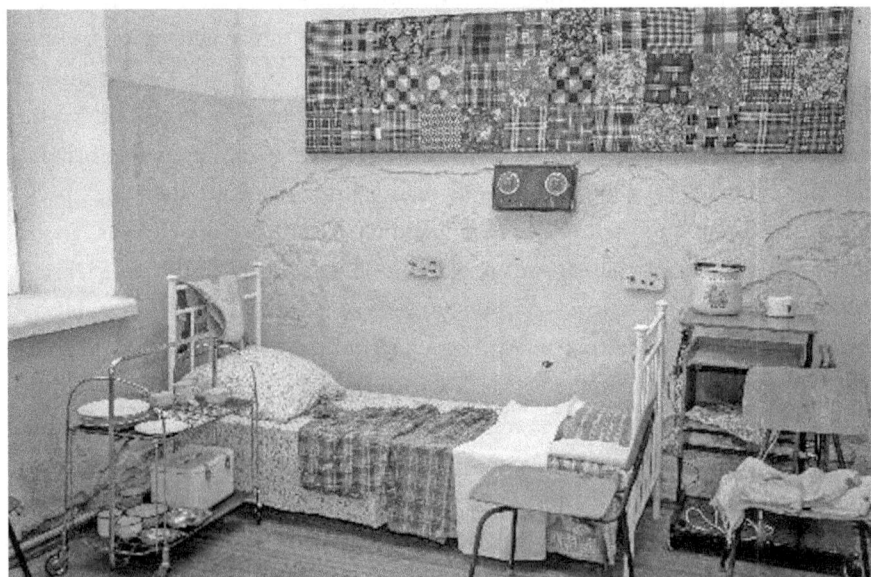

Figure 9.1 Reconstructed birthing room, Latvian Medical Exhibition, Latvia.

stated that birthing wards in the Soviet Union contained six to ten beds,[16] but all the related exhibits present a luxurious version with single-bed birthing wards. The Pauls Stradins Museum and the Latvian Medical Exhibition also both include incubators for newborn babies, which would have been used in the most complex and complicated cases.

Development: From healthy children to healthy citizens

In the early years of the Soviet Union, health consciousness was very low and sanitary conditions were poor. Therefore, to raise healthy grown-up citizens, the state authorities conducted extensive social hygiene campaigns. The state aimed to reap the long-term benefits of placing children in nurseries, conducting vaccination drives, developing a blood donation system, curing polio and building a sanatoria system. Hygiene and medicine were considered vital elements of the modern nation, and the state took on medical responsibility for its citizens from the moment of birth. For example, the benefits of breastfeeding were emphasized and promoted in educational campaigns. Several of the museums analysed here contain exhibits documenting this campaign. In Tashkent's Museum of Healthcare an informational card depicts a smiling mother and baby; it reads, 'breastfeed your baby. Your milk is the best food for your child'. Most post-Soviet medical museums also contain general information about childhood development. At the Latvian Medical Exhibition, the National Medical Museum of Ukraine, Tashkent's Museum of Healthcare and Azerbaijan's Medical Museum (Az.: *Azərbaycan Təbabəti Muzeyinin*) – an institution otherwise largely emphasizing local, Eastern and herbal medicine – visitors can see numerous posters, commemorative cards and postcards that present the symbolic triangle of mother-child-system, with the latter represented by the figure of a doctor, nurse or kindergarten teacher. It should be mentioned that the exhibits tend to exclude fathers, whose role appears to have been reduced to providing financial resources for future citizens.

The Soviet Union took responsibility for its nursery system, day-care centres and kindergartens, all of which were state-run and state-funded.[17] Mothers, especially those coming from rural areas, were often reluctant to leave their children in nurseries, but they were encouraged to do so, in order that they were able to go back to work. Additionally, a home visitation system was developed to track and promote children's health and welfare. Tricia Starks has written about contests that were organized to test the care given to children by their mothers, as well as the usefulness of medical consultations.[18] These contests examined everything, including 'physical development, growth, teeth, weight, and, most important, the lifestyle and housing conditions in which the child grew and developed'. A poster held in Tashkent's Museum of Healthcare shows the practices evaluated in these contests. It presents a woman in traditional Uzbek garb, with a child and a nurse examining him with a stethoscope. The poster also provides information on available places in nurseries and kindergartens.

The Soviet Union was the first country in the world to announce a system of free medical care for all its citizens. In addition to preventive medicine, this system also placed great emphasis on social hygiene: this was considered to be both effective and cost-effective.[19] The Soviet Union's policymakers, through exhibitions in museums of hygiene, aimed to influence citizens' social behaviours and everyday choices in ways as to promote long-term health outcomes. Museums of hygiene were built all over the USSR and were made accessible to the public. Very often, the museums organized guided tours for industrial workers, peasants, schoolchildren and teachers, 'thus promoting personal health and community hygiene'.[20] Systems of health and hygiene were institutionalized, and the establishment of museums of health and hygiene was a significant factor in this process. They became, in the hands of national states and local governments, one of the essential tools for public education in health and hygiene, describing the evolution of medical knowledge and technology.

The content included in earlier museums of hygiene has since found a place in post-Soviet medical museums. All the researched museums devote at least one section to hygiene and sanitation. These exhibitions, through the choice of exhibits, moving images, demonstrations, charts, pictures, dioramas, animated models, diagrams and two- and three-dimensional exhibits, set out to demonstrate that a healthy lifestyle, with fresh air, sunshine and physical exercise, has a positive effect on human life, while also instilling the message that cigarettes and alcohol are dangerous. Left unstated in these exhibits was the motivation for this focus on hygiene: unsanitary conditions and shortages of essential medicines and medical supplies in the first decades of Bolshevik rule left Soviet society much more vulnerable to epidemics and infection than in other industrialized and industrializing nations.

At the National Medical Museum of Ukraine there are numerous charts presenting the proper procedures that can help people live healthily and avoid diseases. By way of illustration, one chart demonstrates how to rid oneself of lice. It instructs viewers to observe cleanliness and maintain personal hygiene. A series of posters, also held in the Ukrainian museum, present simple information about typhoid fever, cholera or tuberculosis transmission: it is possible to get infected through dirty water, by eating dirty things or by not sticking to the rules of elementary hygiene. Mothers should avoid kissing their children on the lips and babies should not chew on their blankets. Adults should not cough in other people's direction or drink water from dirty vessels or from open wooden barrels. In addition, as another poster demonstrates, flies can transmit enteric infections, such as dysentery, diarrhoea, typhoid and cholera. Hygiene, basic sanitation and taking personal action to avoid disease were all part of the prophylactic approach to healthcare and health promotion established by the Public Soviet Commissariat of Health under Nikolai Semashko in the 1920s and continued throughout the course of Soviet history.

Vaccines were also among the highly valued prophylactic measures. In a report on Soviet live vaccine development, A. T. Kravchenko and R. A. Saltykov wrote that 'Following the Great October Socialist Revolution, the young Soviet republic was compelled to devote particular attention to the eradication of widespread infectious diseases, including smallpox'.[21] These vaccination campaigns were highly successful and eliminated smallpox between 1936 and 1938, as well as polio in the early 1960s.

At the National Medical Museum of Ukraine, Tashkent's Museum of Healthcare, the Pauls Stradins Museum of the History of Medicine in Riga, the Azerbaijan Medical Museum and the Institute of Experimental Pathology and Therapy of the Academy of Sciences of Abkhazia numerous exhibits document Soviet vaccination campaigns and the measures taken to eliminate diseases. The informal museum-like exhibitions of the Institute of Experimental Pathology, for example, demonstrate the many ways that this and other institutes involved in animal experimentation were related to vaccine development.[22] At the centre of the Institute, there is a statue of a hamadryas baboon sitting on a pedestal with a caption in Abkhaz and Russian noting that this is a monument to the memory of all the experimental animals used in research there. Many human diseases were studied at the institute and were tested on monkeys, leading to vaccines for polio, measles and hepatitis, along with new antibiotics and drugs for many other diseases. At the Azerbaijan Medical Museum, a poster from 1932 depicting a five-year-old child and the nurse vaccinating him reads 'the USSR will get rid of smallpox by the end of the fourth year of the five-year plan'. It also provides statistics that in 1919, 186,000 citizens had smallpox, while in 1929 this number had been reduced to just 5,000. At the Pauls Stradins Museum, visitors can see a set of vaccines against cholera and typhus, packed in small bottles dating back to the 1920s.

An interesting exhibit for visitors to the Pauls Stradins Museum is a device associated with polio, an infectious disease caused by the poliovirus that can affect the central nervous system and cause muscle weakness resulting in flaccid paralysis. The device, commonly known as the 'iron lung', or tank respirator, was invented in 1927 at Harvard University. When the poliovirus paralysed muscles in the chest, patients were unable to breathe. The device was a respirator powered by an electric motor and a pump that changed the pressure, effectively pulling air in and out of the lungs and maintaining respiration artificially for a couple of weeks until the patient was able to breathe independently. The tank was equipped with special windows so attendants could reach in and adjust limbs or change the patient's bedsheets.[23]

Healthy childhood development and prophylactic medicine was meant to create adult Soviet citizens who would be healthy, robust and fit. A young, fit and healthy workforce was a key element of the ideology and success of the USSR, both as a concept and in reality. The Museum of Healthcare in Tashkent, Uzbekistan, has on display an exhibit of great interest to this topic. It is a mannequin made of glass, reflecting a human's anatomical structure. It is a symbolic exhibit, known locally as the 'glass man' or 'transparent man'. This life-size model of a man has transparent plastic skin, through which can be seen the light metal mould of a human skeleton, with artificial internal organs and veins, all coloured and accurately shaped. The glass man was produced in the GDR and brought to Uzbekistan from Dresden in 1973 as a present from the communist comrades in East Germany. The very first version of a similar glass man dates to 1930 and has been on display in the Dresden Museum of Hygiene ever since, changing the way health education was carried out. It was also clearly in line with the Soviet desire to popularize health and hygiene. Visitors can see through the translucent skin to all the vital organs. As the physician and curator Bruno Gebhard wrote: 'The twenty organs are rebuilt in all their anatomical details and in natural colour; the skeleton is real size and the main blood vessels have been reconstructed as naturally as possible.'[24] For several decades, the Dresden glass man was considered a reference model at an international level in popularising and teaching issues related to the human body, hygiene and health education. After the end of the Second World War, the glass man was also exhibited throughout the Soviet Union, quickly becoming a symbol of health education.

As Soviet citizens grew into adults, they were also expected to take care of their health through preventative means, in part by 'active' rest and visiting the Soviet Union's system of sanatoria and rest homes. The word 'sanatorium' in the Soviet Union was not a word reserved (as in some other countries) for establishments where tuberculosis was treated. Instead, it referred to a mixed resort and recreational facility, convalescent home or a rest home. It was an institution, often located near natural hot springs or in the mountains, where Soviet citizens could both rest and actively improve their health through various procedures. Convalescent children were often sent to sanatoria, where they were treated with various forms of physiotherapy, combined with massage, exercise or, in some sanatoria, baths in radioactive water. A poster from the Ukrainian National Medical Museum, for example, presents a group of children sunbathing in a sanatorium, under the supervision of qualified staff. Another museum, the Museum of Traditional Medicine in Isfara, Tajikistan, was in fact built on the premises of one of the sanatoriums, Zumrad, which is still working. While the exhibitions at the museum are rather small, the museum and attached sanatoria attest to the emphasis placed on active rest and healing in the USSR, as well as the links between these practices and earlier traditional modes of medicine.

Other museums contain information and materials related to practices meant to improve other adult medical conditions. Both the Pauls Stradins Museum and the Black Eagle Pharmacological Museum in Lviv, Ukraine – an institution dedicated to documenting the worldwide history of pharmacology, and which was established in 1966 – there are exhibits referring to methods of curing blood-related illnesses in the Soviet Union. At the Black Eagle Museum, for example, visitors can even purchase the famous 'Iron wine' said to cure anaemia. Despite its name, the drink does not contain wine or any form of alcohol, but it was claimed to improve the appetite and raise the blood's haemoglobin levels. The product was very popular in the USSR, especially after the Chernobyl disaster. The exhibit at Pauls Stradins Museum presents ampoules of dried plasma, dating back to the late 1940s. The Soviet Union, it should be noted, developed an efficient system of blood donation. There were more than 1,400 blood donation stations all over the country and by 1944, this had an important military impact as well: 860 tonnes of blood and three tons of frozen serum had been sent to the front. In peacetime, too, the USSR continued to develop its blood donation service, creating an effective and efficient Union-wide network of stations and research institutes.

The ultimate spoiler: Old age, mortality and causes of death

Discussions over what constitutes a 'natural' death can become quite intense, as definitions can be unclear and problematic. According to WHO, 'natural' deaths include death caused by disease but not due to external injury, whether from unintentional accident or intentionally caused wounds.[25] (At the same time, however, every medical procedure that prolongs life and postpones death, including the treatment of cardiac infarction, hypertonia, diabetes mellitus, arteriosclerosis or intensive medical care, could be understood as an external factor, leading to questions about the *absence* of external elements in the causes of death.) In addition, a lack of technical resources or simple human error can also result in the untimely death of people who would otherwise be alive. In 1989, the German pathologist Wilhelm Doerr suggested that a 'pure' death from old age was the only 'natural' death,[26] building on the definition by Friedrich Husemann, a psychiatrist who had written about 'natural' or 'physiological death from ageing'.[27] While this discussion goes beyond the immediate scope of this paper, with its focus on medical museums, it is useful to consider when analysing the Soviet life cycle and its depiction in these museums.

Several of the museums contain various exhibits, posters, reconstructions and dioramas presenting people dying from diseases, or suffering from accidents and wars. To give one example, at the National Museum of Medicine of Ukraine there is a three-dimensional living scene presenting the interior of a village hut with the whole family gathered there and the figure of Anton Chekhov – a Russian physician (and famous author) – sitting at the bedside of a dying child. The museum in Ukraine also has on display a model reconstruction of an autopsy. A surgeon is shown conducting the autopsy of a young man, with two other surgeons observing the procedure. At Azerbaijan's Museum of Medicine, a diorama presents very young soldiers, bloody and

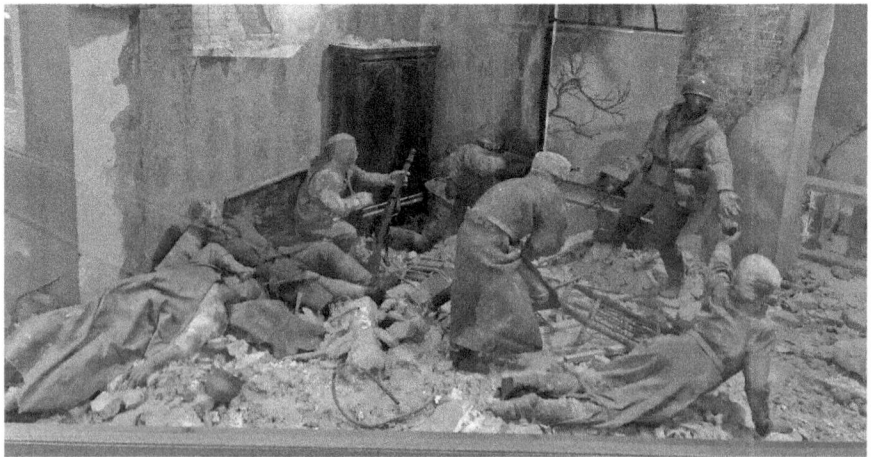

Figure 9.2 Diorama of dying soldiers, Azerbaijan's Museum of Medicine.

dying of bullet wounds (Figure 9.2). However, the diorama is not focused on death as such, but on the heroic feat: with the young heroes firmly in the foreground. A very similar living scene is displayed at the Ukrainian museum, with young war heroes also shown sacrificing their lives for the fatherland at the centre of the exhibit. David Campbell has argued that the presence of the dead in representations of war is crucial, as images leave a lasting impression.[28] The visitor should see the dead and injured, as it is a form of witnessing that can foster an ethical responsibility in the face of crimes against the nation. In none of the life scenes or dioramas in the analysed museum, however, is death presented as a medical issue.

In the Soviet and post-Soviet museums analysed here, surprisingly enough, nobody dies of natural causes – that is, of old age or from disease. Unlike in various Western medical museums, there are no exhibits that attempt to explain the phenomenon of death. Neither are there direct explanations about the complete cycle of human life (ontogenesis) from birth to death. In the analysed museums, natural death does not exist as a natural part of life; it is instead an aberration brought about by war or accident alone. The absence of death stands in stark contrast to much more developed parts of the museums' narratives presenting life. Death is a natural process that occurs in old age, but old age also does not seem to exist in the museums' life-cycle narratives. Depictions of older people, as seen through the narratives of the museums, are doctors, shamans, *znakhorkas* (traditional healers) and museum founders. A curious fact is that doctors and medical authorities are usually depicted as older people. Azerbaijan's Museum of Medicine has an interesting example of this: a sculpture of Ivan Petrovich Pavlov, winner of the Nobel Prize in Physiology or Medicine, which presents Pavlov as an older man in his late seventies, although in fact he was awarded the Nobel prize when he was fifty-four. Old age, as seen at the museums, is allowed when it is associated with wisdom, respect and honour from society, but death from old age seems taboo.

There are no exhibits referring to those illnesses largely associated with old age, such as cardiovascular diseases, arthritis, Alzheimer's or osteoporosis; neither are there exhibits presenting how to take care of or treat older people. Even though the museums in question present the figures of numerous prominent medical scholars, there is not a single figure whose work was dedicated to the problems of ageing, or whose work contributed to the development of gerontology, such as Aleksey Ivanovich Abrikosov, one of the founders of pathological anatomy in Russia, or Nikolay Nikolaevich Anichkov, who discovered the significance and role of cholesterol in atherosclerosis pathogenesis, to name just a couple.

Medicine, as seen through the museums' collections, does not aim to resolve the problems of ageing – or, for that matter, the practical medical problems of older people.

Nor are there any exhibits in the analysed museums referring to longevity, despite the Soviet Union having spent decades making claims about the extraordinary longevity of some of its citizens, notably in the Caucasus region – in Georgia, Azerbaijan and Armenia. Other sources include numerous accounts of Soviet centenarians, with the National Museum of Abkhazia even devoting a whole exhibition to the republic's super-centenarians: those said to be living up to 150, often still in good health and vigour. Yet the Institute of Experimental Pathology and Therapy of the Academy of Sciences of Abkhazia in nearby Sukhumi does not include any information about these centenarians or super-centenarians, even though the institute participated in 1970s and 1980s research into their ageing and health.[29] Although the exceptionally high proportion of centenarians in the Soviet population has been proven to be significantly overstated, the myth of extreme longevity is still alive in the populace of the former USSR, and in some national museums. Yet it is not generally recognized by post-Soviet medical museums.

This lack of older people's representation may have resulted from a general reluctance to present vulnerable groups, such as the disabled and mentally ill. In the Soviet bloc, these groups were stigmatized and hidden away from the public eye. As people in old age are statistically more likely to have impairments – more than 46 per cent of people aged sixty years and over experience physical and mental limitations in some form – in the Soviet Union they were ignored and treated as invisible.[30] It is also the case that 'propaganda argued that the perfected individual, as both a citizen and a worker, could streamline government, increase production, and speed the transition to communism'.[31] Non-perfected individuals, whether impaired or older or both, were left with a lack of clarity as to where they fit into the state's vision. As the museums clearly show, an older citizen who was no longer able to increase production and whose body was no longer perfectly fit, but wrinkled, weak and impaired, did not deserve to play a role in the museums' narratives.

While analysing the reasons why natural death is swept under the carpet in these museums, two somewhat contradictory hypotheses can be drawn from the way in which the human lifecycle is depicted. Firstly, this may result from the widespread modern denial of 'natural' death or the concept of death as a natural part of life. The British anthropologist Geoffrey Gorer observed that conversations about death in the contemporary world, notably in Western cultures, have come to constitute a taboo, making death more and more 'unmentionable' as a natural process.[32] In addition, Ernest Becker, the author of the highly acclaimed publication *Denial of Death*, states that 'the idea of death, the fear of it, haunts the human animal like nothing else; it is a mainspring of human activity, activity designed largely to avoid the fatality of death, to overcome it by denying in some way that it is the final destiny for the man'.[33] Modern medicine, for its part, has accepted the mission to eradicate pain, sickness and even death. Death can be postponed or even avoided.

The other contradictory but parallel conclusion to be drawn from museums described here is that death is not considered to be a medical issue. It is a natural process, not something medicalized. It is simply a natural part of the life cycle. In the Soviet Union, there were only a few specialized hospitals for geriatric patients. As Susan Grant describes elsewhere in this volume, the primary providers for care to geriatric patients were nursing homes, run under the auspices of the All-Union Ministry of Health and the Ministries of Social Security of the Soviet Republics. However, due to shortages of space in these institutions, geriatric patients very often stayed at home and were supported mainly by their families. In the Soviet Union, older people usually died at home; they were familiar with the fact that they would die one day, generally preparing their burial clothing before they died. After a natural death, the deceased remained in the house for three days before burial.[34] Analysing the issue of dying from this perspective, it could be argued that death did not belong to medicine, and therefore did not belong in a museum of medicine.

Concluding comments

In the researched museums, life as a whole entity is not the main narrative. It is possible to reconstruct its particular stages; however, not a single museum presents life from birth to natural death. A visitor who enters the museums' premises will not find the answer to the burning question posed by Monty Python 'Why are we here, what's life all about? [...] What's the point of all this hoax? [...] are we just simply spiralling coils of self-replicating DNA? [...] Is mankind evolving, or is it too late?'[35]

As seen through the museums' narratives, the cycle of life is uneven, with an emphasized beginning and blurred or rather shyly hidden final stage and end. These observations are undoubtedly limited to specific museums that exist in a particular context. Based on more extensive research, it might be possible to verify whether the observations are universal. It seems necessary to examine whether they also apply to other types of museums or whether they apply on a larger scale. Otherwise, it would be impossible to determine whether the narratives in the researched museums are local or paradigmatic.

Notes

1   Jerzy Trzebiński, *Narracja jako sposób rozumienia świata* (Gdańsk: Gdańskie Wydaw. Psychologiczne, 2002), 15.
2   Fieldwork was conducted in the following museums: the Museum of the History of Lithuanian Medicine and Pharmacy in Kaunas, Lithuania; the Museum of Healthcare in Tashkent, Uzbekistan; the 'Medical exhibition with an exposition of birth control items', organized in the post-Soviet period in Daugavpils, Latvia; the National Museum of Medicine of Ukraine, in Kyiv, Ukraine; the Pauls Stradins Museum of the History of Medicine in Riga, Latvia; Azerbaijan's Medical Museum in Baku, Azerbaijan; the Institute of Experimental Pathology and Therapy of the Academy of Sciences of Abkhazia in Sukhumi, Abkhazia; Museum of Traditional Medicine in Isfara, Tajikistan; and the Black Eagle Pharmacological Museum in Lviv, Ukraine.
3   Tricia Starks, *The Body Soviet* (Madison: University of Wisconsin Press, 2009).
4   Nikolai Krementsov, *A Martian Stranded on Earth: Alexander Bogdanov, Blood Transfusions, and Proletarian Science* (Chicago: The University of Chicago Press, 2011); Nikolai Krementsov, *Stalinist Science* (Princeton: Princeton University Press, 1997); Nikolai Krementsov, *Revolutionary Experiments* (Oxford: Oxford University Press, 2013).
5   Loren R. Graham, *Science in Russia and the Soviet Union; a Short History* (Cambridge: Cambridge University Press, 1993), 248.
6   Susan Grant (ed.), *Russian and Soviet Health Care from an International Perspective* (Palgrave, Macmilian, 2017).
7   Alexander Grando, *Ochyma khudozhnykiv: medytsyna v Ukrains'komu obrazotvorchomu mystetstv* (Kyiv: RVA Triumf, 1994).
8   Velma Gudiene, 'Medicines Produced in Telšiai Pharmacy (Vilnius Governorate): Analysis of Prescription Book from 1830', *Pharmazie* 69, no. 1 (2014): 76–80.
9   Anatoliju Kostukijukievicus and Tauras Mekas, 'The Lithuanian Museum of Pharmacy: Tales from behind the Iron Curtain', *The Pharmaceutical Journal* 277, no. 23/30 (2006): 789–90; Taras Mekas, 'The Museum of the History of Lithuanian Pharmacy', *Medicina nei secoli. Arte et Scienza* 21, no. 1 (2009): 245–55.
10 'Maternal and Child Health in the USSR. Report Prepared by the Participants in a Study Tour Organised by the World Health Organisation' (Geneva: World Health Organisation, 1962), 9.

11 Igor Kon, *The Sexual Revolution in Russia: From the Age of the Czars to Today* (New York: The Free Press, 1995).
12 Melanie Ilic, *Soviet Women – Everyday Lives* (London: Routledge, 2020).
13 A.N. Shibaeva, 'O nekotorykh formakh propagandy protivozachatochnykh sredstv', *Fel'dsher i akusherka* XXVII, no. 5 (May 1962): 50.
14 Vyacheslav Karpov and Kimmo Kääriäinen, '"Abortion Culture" in Russia: Its Origins, Scope, and Challenge to Social Development', *Sociological Practice* VII, no. 2 (Fall–Winter 2005–2006): 13–33.
15 'Edit of Supreme Soviet of USSR on the increase of State aid for mothers and children', *Embassy of the Union of Socialist Republics Information Bulletin* 4, no. 84 (Washington, DC, 1944): 2.
16 'Maternal and Child Health in the USSR', 25.
17 For the development of (and background to) Soviet pedagogical thought and childcare institutions, see Andy Byford, *Science of the Child in Late Imperial and Early Soviet Russia* (Oxford: Oxford University Press, 2020).
18 Starks, *The Body Soviet*, 150.
19 Susan Gross Solomon, 'Social Hygiene and Soviet Public Health 1921–1930', in Susan Gross Solomon (ed.), *Health and Society in Revolutionary Russia* (Bloomington: Indiana University Press, 1990), 175–99.
20 Bruno Gebhard, 'Art and Science in a Health Museum', *Bulletin of the Medical Library Association* 33 (1945): 41.
21 A. Kravcheno and T. Saltykov, *Development of Life Vaccines in Soviet Union* (Washington: US Army Foreign Science and Technology Center, 1969), 1.
22 For more information on this point, see Krementsov, *Revolutionary Experiments*.
23 Since acquisition records were not kept, it is impossible to know the origin of this iron lung, although it was most likely produced outside of the USSR and brought to the country as part of a medical exchange programme or simply purchased abroad. For more on Polio and the USSR's medical exchanges with the West, see: Saul Benison, 'International Medical Cooperation: Dr. Albert Sabin, Live Poliovirus Vaccine and the Soviets', *Bulletin of the History of Medicine* 56, no. 4 (1982): 460–83.
24 Gebhard, 'Art and Science in a Health Museum', 45.
25 *International Guidelines for the Determination of Death – Phase* (Montreal: World Health Organization, 2012), 14.
26 Wilhem Doerr, 'Arzt und Tod', in H.H. (Hrsg) Jansen (ed.), *Der Tod in Dichtung Philosophie und Kunst* (Berlin- Heidelberg: Springer Verlag, 1989), 1–13.
27 Friedrich Husemann, *Vom Bild Und Sinn Des Todes: Entwurf EINER GEISTESWISSENSCHAFTLICH Orientierten Geschichte, Physiologie Und Psychologie Des Todesproblems* (Frankfurt am Main: Fischer-Taschenbuch-Verlag, 1982).
28 David Campbell, 'Horrific Blindness: Images of Death in Contemporary Media', *Journal For Cultural Research* 8, no. 1 (2004): 55–74.

29 For the history of the Sukhumi institute, see Krementsov, *Revolutionary Experiments*; on the Institute's work related to 'super-centenarians', see Sula Benet, *Abkhasians: The Long-Living People of the Caucasus* (New York: Holt, Rinehart, and Winston, Inc., 1974); S.D. Gogokhia, N. Sh. Basilaya, and V.V. Pustalov, 'On Some Results of Longitudinal Studies of the Abkhazian Centenarians', in S.M. Dalakshivili (ed.), *Mechanisms of Aging and Longevity: Materials of the Conference, Sukhumi, June 19–21, 1991* (Tblisi, 1991).

30 Stephen Dunn and Ethel Dunn, 'Everyday Life of the Disabled in the USSR', in William O. McCagg and Lewis Siegelbaum (eds.), *The Disabled in the Soviet Union Past and present. Theory and Practice* (Pittsburgh: University of Pittsburgh Press, 1989), 199–234; Sarah D. Phillips, '"There Are No Invalids in the USSR!" A Missing Soviet Chapter in the New Disability History', *Disability Studies Quarterly* 29, no. 3 (2009).

31 Starks, *The Body Soviet*, 163.

32 Geoffrey Gorer, 'The Pornography of Death', in G. Gorer (ed.), *Death, Grief, and Mourning* (New York: Doubleday, 1955), 193.

33 Ernest Becker, *The Denial of Death* (New York: Free Press, 1997), xvii.

34 Jeanmarie Rouhier-Willoughby, 'Contemporary Urban Russian Funerals: Continuity and Change', *Folklorica* 12, no. 0 (February 2010): 110; Sergei Mokhov, 'Care for the Dying in Contemporary Russia: The Hospice Movement in a Low-Income Context', *Mortality* 26, no. 2 (March 2021): 202–15.

35 Terry Jones and William Terry (dirs.), *Monty Python's the Meaning of Life* (Elstree Studios, 1983).

Part Four

International contexts

10

The burden of old age: The fate of older people in the People's Republic of Poland

Ewelina Szpak

In 1954 in Zakopane, two older people – she sick and infirm, he a retired engineer who was incurably ill and therefore unable to work – had neither family nor means of subsistence. They decided to poison themselves. When the ambulance came to take them away, they found a note: 'We poisoned ourselves because we had no means to live and no physical ability to work. We had the poison from the occupation because we were always prepared for death. What happened now we did consciously, we did not want to be a burden for the People's Poland.' This was quoted in a letter to the editor of Polish Radio by a resident of southern Poland. In his comment the resident also added, 'The government of People's Poland is to be blamed for their deaths, treating us as if we were not important enough, pouring millions into unnecessary investment'.[1] That same year, in a collective letter to the editors of Polish Radio, a group of pensioners wrote: 'Comrades full and clothed. Let us eat. Do you know that there are wretched people living next to you who are dying of malnutrition, hunger, poverty and cold? They are pensioners, old people who have worked almost their whole lives. ... Where is the social justice or care for people?'[2]

Both of these moving letters were sent by ordinary citizens in the mid-1950s, about a decade after the end of the Second World War. Both illustrate an enormous sense of social injustice and ignorance, as well as the local scale of poverty and destitution. However, was the picture of old age emerging from these descriptions true and representative? Can it be considered a symbol of the fate of older people in communist Poland? Starting from this main question I will try to show how both older people and the phenomenon of the ageing of society were perceived in the socialist state, in which slogans of equality, care and social welfare dominated public discourse. Then, in more detailed questioning, I will try to determine to what extent the situation of older people, mostly women, referred to in the above-mentioned letters was conditioned by the economic difficulties of the country and to what degree it resulted from the deliberate policies (biopolitics[3]) of the communist state. What place and meaning were given to old-age pensioners in terms of the state's social and health policy (including in public and expert discourse) and how was the ageing process of Polish society – which accelerated from year to year – translated into social relations and the practice of older people's everyday life, in both rural and urban settings?

Designed in this way, the analysis is based on diverse source material, in which epistolary sources play a special role, especially letters, applications and complaints written by older people to the communist authorities throughout the communist period. The growing number of these letters and the scope of the problems they dealt with, juxtaposed with the social, cultural and economic context of the People's Republic of Poland, show both the complexity of the issue of old age in the People's Republic of Poland and its everyday and emotional aspect. Another important supplement to epistolographic materials are sources that reflect both the official public (and expert) discourse and the social perception of old age, which consist of press materials, reports and films, among other things.

Post-war background and realities

As a result of its enormous war losses, Poland was one of the youngest European countries in demographic terms. A decade after the Second World War, in 1956, the national ratio of people over sixty (women) and sixty-five (men) years of age amounted to slightly over 7 per cent, while in the neighbouring German Democratic Republic it had reached 20 per cent, hovering at a similar level in Western European countries as well (e.g. in Belgium and France at the time it was 17–18 per cent).[4] According to the calculations of Polish demographers, by 1950 the total number of people in the post-working age group in Poland reached approximately 2.6 million, while by the mid-1970s this number had doubled to 5.4 million, constituting approximately 16 per cent of the population and significantly approaching the Western European levels of that time.[5] Thus, over those three decades the ageing of Polish society accelerated significantly, but at the same time the social structure itself also underwent profound transformations, which, as I will demonstrate in this chapter, also had a significant impact on the fate of older people in the People's Republic of Poland.

Shortly after the war, in 1945, Polish society was predominantly agricultural. Nearly 70 per cent of the Polish population lived and worked in the countryside. As a result of spatial migrations (resulting from post-war territorial transfers and rapid industrialization and urbanization), this disproportion changed noticeably; in 1970 the urban population began to dominate, reaching 52 per cent.[6] Despite the communists' systematic efforts to nationalize and socialize agriculture (e.g. through the creation of State Agricultural Farms [PGRs] and the collectivization of agriculture by creating Collective Farms), throughout the entire communist period the majority of people living in the countryside maintained their own farms.[7] Private owners of farms (especially large ones) were however considered ideological enemies of the system, which was particularly brutally expressed in the Stalinist period through the high taxes imposed on farmers, compulsory deliveries and the exclusion of farm owners from the system of free state healthcare and other social benefits, including pensions. The right to such benefits, according to a law introduced in 1950, was granted only to persons employed in the state economy (state-owned enterprises or PGRs). Until the end of the 1960s, peasants (farmers) secured old-age support through the traditional system of 'life annuity' (*wycug*),[8] which, as I will show later, often completely failed to fulfil its function in practice. The enormous scale of migration from rural to urban areas, the most intensive period of which took place in the 1950s, involved the youngest generations, leaving the oldest ones in the countryside and initiating the rapidly progressing process of ageing and depopulation in the Polish countryside over the following decades.[9]

Legal framework for pension policy

The letters cited at the beginning of this article come from the 1950s, a period of huge economic crisis, when poverty, food shortages and terrible sanitary and housing conditions were experienced by most citizens of post-war Poland. It was at this time, while the country was recovering from post-war ruin and destruction, that the process of creating new state institutions and legal systems began. This also applied to the system of old-age benefits and pensions, which until the end of the 1950s was very complicated, inconsistent and frequently adjusted to fit with the ideological and practical goals of the state. At least until 1953 (and hence until the end of Stalinism), almost all the state's efforts were concentrated on industrial investment driving the pace of forcible industrialization. State social policy was almost completely marginalized, and a reluctance to expand the system of social benefits prevailed among policymakers.[10]

Before 1953, preferential benefits and assistance were available to 'those who contributed to the establishment of the new system' and to their relations (orphans and widows), as well as to those who, after the war, 'stood guard over the new system of power', i.e. officers of public security (UB) and uniformed services (militia, soldiers of the Polish Army, etc.).[11] Simultaneously, the insurance system was meant to 'punish' the so-called undesirable elements or those who were considered enemies by the state authorities. In addition to peasants, this group also included the German population living in the Regained Areas – territories annexed to Poland in 1945.[12] In the years after the war, the amount of pension benefits was a flat rate and not dependent on the type of employment or length of service. Those who were entitled to claim these benefits (and did not belong to a privileged group) could count on symbolic amounts, fluctuating well below the poverty line as the ratio of the average pension to the average wage was between 15 and 20 per cent in 1951–4. It is no wonder, then, that the majority of people of post-working age, including invalids – regardless of their burdens and physical infirmities – continued to work. According to research on the 1950s, only 22 per cent of people in the post-working age group were covered by benefits, although, as other studies suggested, a majority of them supplemented their benefits with additional paid work.[13]

The first long-term reform came in 1954, i.e. during the first year of de-Stalinization.[14] It was then that old-age benefits, disability benefits and family benefits were differentiated. At that time, three hierarchies of pensioners emerged. The first was based on occupational affiliation, the second on the provisions of the application for benefits in force at the time (the 'new wallet') and the third included persons who had been granted benefits before 1954 (the 'old wallet').[15] The first and most privileged group of pensioners was made up of workers in heavy industry and miners. However, civil servants, military personnel and militia and Department of Security officers also retained their separate social programmes and the possibility of early retirement. Other workers – usually in trade, transport and services – received much lower benefits. In 1955, only 7.6 per cent of the 1.1 million pension beneficiaries received the top level of support allowed by the 'new wallet', while the rest received on average 40 per cent lower benefits.[16] The consequences of this classification became visible two years later in 1956, when several improvements were introduced as part of further work on the pension system aimed at improving the living conditions of older people.[17] However, these changes concerned only younger pensioners, belonging to the 'new wallet', or those who had obtained the right to benefits after 1954.

The bitterness, anger and sense of injustice were reflected in hundreds of letters, complaints and grievances sent by senior citizens to the central government. The 1958 reform was supposed to help alleviate the growing social discontent and was an attempt to weaken the division between the old and new 'wallet', but it failed to remove all differences.[18] The 'old wallet' pension base was only partially revalued. The sense of income inequality was still clearly palpable, as reflected in a letter from the pensioners at the time:

> Such inequality and such privileging of some at the expense of others did not exist before 1958. There were low pensions and things were bad, but for everyone equally; the differences in pensions were minimal. This matter hurt and irritated disadvantaged people who still lived miserably (on 500 zlotys) and look at the better life of [other] pensioners, who were privileged, although the former worked the same amount as the latter.[19]

Pensioners' problems did not end with the unequal, often starvation-level, rates of pensions.[20] In 1958 the problem of unemployment and lack of jobs for young people began to emerge locally. In response to this, drastic restrictions were placed on combining paid work with the provision of old-age benefits. For pensioners – in both 'wallets' – employed part-time or on a casual basis (and in 1956 such people still made up more than 38 per cent of the pension-age population),[21] a limit on permissible monthly salaries was introduced.[22] Exceeding this limit resulted in a reduction or suspension of the individual's pension. In practice, especially for highly qualified people and those with high earnings thanks to additional work, this meant a significant degradation in their standard of living.

The new regulation also introduced complications into the labour market itself, since in many sectors the experience of retired people working extra hours was invaluable and could by no means be replaced by the enthusiasm of new employees. This resulted in successive amendments to the law, which introduced special rules for select occupational groups representing priority industries (e.g. steelworkers and railwaymen), making the disability benefit system more complicated as it introduced new inequalities and caused further bitterness and disappointment among the oldest Poles.

The pessimistic mood among pensioners continued in subsequent years. The somewhat increased old-age pension benefits, partly revalued in 1958, were not adjusted to the growing inflation in the following years. Their real value therefore grew slowly, reaching no more than 40 per cent of the average salary between 1964 and 1968 (in the case of invalidity pensions, the level was around

23 per cent).[23] The lack of regular wage indexing affected the entire social security system, including family benefits. It only bypassed the pension benefits of selected and privileged professional groups, such as the aforementioned militia officers, security services officers, military veterans and miners. The scale of inequality was evidenced, for example, in the year 1970, when, due to an economic crisis, expenditure on family benefits was halved. However, according to researchers' findings, at the same time the Social Insurance Institution spent 50 per cent more money on benefits for 38,000 retired military officers and militiamen than on all benefits for working mothers combined.[24]

Such an inconsistent and instrumental treatment of the system of social benefits and the idea of the welfare state was the result of Władysław Gomułka's post-Stalinist policy of belt-tightening and investing resources in industrialization at the expense of social programmes. In December 1970, however, the decision to raise prices in the middle of a recession and the use of force against the participants of workers' protests on the coast led to Edward Gierek's appointment as the new General Secretary of the Central Committee of the Polish United Workers' Party (PZPR), and marked the beginning of a new direction in social policy. According to Tomasz Inglot, the push for changes came from the USSR, where 'a new and consumer-orientated model of welfare state authoritarianism – a kind of informal "social contract" between the authorities and society – became a pillar of the policy pursued by Leonid Brezhnev'. In 1971, during a hastily convened meeting with Gierek, Brezhnev advised the new Polish party leader 'to follow the example of other "socialist" states and build social support for the system by modernizing social policy and improving the living conditions of working people'.[25] A Soviet loan of 100 million dollars was supposed to make it possible to achieve this goal and to overcome the ongoing economic crisis (by lowering prices and raising salaries).

Despite ad hoc measures that legitimized the new government (an increase in salaries and benefits, as well as the extension of the full range of pension benefits to additional occupational groups – including farmers and artists), maintaining the steady increase in salaries, pensions and disability benefits planned at the beginning of the decade proved unrealistic. The short-lived revival of the economy and the fast growth of salaries, again as in the previous decade, were not accompanied by a steady indexing of benefits for senior citizens, which in the second half of the 1970s led to a decline in their value below 40 per cent of the average salary. Just as before, the decline did not apply to pensions of privileged groups and professions, whose benefits were steadily increasing. It did, however, affect at least 74 per cent of senior citizens collecting benefits under the general old-age pension law, whose monthly income in 1980 was below the then postulated social minimum.[26] According to research carried out by the Institute of Labour and Social Policy, moreover, in the period of 1975–9 almost 4 million people (excluding the agricultural population) did not receive subsistence-level income. Three social groups predominated: pensioners, families with many children or single-parent families (usually single mothers) and persons affected by unpredictable life tragedies.[27]

Another, larger, reform of the old-age pension system appeared at the beginning of the 1980s. The reform introduced minimum pension benefit rates of 90 per cent and 75 per cent of salary. However, these provisions only applied to those who retired in the year in which the new legislation came into force (1982). Similarly, like the reform from the first half of the 1950s, this legislation introduced a division into better- and worse-off pensioners, thus once again evoking a sense of disappointment, negligence and social injustice.[28]

The inadequate and devaluing benefits of pensioners condemned them to an extremely poor life, or to living on the verge of poverty. The latter was particularly true of married couples without children or single and infirm people. (It is calculated that on average these salaries were spent in 60–65 per cent on basic daily food and about 15 per cent on housing, 5–6 per cent on medical care and medicines and another 5–6 per cent usually on clothing and other necessities.)[29] Theoretically – in accordance with the law and the regulations being introduced – the poorest seniors could apply for public assistance, both financial and material. However, the allocation of aid from the social fund required the fulfilment of a number of conditions and official approval. It also required that the appropriate resources be available and that individual municipalities and voivodeships[30] were able to set aside funds for this purpose. As most documents show, the local administration did not always have adequate funds to cover these needs. In practice, for almost all of the history of People's Poland, this resulted in local officials refusing to provide assistance to senior citizens (or providing them with ad hoc or symbolic aid), condemning them to a life of difficult conditions.

Expert and public discourse

In the first years after the war and during the Stalinist period, the difficult situation of older people was not a subject of public debate or wider public interest. Old age, as an element incompatible with the image of the new socialist

Poland built in the shadow of Joseph Stalin's Soviet Union, was tabooed as a social problem. As noted by Katarzyna Stańczak-Wiślicz in her analysis of the press discourse of the immediate post-war period, at the end of the 1940s old age and older people were grouped together with invalids, and as such were counted among the people who were 'redundant, unproductive and thus burdening the economic capacity of the state rebuilt from material ruins'.[31] In the second half of the 1950s, along with the programme of de-Stalinization, more and more information about the difficult fate of Polish seniors began to filter into the press. More articles were also written about the terrible conditions in which they lived, about starvation wages and abandonment by their relatives.[32] It was also at this time that the letter offices of central institutions (including the PZPR) began to receive more and more dramatic reports and requests from desperate senior citizens. In the following years, the problem only grew, and with it the number of letters, which in the case of the Central Committee of the PZPR, amounted by the end of the 1960s to around 10 per cent of all letters with complaints and requests received from citizens.[33]

In 1965 one of the officials responsible for reporting cases of complaints sent to the State Council Chancellery wrote:

> Among the cases received by the State Council Chancellery, a large group are applications demanding changes in the pension regulations, which under the current system create difficult living conditions for many pensioners (…) Some of them ask for a special pension, trying to prove their political and social merits, others ask for a state distinction entitling them to a 25 per cent supplement to the pension, and finally there are those who ask for an increase in their disability group, automatic pension rises, or to be sent to a pensioners' home.[34]

Two years later, the same official reported that:

> compared to previous years, the number of applications for an increase in pensions has risen significantly. Such applications were motivated by a general rise in prices, indicating at the same time that the previous increases in pensions did not compensate for the rising cost of living. … The number of applications for material assistance and social care has especially increased recently. Such applications were motivated by the lack of any means of subsistence, the inability of persons obliged by law to provide maintenance for the elderly, or, in the case of pensioners, by the inadequacy of the pension to meet their basic living needs, especially in autumn and winter.[35]

Many, if not most, of these applications were rejected, mainly due to a lack of funds.

In the 1960s and 1970s, experts – sociologists, physicians and social workers – more frequently spoke out about the problems resulting from the accelerating ageing process. Apart from proposing ways to help older citizens stay active (which would minimize their sense of loneliness, uselessness and social deprivation), they usually emphasized the importance of support from close family and neighbours, condemning the indifferent and cold treatment of older people observed at that time.[36]

The widespread press and expert discourse sensitizing society to the needs of older persons and appealing to their conscience and to social responsibility for the fate of seniors was undoubtedly a form of shifting responsibility from the state (which, as some wrote, 'was yet to mature for great reforms') onto society. But it was also a form of response to the immense social immaturity and unpreparedness for the scale of the phenomenon, as emphasized in many texts. The climate of the era and immediate post-war perception of old age as an economic and social burden were also significant here. In a society where, for at least two decades, posters, banners and the walls of public buildings had been displaying the slogan of 'work as the basic measure of social value and usefulness', old age understood as infirmity and inability to work could often become doubly disqualifying. This was true of both urban and rural areas, although, due to the earlier ageing of the countryside mentioned in the introduction, the problem was greater and more visible earlier there.

Rural ageing

In 1960 the total number of seniors (women and men) in Poland amounted to 3.38 million people.[37] However, there were over 200,000 more of them in rural areas than in cities, which illustrated well the dynamics of the ageing phenomenon.[38] Old-age pension benefits of any kind were available only to those farmers who decided in the 1950s to incorporate their lands into a production cooperative or who took up employment in the State Agricultural Farms. In fact, the percentage of rural seniors who were covered by state pension benefits in the early 1960s did not exceed 0.01 per cent.[39] The rest of the older farmers either worked until the end of their lives, trying to carry out agricultural work with the last of their strength (especially if their children had moved away to more distant towns), or – if they had successors – they concluded a 'life contract' for an annuity (*dożywocie* or *wycug*) with them. These agreements, despite the fact that they were between family members, specified in great detail the scope of obligations of both parties. At the same time, however, after the formal transfer of the farm to its young heirs, the position and social status of the former owner tended to fall dramatically, which often translated into a disrespectful or contemptuous attitude towards him or her.[40]

In the 1960s and 1970s, the need to care for and maintain for many years an ill parent who required time and care was in many cases seen as both an obligation and an additional hardship or burden. Of course, this burden was borne in different ways by members of the immediate family, which undoubtedly was rooted in the strength and nature of the familial bonds and relationships formed earlier. These were not always simple or proper, which gave rise all the more to the fear of old age expressed in the letters of many rural senior citizens. A female author of a letter addressed to the editor of Polish Radio put it very bluntly in 1971: 'People from the countryside will not be taken care of. They have worked all their lives, and in their old age they are 99 per cent deprived of basic conditions. People in the countryside are often heartless. If you don't work, you are useless.'[41] Her words were also confirmed by another letter sent to one of the central institutions, in which the reporting author described the fate of a neglected and lonely 82-year-old mother of four adult children. She was living in a separate room of a family house inherited by one of her sons, in conditions that did not allow her to function. As the author added, 'the son with whom she lives does not give her food because his wife, a monstrous daughter-in-law, does not allow it, wanting the old woman to meet her end sooner.'[42] As a result of the letter, the intervention of the local social services contributed to a relative improvement in the situation of the old woman, extending – at least temporarily – the state's control over her neglectful close family.

The progressive ageing of the rural population, together with the widespread exodus of rural youth to the cities in the 1960s, quickly resulted in an increased number of farms that were neglected and unable to meet their obligations to the state. The possibility of handing over a farm (the land as well as the buildings belonging to it) to the state was introduced in 1968, but only slightly changed the situation. To take advantage of the new regulation it was necessary to fulfil a number of formal conditions, which did not always depend on the landowner in question. For example, if the land was in an inconvenient location or far away from state farms, the chances of handing it over in exchange for an old-age benefit pension fell almost to zero. One example of this is a letter from a 79-year-old woman, childless and single, who owned a nine-hectare farm that she unsuccessfully tried to hand over to the State Treasury in exchange for a pension. Each of her applications was refused because her land was located off the grid and was too small. In her moving letter, the desperate woman wrote: 'And now I have no idea what to do with myself. Somehow, I don't dare to poison myself, and it is very hard to die of starvation, because a man wants to eat while he is still alive. In view of the above, I kindly ask you to grant my request.'[43] Although her letter, after being sent to a Warsaw radio station and examined, resulted in state support (she was granted a temporary benefit for the time needed to arrange the formalities related to the transfer of ownership rights to the farm), in many other similar cases the applicants were out of luck and received refusal letters.

Although there was a long tradition of writing letters, petitions, requests and complaints in the Polish countryside, this did not apply to everyone. Many inhabitants were characterized by fatalism and acceptance of their fate. Epistolographic sources also show such examples. One of the letters sent to the central authorities by a desperate local social worker describes the story of a lonely, illiterate 70- or 80-year-old woman, without any family and completely unable to work, whose 'arms and legs, twisted by rheumatism, made it impossible to move from place to place. ... The old woman has an old hut [without a floor] in which other people would not even want to keep animals, as they were afraid that the remains of the old straw roof would collapse'.[44] The intervention initiated by the above-mentioned letter resulted in the old woman being granted a permanent pension, as reported by a social worker from Lomza in her letter of thanks: 'As soon as her case was settled, [the woman] came to me and said only these words: "The postman has already come and brought ..." and she could say no more, she just burst into tears and sobbed for a long time. I barely calmed her down'.

In view of the still growing problem of rural old age (and neglected farms), in 1977 additional facilitations were introduced for the handing over of land in exchange for an old-age pension, improving the position of at least some of the rural senior citizens. However, as research shows, it was only in the 1980s, after the right to an annuity was also extended to spouses or close relatives working on the farm, that the process of transferring land for a pension accelerated, raising the number of people in rural areas benefiting from the pension system from 13 per cent (in 1977) to 50 per cent (by 1982).[45]

Although the idea of nationalizing and socializing agriculture had been one of the priorities of rural Polish policy since 1948, as in the case of urban areas, it did not include investment in rural social policy. The availability of social welfare homes for the rural population was very limited, and the few institutions that existed in urban areas at the time were treated as a last resort. In such a situation, the only chance for rural older people to improve their situation was to be granted either a pension or social assistance. In many cases, as I have shown above, this required additional effort or assistance and was not always met with success.

Urban ageing

The 1980s demonstrated significant change in the ageing of Polish society. By 1982, the demographic proportions had reversed, and it was the cities that had more people of post-working age. Their financial situation and social status after retirement was most often associated with social degradation, although its practical consequences were slightly different than in rural areas.

Due to the difficult housing situation in Poland, most urban seniors lived with their families (63 per cent),[46] which meant that loneliness, in the sense of absolute social isolation, theoretically affected them less than rural seniors. The meagre and devaluing salaries of old-age pensioners sharing a flat with family members, moreover, usually constituted an additional source of income for the whole household. Grandparents, and especially grandmothers, also often played an important role in the process of bringing up the younger generation (grandchildren). Even if they were not childcare providers (most urban families made use of state or private nursery schools and kindergartens),[47] they participated in the rearing of children. During the economic crisis (1980s), the generation of grandmothers and grandfathers, having extra time at their disposal, also played the role of 'queuers' – people who, by virtue of standing in queues for hours, were able to acquire scarce products (they could later be resold, which also ensured additional income).[48]

However, the function of 'scarce goods conqueror' concerned more energetic and physically fit seniors, and usually also the younger ones, who used their enterprising skills to defend themselves from being seen as useless or unproductive people fully dependent on the support and help of others. Advanced age and the attendant deterioration of their physical condition greatly changed the situation of older people and added to their plight, as evidenced by their hundreds of letters, complaints and requests addressed to the Party or the central authorities, which were often treated as a last resort.

One outstanding symbol of the fate of older people in the 1970s was the fate of Eleonora P. – a senior from Łódź and the heroine of the 1970 documentary movie entitled *The Atrophy of the Heart*. The story of her life and the circumstances of her death, depicted in the film, triggered a broad media discussion about society's attitude towards old people in Poland. The eighty-year-old Eleonora lived with her daughter and two granddaughters and had been struggling with a festering leg wound since the end of the war. When her granddaughters were small, she looked after them.[49] She did not work. However, her advanced age, the increasing difficulty in coping with her own illness (the increasingly foul wound) and her increasing dependence on her family members gradually meant that she also became more and more of a nuisance to them. Her behaviour and appearance embarrassed and irritated her growing granddaughters and their peers. Neighbours complained about the increasingly strong smell of her wound spreading in the stairwell, and her daughter was more and more irritated by her ageing mother's needs – especially her presence and constant need for contact and increasing infirmity. The old lady, eventually placed in an isolated room (adapted from a former laundry room) – 'for her own good' – was initially allowed to leave the isolated premises on her own, but after some time she became completely incapacitated and was locked up. Starved, deprived of access to water and forced to defecate in the same room where she lived, she repeatedly asked the surrounding neighbours for help, wailing loudly from her cell. When, after several weeks of torment, the neighbours finally called for help, it was too late. The old woman had died from exhaustion and dehydration, and the public prosecutor's office initiated proceedings against the daughter, accusing her of abusing her mother.

And although Eleonora's story is extreme and shows, above all, family dysfunction, it also says a good deal about the general situation of older people in communist cities. This is illustrated by the statements of witnesses recorded on camera: neighbours, the family of the deceased and the local militia. All the 'actors' and 'witnesses' of the drama refuse to take any responsibility for the tragedy. For the family of the deceased, the blame was on the deceased herself, as she could not sit alone in the 'room' she occupied, and on a social worker, whose 'duty' it allegedly was to help the old woman in need. A negative role according to the granddaughters was also to be played by the neighbours themselves, who – due to constant complaints about the stinking wound – 'forced' the daughter of the deceased woman to put her in a closed and isolated room. According to the neighbours, who eventually reported the case to the relevant services two months before the old woman's death, the deceased's family was entirely responsible for the situation.

However, the authors of the documentary, quoting the sometimes quite ethically ambiguous statements of the next-door neighbours, demonstrated that among the neighbours there was a certain degree of consent for the way the old woman had been treated. Her isolation was convenient for them since it guaranteed a relatively comfortable life far from the stench of her decaying old wound and the screams of the family in conflict. The problem was partly explained by the militiaman speaking in the film, 'When I asked them why someone took steps so late to inform us and to change the situation, people could not find an answer. It's only when the case becomes sensational and loud that everyone somehow wants to participate in the drama, wants to act as someone who can say something.'

The desire to cut oneself off from someone else's problem and concentrate on one's own everyday matters, as well as a kind of indifference to the needs of a helpless old woman, seemed to be the most universal symptom of the attitude of city dwellers towards older people living in their close proximity (or in their households) in the late 1960s and early 1970s. This was also pointed out – although beyond the context of this film – by a publicist:

> The family cell – for reasons entirely beyond its control – brings bad prospects for the increasing demographic ageing of the population. Every street and every household in it has at least one gloomy flat, where ageing eyes mourn their plight. The desks of care departments are crammed with letters from those who appeal to what we used to call the social conscience. To a large extent they remain just appeals. ... In recent years there has been a proliferation of reflections on ways of alleviating the plight of the older person. ... Ageing people, dependent on our loyalty, cannot wait for great reforms to mature.

The counterpoint to the 'immaturity' and inability of the state to take responsibility for the fate of older citizens that emerges from this statement is the social conscience or the expected social (family) readiness to face the problem. What does not appear in any of the above quotations, however, is the livelihood and economic context of the fate of seniors and their families.

Poverty in communist Poland was a common phenomenon and problems with provisions and housing (in cities) affected almost everyone. In practice, this translated into overcrowded flats, growing frustration resulting from the inaccessibility of a range of goods and the constant focus of families on their economic difficulties. As the letters also show, many requests for material or financial assistance from older citizens were motivated by a desire to help their adult children or to relieve them of the burden of supporting an infirm parent. This usually involved older women, who, due to the early termination of their employment (usually after the birth of their first child), had not acquired the right to any pension benefits. In their cases, the only solution suggested by social workers was to collect alimony from their children. The vast majority of older women, however, out of concern for their children, in such cases withdrew their claims or were quite selective in their approach.

Family conflicts and old grudges also cast a shadow over the relationship between ageing parents and their children. The emotionally charged refusal of adult children to take responsibility for the fate of an older parent was evident in many of the stories in the significant collection of letters from this period.[50] Importantly, however, the desire to reduce the time spent caring for older parents as quickly as possible – or to transfer this duty to state institutions – did not necessarily characterize only dysfunctional families at the time. An interesting example of this was the case of a woman in her sixties who, because of her age, professional work, and desire to care for her granddaughter, took steps to place her now older parents (aged ninety and eighty-one) in a pensioners' home near Warsaw. According to archived correspondence, despite her application for placement in the facility being approved, in the end the parents themselves did not agree to stay there, resigning voluntarily (and without the daughter's knowledge) from the placement.[51]

Although in this case the daughter managed to work out a compromise with her parents (they agreed to stay in a smaller home), it is worth stressing that a stay in an institution dedicated to lonely and infirm persons was often treated by older urbanites in the same way as by rural old people – as a last resort. These institutions also did not have a very good reputation and were perceived by many as the repository of 'abandoned parents'.

As shown by the accounts of residents of one such facility in Łódz, staying in a pensioners' home was, for many, associated with a specific trauma, the origin of which lay in the experiences from their family home or circumstances accompanying their admission to the centre. As some of the older residents reported: 'She [the daughter] left me here. And, sir, when she brought me in, she immediately took everything off me – she took my stockings and shoes and left. She didn't even say goodbye to me. At night I keep walking in the corridor because I can't sleep.'[52] 'That older son, the one I lived with, he used to beat me a lot. He strangled me three times, mistreated me.' 'They started to poison me. ... I lost consciousness. ... I don't want to go home, because they'll poison me again.'[53]

In addition, the number of beds available in pensioners' homes was insufficient throughout the entire communist era.[54] Many times, hospitals were used as a shelter for abandoned older people, as doctors' recollections from the 1980s testify.[55] Until the end of the People's Republic of Poland, long-term stays of older people who had nowhere to go after finishing their treatment were a kind of norm among all inpatients. Such stories can also be found in letters and requests sent to the central authorities.[56] From the early 1970s, however, a system of specialized social organizations aimed at helping the old people also gradually developed. Social welfare centres were established at district health centres, replacing the voluntary system of social workers which had existed since 1959.[57] The number of 'Seniors' Clubs', i.e. facilities providing opportunities for the daily socialization of older people, was slowly increasing.[58] However, as most of these facilities were located in larger cities, they were inaccessible to many older Polish citizens.

The loneliness and economic poverty of older Polish people was therefore a fairly common occurrence. As statistical data from 1950 to 1970 show, throughout the entire communist period this also affected women to a much greater extent. Throughout these decades the proportion of women among seniors was significant and remained approximately 70 per cent.[59] This was undoubtedly a reflection of the 'premature mortality of men aged 25–60 years', which has been described by some researchers of Polish health policy.[60] In the urban context it was also a result of changes in the policy of including women in the workforce, which had been liberal in the Stalinist period and was significantly curtailed after the 'October Thaw' (de-Stalinisation).[61] After 1956 women not only worked in lower-paid and less prestigious jobs, but also worked for shorter periods of time, and after giving birth to a child they often did not return to gainful employment, which in old age often translated into an inability to apply for retirement benefits and condemned them to full financial dependence on having a husband, raising children or relying on the state. Eleonora P., referred to earlier, was just one such an example.

Conclusion

Ageing in post-war Poland was associated with economic and social degradation, a sense of injustice and the growing loneliness of older citizens, not infrequently aligned with the beliefs present in public discourse about the redundancy/uselessness of old and infirm people. In a country where for decades the public space and public discourse had been dominated by the slogan of work as the supreme human value, this was all the more poignant. The difficult and sometimes dire fate of thousands of senior citizens exposed the complete lack of preparedness of both the state and society to face this growing social issue.

The state's immaturity was reflected in the long marginalization of social policy resulting in the inadequate systemic reforms and inequalities that gave rise to a sense of injustice and segregation, forcing older people to live in poverty or destitution, or to live in total economic dependence on their relatives. The complete transfer of responsibility for the fate of the old people onto their families was also expressed in the almost complete inaccessibility of institutions, i.e. facilities providing both safe places to stay for the neediest and most lonely seniors (retirement homes) and facilities enabling them to socialize and counteract or minimize social deprivation, loneliness and their sense of superfluity. Locked in tenements, or in decaying country houses, older Polish citizens and their needs disappeared from the public space of Polish villages and cities, appearing in the latter only as useful 'queuers' and acquirers of scarce goods or as the protagonists of dramatic news reports and documentaries.

Funding acknowledgement

The research was financed by the National ScienceCenter in Poland pursuant to Decision no DEC-2015/17/B/HS3/00170.

Notes

1   Archive of the Centre for Documentation and Programme Collections of TVP SA, Radio Committee 'Polskie Radio', Letter Office, [Hereafter: ACDPC TVP] ref: 1050/17, Bulletin No. 54 (8 September 1956). Cited in Dariusz Jarosz, *Rzeczy, ludzie, zjawiska. Studia z historii społecznej stalinizmu w Polsce* (Warsaw: IH PAN, 2013), 70.
2   ACDPC TVP, ref: 1050/37, Bulletin No 1. See also: Jarosz, *Rzeczy, ludzie, zjawiska*, 69–70.
3   The concept of biopolitics described by Michel Foucault is largely derived from his notion of 'biopower' and can be understood as the state's practical application of practices meant to organize and control people as bodies, the purpose which is 'to ensure, sustain and multiply life to put this life in order'. See Michel Foucault, *Narodziny biopolityki* (Warsaw: PWN, 2011), 22, 42.
4   Dariusz Jarosz, 'Życie niewesołe. Ludzie starzy w krajobrazie społecznym PRL', in A. Janiak–Jasińska, K. Sierakowska, and A. Szwarc (eds.), *Ludzie starzy i starość na ziemiach polskich od XVIII do XXI wieku (na tle porównawczym)*, vol. 2, 153 (Warsaw, 2016): DiG; S. Klonowicz, 'Starzenie się ludności', in I. Borsowa et al. (eds.), *Encyklopedia seniora* (Warsaw: Wiedza Powszechna, 1986), 45; Jarosz, *Rzeczy, ludzie, zjawiska*, 72.
5   J. Kurczab, 'O spokojną starość', *Przekrój*, 16 June 1968, 5.

6   *Mały Rocznik Statystyczny* (Warsaw: GUS, 1974), 15.
7   *Mały Rocznik Statystyczny*, 25 (after 1956, about 70–80 per cent of residents in rural areas made a living by working on individual farms).
8   An annuity was a traditional form of retirement security for the rural population, dating back to the Middle Ages. It was a written or oral agreement (signed in front of witnesses or with a notary), according to which the transferor of land specified the conditions of its transfer and defined in detail the scope of services and securities which the recipient of land undertook to provide to the farmer until his death (usually it came down to a guarantee of accommodation, food, provisions, etc.). Jarosz, *Życie niewesołe*, 153; Barbara Tryfan, *System emerytalny w opiniach ludności wiejskiej* (Warsaw: PAN, 1978), 6; B. Tryfan, *Problemy ludzi starych na wsi. Studium porównawcze sytuacji w Polsce i we Francji* (Warsaw: PAN, 1971), 127–44.
9   It is estimated that around 1 million young inhabitants emigrated from the rural countryside between 1950 and 1956. In the entire period of the People's Republic of Poland, migration from the countryside to the cities was to involve around 6 million people, Dariusz Jarosz, *Polacy a stalinizm 1948–1956* (Warszawa: Instytut Historii PAN, 2000), 65 and Jarosz, *Rzeczy, ludzie, zjawiska*, 224.
10 Tomasz Inglot, *Welfare States in East Central Europe, 1919–2004* (Warszawa: Elipsa, Wydawnictwo Wyższej Szkoły Pedagogicznej TWP, 2010), 196.
11 Jarosz, *Rzeczy, ludzie, zjawiska*, 80–1.
12 Ibid.
13 Ibid., 85; In 1958, 40 per cent of pensioners were employed, of which more than half were people 70–80 years of age. See: W. Muszalski, *Zatrudnienie a ubezpieczenie społeczne* (Warsaw: PWN, 1992), 158.
14 T. Gortat, 'Zaopatrzenie emerytalne w Polsce', in E. Rosseta et al. (eds.), *Problemy ludzi starych w Polsce* (Warsaw: PWE, 1974), 167.
15 Jarosz, *Rzeczy, ludzie, zjawiska*, 70.
16 Ibid.
17 These improvements included recognizing periods of war service and time spent in camps and prisons as counting towards 'length of service', as well an increase in benefits.
18 Ibid., 70.
19 As quoted in D. Jarosz, 'Emeryci w przestrzeni publicznej Polski gomułkowskiej', *Polska 1944/45–1989. Studia i Materiały* 11 (2013): 86.
20 In 1950 the average pension was 17 per cent of the average wage; in 1958 it rose to about 30 per cent.
21 Jarosz, *Rzeczy, ludzie, zjawiska*, 93.
22 Ibid., 102.
23 Inglot, *Welfare states in East Central Europe*, 206; For example, in 1970 the average monthly pension from the general pension insurance amounted to 1,080 zlotys (the 'old wallet'), while newly awarded pensions were at the level of 1,340 zlotys

(the 'new wallet') and benefits for privileged groups (e.g., miners) oscillated around 2,000–2,500 zlotys. At the same time, the average monthly earnings of employed people fluctuated around 2,000–2,700 zlotys).

24 Ibid.
25 Ibid., 211.
26 Lucyna Frąckiewicz, *Karta praw człowieka starego* (Warsaw: Instytut Wydawniczy Związków Zawodowych, 1985), 90.
27 Ibid.
28 Pensions received before 1982 were several times lower than for those who switched to it in 1985, Michał Zawisza, 'Problemy bytowe ludzi starych', in N. Jarska and J. Olaszek (eds.), *Społeczeństwo polskie w latch 1980 – 1989* (Warsaw: IPN, 2015), 132.
29 Frąckiewicz, *Karta praw człowieka starego*, 90.
30 The pension system was administered locally, under the supervision of voivodeships and municipal councils.
31 Katarzyna Stańczak-Wiślicz, 'Największy problem to starcy, kaleki i dzieci. Obrazy starości w dyskursach o odbudowie Warszawy po II wojnie światowej', in A. Janiak Jasińska, K. Sierakowska, and A. Szwarc (eds.), *Ludzie starzy i starość na ziemiach polskich od XVIII do XXI wieku* (Warsaw: DiG, 2016), 387–95.
32 O. Budrewicz, 'Pomóżcie starości i samotności', *Przekrój*, 22 December 1963, 7; J. Bujak, 'Oddam klucze', *Polityka*, 18 April 1970, 7; J. Lesseman, 'Samotni bez samotności', *Przekrój*, 22 September 1974, 11; W. Grochola, Jak być starym, *Polityka*, 25 January 1975, 4–7; W. Kopaliński, 'Uwaga seniorzy nadchodzą', *Polityka*, 8 March 1975, 3; H. Szwarc, Zachować siły witalne, *Przekrój*, 19 November 1978, 5, 11.
33 M. Karczewski, 'Rola i miejsce pomocy społecznej', in E. Rosseta et al. (eds.), *Problemy ludzi starych w Polsce* (Warsaw: PWE, 1974), 153–7.
34 Archive of Contemporary Records – [hereafter ACR], Kancelaria Rady Państwa [Chancellery of the Council of State – hereafter CCS], ref. 89/1, Sprawozdania roczne i analizy anonimów w 1962–1965, 174.
35 ACR, CCS, ref. 89/2, Sprawozdania roczne i analizy anonim w 1966–1969, 72.
36 A. Kamiński, 'Wychowanie do starości', *Kierunki*, March 1970, 1, 6; Grochola, 'Jak być starym', 2, 4, 7; M. Gumińska, 'Starości sny niewesołe', *Więź* 11, no. 9 (1968): 69–75; Piotr Krasucki, *Praca ludzi starszych* (Warsaw: Instytut Wydawniczy CRZZ, 1979); J. Piotrowski, 'Miejsce człowieka starego w społeczeństwie', in I. Borsowa et al. (eds.), *Encyklopedia seniora* (Warsaw: Wiedza Powszechna, 1986), 71–165; Jadwiga Różycka, *Psychologia zachowań kobiet w wieku starszym* (Wrocław: Ossolineum, 1971); Irena Gumowska, *Życie bez starości* (Warsaw: Wiedza Powszechna, 1962).
37 Jarosz, 'Emeryci w przestrzeni publicznej Polski gomułkowskiej', 69, 70.
38 In 1989, however, there were around 250,000 more senior citizens living in cities.

39 J. Łopato, 'Społeczna kwestia ludzi starych na wsi', in B. Rysz-Kowalczyk (ed.), *Społeczne kwestie starości* (Warsaw: Ośrodek Badań Społecznych, 1991), 52.
40 Ewelina Szpak, *Mentalność ludności wiejskiej w PRL. Studium zmian* (Warsaw: Scholar, 2013).
41 Archiwum Ośrodka Dokumentacji i Zbiorów Publicznych [Archive of the Centre for Documentation and Public Collections – hereafter ACDPS], Biuro Listów – Komitet ds Radia i Telewizji [Office of Letters of the Radio and Television Committee– hereafter OLRTC], ref. 1231/2, Internal Bulletin 1971: *The Atrophy of the Heart* continued ..., (10) 2.
42 ACDPS, OLRTC, *The Atrophy of the Heart*, continued, 10.
43 Ibid., 14.
44 Ibid., 15.
45 Zawisza, 'Problemy bytowe ludzi starych', 131.
46 Research shows that the 1960s around 63–67 per cent of Polish seniors lived in their own home, together with their spouse and/or children or other family members; less than 17 per cent lived alone; Archiwum Badań Opinii Publicznej [Archive of the Public Opinion Research Centre] – hereafter ACDPS, Henryk Stasiak, Sprawy ludzi w wieku emerytalnym – ankieta z 1960 r., Warsaw: 1961, 15; Jarosz, *Życie niewesołe*, 177.
47 ACDPS, Henryk Stasiak, Sprawy ludzi, 10.
48 Zawisza, 'Problemy bytowe ludzi starych', 137.
49 Krzysztof Gradowski (dir.), *Zanik serca* [*The Atrophy of the Heart*] (Film; Poland: Wywórnia Filmów Dokumentalnych, 1970). Additional sources of information concerning Eleonora's P. fate are archival documents and press releases: ACDPS, OLRTC: *The Atrophy of the Heart*, continued ..., 10; 'Kronika sądowa', *Życie Warszawy*, 11–12 January 1970, 11; 'Więziły matkę w okratowanym mieszkaniu', *Głos Robotniczy*, 9 Februrary 1970, 4.
50 Anna Adamus, Dariusz Jarosz, Grzegorz Miernik, and Ewelina Szpak, *Letters to the Central Authorities in Poland, 1945–1989 (A Guidebook)* (Warsaw: Instytut Historii PAN, 2019).
51 Archive of the Chancellery of the President of the Republic of Poland, Chancellery of the State Council, Complaints Division, ref. 763/5 (1).
52 *The Atrophy of the Heart*.
53 Ibid.
54 In 1960 there were only forty-two retirement homes in Poland (providing 3,500 beds); in 1973 the numbers rose to eighty-seven houses (with 8,500 beds), *Mały Rocznik*, 265.
55 Anita M. Magowska, 'Medicine in the Polish People's Republic', in A. Bochen et al. (eds.), *Polish Medicine* (Bydgoszcz: Quxi Media, 2018), 172. Available online: http://redakcja.quixi.pl/link/Medycyna.pdf, accessed 20 July 2021.

56 ACR, CCS, ref. 101/40, Akta skarg w sprawach rent i pomocy społecznej 1972, 206–7.
57 Janina Szumlicz, *Pomoc społeczna w polskim systemie zabezpieczeń społecznych* (Warsaw: IPPiS, 1987), 51.
58 Frąckiewicz, *Karta praw człowieka starego*, 91.
59 Jarosz, 'Emeryci w przestrzeni publicznej Polski gomułkowskiej', 69.
60 Witold Zatoński, *Rozwój sytuacji zdrowotnej w Polsce na tle innych krajów Europy Środkowo-Wschodniej* (Warsaw: Maria Skłodowska-Curie: Institute of Oncology Anta, 2001), 7.
61 Natalia Jarska, *Kobiety z marmuru. Robotnice w Polsce w latach 1945–1960* (Warsaw: IPN, 2015).

11

Ageing and gerontology in Britain after 1945: The 'menace' of an ageing population

Pat Thane

In 1945 Britain was experiencing a panic about the ageing of society, similar to present concerns in the early twenty-first century. From the 1870s the birth rate underwent an unprecedented decline, reaching its lowest recorded point in 1941–2. At the same time, average life expectancy rose: in 1901 6.2 per cent of the population were of what by 1941 was state pensionable age (males sixty-five, females sixty), by 1941 the figure was 12 per cent. These trends were expected to continue indefinitely. From the 1920s there were growing concerns about the risk to the economy from a declining working-age population required to fund the increasing costs of pensions and care for retired people, views expressed at the time by, among others, the internationally respected economist and government adviser, John Maynard Keynes, and William Beveridge, expert on social insurance and wartime government adviser, whose work is discussed later. Similar concerns were heard in France, Germany, Italy and other European countries which had similarly declining birth rates. The international concern stimulated the growth of the science of demography, driven by the desire to understand why birth rates rise and fall and the social and economic implications of changing population structures.[1]

In Britain there were fears about an assumed threat to international and race relations and Britain's position in the world. William Beveridge suggested in 1924, and was echoed by others, that the declining birth rate could:

> Bring about a stationary white population after or long before the white man's world is full ... [and] ... leave one race at the mercy of another's growing numbers or drive it to armaments or permanent aggression in self-defence.[2]

There was scepticism in Britain that the problem could be solved by providing material incentives to women to have more children, as was being attempted in fascist countries. Britain had an active women's movement enthusiastic about birth control and the value of fewer births for women's health and freedom. Feminists favoured the falling birth rate. The thoughts of politicians and reformers turned towards recognizing and assessing the potential of older people to make positive contributions to society and the economy rather than perceiving them simply as costly burdens. The influential sociologist, David Glass, argued in the late 1930s that the work capacity of older people was unknown but could potentially be extended by new technology or changes in the organization of work, together with continued improvement in standards of health and health care.[3]

The debate about the ageing population was muted during the Second World War, when people had other concerns, although William Beveridge, in his influential 1942 report on social insurance, recommended that the improved pensions scheme he proposed should include a built-in incentive for older people to stay at work for as long as possible by receiving a higher pension for each year worked past the official retirement age.[4] The post-war Labour government implemented this in only a token way, however, with small increments to pensions for each additional year worked. This was one of Labour's many modifications to Beveridge's proposals due to post-war financial difficulties and their prioritizing the rebuilding of the economy over social expenditure. In fact the birth rate rose unexpectedly from 1942, leading to the post-war 'baby-boom', but not until the 1950s was it widely recognized that a sustained rise in births was under way. Until then, panic about long-term decline revived after 1945, further stimulated by the fact that by 1947 Labour had achieved full employment and there was a labour shortage.

Older people and work

From 1947 the independent Nuffield Foundation invested heavily in research into the work capacities of older people, to test and counter commonplace negative assertions based on prejudice rather than knowledge.[5] The outcome in the 1950s was a series of impressive, innovative studies by industrial anthropologists and industrial psychologists, the first to study older people at work and their work capacities. These were overwhelmingly male workers and rarely women, who were assumed to be less vital to the economy. They found that men could work efficiently at least into their later sixties in a wide variety of occupations, including heavy manual labour, if they could control their pace of work. A study of miners found that older men could cut coal as efficiently as younger men: what caused them the most strain was the walk through the mine to the coal-face when younger men set a fast pace.[6] It was found that the work efficiency of older people deteriorated fastest when the pace was controlled by machines or time stipulations. Such work could be adapted to the needs of older workers without sacrificing productivity. It was concluded that whatever older workers lost in speed, adaptability or the capacity to learn new skills (which was much less than commonly assumed) was compensated in most occupations by experience, skill and reliability. Most younger workers were under-stretched and had reserves to call upon as they aged. It was emphasized that where older people appeared to be conservative and inflexible at work, this was often due to socialization and their internalization of widespread low expectations and assumptions of decline, rather than reflecting their actual potential. Due to low expectations, employers rarely offered further training to people over forty.[7]

Labour, then Conservative, governments in the late 1940s and 1950s tried to convey this positive image of older workers to employers, who were exhorted to keep them at work, with little success because most employers shared the pervasive negative image of older people. Also few employers were seriously affected by a shortage of labour as more women entered the workforce (though rarely in normally male jobs) and increasing numbers of young immigrant workers arrived with government encouragement and support and were directed into shortage areas.[8] And older people themselves preferred to retire if they could afford it on their pensions and savings. State pensions improved from 1946 but were still low – lower than Beveridge had recommended – but more people retired at the official pension ages than ever before. The percentage of men aged 65–69 who were retired rose from 32 in 1931, to 48.8 in 1951, to 62.7 in 1961.[9] Very many of them, having worked hard since their early teens, welcomed a period of leisure.[10] Also many adult children became better-off due to full employment and could give their parents more support. Retirement became a recognized phase of life for most working-class people for the first time.

The positive findings of the research about work capabilities in later life were largely forgotten when the ageing panic in Britain subsided from the 1950s, but the previously limited understanding of old age had begun to expand.

The emergence of geriatric medicine

A longer-lasting shift to greater understanding and more positive thinking about old age had begun in the mid-1930s with the initiation of geriatric medicine in Britain.[11] It was already developing in the United States, France, Russia and Germany. From 1929 the long-established system of Poor Law relief, including workhouse hospitals, was merged into the local government system. Marjorie Warren, a doctor in a local authority hospital in London, was shocked to discover the neglect of older patients in the Poor Law hospital for which she gained responsibility. Poorer old people often ended their lives in these institutions when other hospitals would not accept them because they believed them incurable, and, unlike better-off people, they could not afford private care. She found 700 bedbound older people in large, dismal wards, with poorly trained nurses and largely ignored by doctors. Victims of heart attacks, strokes or other severe conditions were left in bed awaiting death. Warren had the wards attractively painted, provided dayrooms and activities, creating incentives to get out of bed. She seriously diagnosed patients' conditions and promoted physiotherapy and other forms of rehabilitation, enabling 200 of the initial patients to leave hospital to live with relatives or in care homes. She was among the first in Britain to recognize that diagnosis of older people could be difficult because they often suffered from multiple conditions including physical, mental and social ailments. But, as long as remained the case with geriatrics, her innovations were not recognized or well-regarded even at her own hospital.[12]

Over time, however, her work attracted the attention and support of the Ministry of Health and the British Medical Association (BMA), especially after the foundation of the National Health Service (NHS) in 1948. The British Geriatrics Society was formed in 1947 to promote the specialism and research and treatment gradually expanded, but it long remained a low-status field of medicine, in a highly status-conscious profession, especially concerning the mental health of older people which received particularly little attention, as historian Claire Hilton has described.[13] In 1975 a leading British geriatrician could still comment:

> There are few doctors with special knowledge of disease in the elderly; there are no nurses deliberately trained to care for the elderly ... Geriatrics is more a state of mind than a branch of medicine or a mode of treatment. It is a reaction against the belief that after sixty a patient is too old to be medically interesting or therapeutically rewarding.[14]

Progress was faster in Scotland with its tradition of high-quality medical training – although as late as 1958 Glasgow teaching hospitals still banned patients over age sixty-five. The development of geriatrics in Scotland was led by W. Ferguson Anderson, Britain's first Professor of Geriatrics at Glasgow University from 1964, who had been inspired by Warren. He made geriatric training obligatory for medical students in Glasgow. Not until the mid-1970s did the BMA urge it on all British medical schools.[15]

Nevertheless older, and many younger, people gained from Labour's introduction of the NHS, providing comprehensive free healthcare for the whole population. For the first time poorer people of all ages had access to free dental care and, of particular value to older people, free sight tests and spectacles and hearing aids. Previously many of them had resorted to spectacles bought second hand or passed on by relatives, or they had been left helplessly deaf. But the new services were imperfect and locally variable in quality. Gradually the NHS revealed older peoples' needs, but still in the early 1960s a high proportion of them had not accessed one or more of the services despite acute need, because they were locally inadequate or they were unaware of their rights or how to access them and they lacked advice.[16]

Age discrimination

Medical care for older people began to improve seriously only in the 1980s, when the birth rate was again declining and panic about the ageing population revived, again internationally. It had been assumed that the birth rate would remain satisfactorily high, until it began to decline again from c. 1968 following the introduction of the birth control pill and the revival of feminism. From the 1960s onwards medical research made breakthroughs especially valuable to older people, including cardiac pacemakers and kidney dialysis, from the 1970s there were quick developments in cataract, joint and organ replacement surgery. Evidence continued to emerge of age-based rationing of treatment, with younger people receiving precedence for these treatments. As late as in 1994 the Medical Research Council complained that there was too little research on health and illness in old age and that older people were normally excluded from clinical trials of the drugs, cancer therapies, coronary bypass surgeries and other treatments they were highly likely to need.[17] They were also often excluded from access to diagnosis and treatment for these and other conditions: universal free screening of women for breast cancer by the NHS stopped at age seventy, although women were/are more likely to suffer from breast cancer after the age of seventy. Even in 2021 women over seventy are not automatically invited for this screening, although they may request it.

There had long been discrimination against older people in healthcare as in employment and other areas of life. The underlying thinking was expressed in a comment made by William Beveridge in his 1942 report: 'It is dangerous to be in any way lavish to old age until adequate provision has been assured for all other vital needs, such as prevention of disease and the adequate nutrition of the young.'[18] Such thinking has certainly not gone away, as was evident from the treatment of older people by the NHS during the Covid-19 pandemic. Patients over the age of sixty suffering from Covid-19 were too often denied treatment due to the prioritization of younger people. Many with other conditions were moved from hospitals into care homes to free beds for younger Covid-19 patients, without being first tested for Covid-19, adding to the high rates of infection and death in these homes.

Until late in the twentieth century older people rarely protested against age discrimination, apparently internalizing popular assumptions that they did not deserve equal treatment with younger people who still had their lives ahead of them and much to contribute to society, whereas their own lives and contributions were almost over. But as the 'baby-boom' generation grew older, many of them better educated, more prosperous, healthier and more active at later ages than their predecessors and more accustomed to public protest – they were also the 1968 generation grown older – they organized against what became known as ageist discrimination in healthcare, employment and much else. This led to some of the first research into age discrimination, including studies sponsored by the official Equality and Human Rights Commission (EHRC), established in 2007, which included age discrimination in its brief.[19] The first legislation against age discrimination was introduced more than forty years after the first UK legislation against Sex and Race discrimination. Age discrimination in health and social care became illegal under the Equality Act, 2010, implemented in 2012, but it has not been eliminated in practice.

The emergence of a more assertive, active older generation stimulated efforts to promote more positive attitudes to later life, stressing that old-age frailty could be prevented or delayed through physical and mental exercise and healthy eating, and that experiences in later life were not inevitable but could be shaped in positive ways.[20]

Social care

Many older people living in the community alone or with families or others, or in residential care homes, needed social care services but, like healthcare, these were never fully adequate. They expanded from 1948 with government funding, provided by local authorities or by voluntary organizations supervised by local authorities. These public and private institutions employed social workers to support older people and their carers, home helps (as they were known) to perform housework and district nurses to care for the sick, while the voluntary Women's Voluntary Service (WVS) provided 'meals on wheels', free, ready-made meals delivered to the home. But these services received limited funding amid post-war austerity and local authority services were charged for and means-tested as healthcare was not. They were unevenly available across the country. The social researchers, Peter Townsend and Dorothy Wedderburn, found that still in the early 1960s many older people did not have access to the services they needed. Family and friends provided more support. The researchers found no evidence for the persistent rumour that the growth of public welfare services had displaced family care, rather they concluded that 'In illness and infirmity the role of the family dwarfs that of the social services'.[21] But families and friends could not always provide adequate care without suitably skilled assistance and the researchers advocated more intensive enquiry into family care which their research indicated was of highly variable quality. Better-off people, as ever, could pay for private care. The administrative separation of health and social care caused lasting problems because many older people needed social as well as healthcare, in the community or in institutions, due to physical or mental health conditions, such as dementia. This separation and the inadequacy of social services were persistently criticized, including by official reports, from the 1960s to the present, but with little response from successive governments for whom the needs of older people have had low priority.

After 1948 much local authority institutional care was of poor quality, often in former Poor Law workhouses in grim conditions because there was no funding for new buildings, conditions exposed by Peter Townsend in research conducted in the late 1950s and published as *The Last Refuge* in 1962. Townsend described his first visit to such an institution, which had stimulated the wider study:

> The first impression was grim and sombre. ... Several hundred residents were housed in large rooms on three floors. Dormitories were overcrowded, with ten or twenty iron-framed beds close together, no floor covering and little furniture

other than ramshackle lockers. The day-rooms were bleak and uninviting. In one of them sat forty men in high-backed Windsor chairs, staring straight ahead or down at the floor. They seemed oblivious of what was going on around them. ... They had the air of not worrying much about their problems because of the impossibility of sorting them out, or the difficulty of getting anyone to understand or take notice ...

The staff took the attitude that the old people had surrendered any claim to privacy ... They also admitted that improvements in staffing standards and in the conditions of the buildings had been small [since the days of the Poor Law].[22]

Townsend calculated the extent and variety of institutional provision (Table 11.1).

Table 11.1 Number of institutions and homes of various types in England and Wales

Type of institution	Number of institutions	Number of beds
Former public assistance	309	36,934
Other local authority	1105	36,699
Voluntary	815	25,491
Private	1106	11,643
Total	3335	110,767

Peter Townsend, The Last Refuge: A Survey of Residential Institutions and Homes for the Aged in England and Wales (London: Routledge and Kegan Paul, 1964), 24.

Townsend found no evidence for assertions that careless families increasingly abandoned older relatives into care homes. He and Wedderburn later found that most care home residents had no close relatives, or needed skilled, specialized care beyond the capacity of their relatives to provide.[23] When *The Last Refuge* revealed how little had changed in ten years since the system was reformed in 1948 it caused such shock and concern that it led in the 1960s and 1970s to increased public funding, the gradual improvement of publicly provided institutions and increasing emphasis upon community care provided by social workers to support and encourage independent living, though it remained means-tested, locally variable and far from meeting the needs of all older people. Sheltered housing, with carers on site, was also increasingly though unevenly provided, also recommended by Townsend.[24] But all social services suffered severe cuts and privatization into the hands of profit-seeking providers under the neoliberal Conservative governments of Margaret Thatcher in the 1980s, a policy followed still more intensely by governments since 2010. Access to and conditions in the already precarious care system deteriorated, severely increasing pressure on family carers who suffered ever more severe stress, exhaustion and risk of breakdown.[25]

Social research

There was an unprecedented amount of research into the lives and experiences of older people in the later 1940s, 1950s and 1960s, part of a general expansion of social research. Townsend and Wedderburn commented: 'Suddenly in the late forties and fifties, or so it may seem to the historian of the written or spoken word, the problems of old age were discovered.'[26] They highlighted a 'selected list' of thirty-three 'Social Surveys of Old People' made across the UK, 1945–64.[27] These focused upon the problems of poorer people, since older people were believed to be the largest group in poverty following the development of the post-war welfare state and full employment, and there was growing concern about their conditions. Further research by Peter Townsend and his colleague at the London School of Economics, Brian Abel-Smith, in the early 1960s revealed considerable poverty among low-income working families with children, though older people remained the largest single group in poverty.[28]

Much of this research reinforced images of older people as a problem group: weak, dependent, lonely, poor and miserable, which was true of some but by no means all, as some researchers revealed. Another Nuffield-funded survey, of older people living alone in Wolverhampton in the late 1940s, concluded that, although many older people lived alone, they did so from choice not as a result of family neglect, because they believed that independent living kept them fit and active. Living alone did not necessarily signify loneliness, as was widely assumed, for most older people surveyed had close contact with family and friends. The researchers pointed out that older women, up to at least age seventy-five, 'give the community more than they take in the matter of domestic responsibility' through caring for grandchildren and sick and disabled children and nursing other sick relatives, neighbours and friends.[29] This point was also later made by Townsend and Wedderburn who concluded that older people 'need to be independent and to be able to play a part as givers as well as receivers'.[30] Older people were shown to be making a significant, hidden, contribution to the economy and to social welfare.[31]

The family lives of older people

Social research steadily extended knowledge and understanding of later life. An influential example was *Family and Kinship in East London* by Michael Young and Peter Wilmot which studied a sample of residents in working-class Bethnal Green in East London in 1953–5.[32] It contributed further to shattering what had been the conventional conviction of sociologists: that in the busy, prosperous, mobile, modern world 'traditional' close family ties had been destroyed, causing familial neglect of older relatives. The researchers found that relationships between ageing parents and their adult children in Bethnal Green were generally close. They often lived close to one another and families were the main providers of care for older people who needed it, far more than the formal social services.

This was reinforced by Peter Townsend's study of *The Family Life of Old People* in Bethnal Green in 1954–5, based upon 203 interviews with people above pension age and week-long diaries kept by twelve of them.[33] This, Townsend's first study of older people, published in 1957, studied working-class people, asking 'How many of them are miserable or poverty-stricken?' Fewer than often believed, he discovered, partly because family obligations were taken more, not less, seriously than before and families were central to the lives of all but a very few older people, even when, as many did, they preferred the independence of living alone. Relatives, mainly daughters, helped them when needed. Townsend was even more surprised and impressed by how often this help was reciprocated, 'through provision of midday meals, care of grandchildren, and other services. The major function of the grandparent is perhaps the most important fact to emerge from this book'.[34] A small minority of older people *were* isolated and lonely. They needed support from public health and welfare services, as did families seeking to provide adequate care of frail relatives, but Townsend found that these services suffered from 'lack of coordination and inadequacy'. He also argued that older people needed more substantial pensions.[35]

Social research at this time tended to focus on the 'lower' classes – perhaps the better-off were more resistant to scrutiny. An exception was Wilmott and Young's study of Woodford, a London suburb of relatively prosperous middle-class and skilled working-class owner-occupiers, which they undertook to establish whether family relationships were more 'modern' and less close than in long-settled, working-class Bethnal Green.[36] They interviewed a sample of residents in 1957–9 and concluded that 'perhaps the greatest surprise of the whole report is that the two places are so alike'.[37] 'The old people of the suburb are plainly as much in touch with their children … as those in the East End'.[38] Adult children rarely lived as close to their ageing parents and they saw each other less often, but neither generation resented this, each valuing their independence. They helped each other when needed and could more easily keep in touch over a distance than in the past or among poorer people by car, telephone or letter-writing.[39] As parents grew older, into their seventies and eighties, they saw more of their children and more often lived with them.[40] In Woodford as in Bethnal

Green 'the family is … the main source of support' and 'the old … are no more neglected than in Bethnal Green'.[41] Only 21 per cent of the minority of older people without children lived alone; most lived with relatives, mainly siblings, others with friends. Very few expressed loneliness.[42]

The diversity of later life

Representations of old age in Britain in the generation after 1945 gradually extended awareness of the diversity of a much stereotyped stage of life, though it remained limited. 'Old age', as it continues to be conventionally defined, stretches from people in their sixties to past 100 – longer than most age groups – and includes the very rich and the very poor, the very frail and marathon runners in their nineties, among many other differences. Also it has long been predominantly a female experience because women tend to outlive men, though they do not necessarily spend more years in good health. In 1951 average life expectancy at birth was 72.7 years for men, 78.3 for women;[43] in 2018 79.6 for men, 83.2 for women.[44] Townsend and Wedderburn rightly commented on how rarely this was noted in studies of old age, or that, as their research showed, older women were more likely to suffer poverty than older men, especially if they were unmarried or widowed early in life, because they earned less and so could save less and often qualified for lower pensions.[45] Also, following divorce, women were generally poorer than men. All of this remains true to this day but it is still rarely noted.[46] Townsend and Wedderburn described the diversity of older peoples' lives more broadly, including in their incomes and living conditions, and challenged popular myths, including evidence further questioning the assumed displacement of family care by state welfare.

Rich, active people were and are less likely to be represented as 'old' – by the media for example – than those who appear to fit the conventional stereotype. William Beveridge was sixty-three when his report appeared in 1942. He remained very active in public life, travelling and writing until close to his death in 1963,[47] at the age of eighty-four. Winston Churchill was sixty-five, retirement age, when he became Premier at the beginning of the war in 1939, seventy-one when it ended; seventy-seven when he became Premier again in 1951, retiring in 1955 at eighty-one following a stroke, though he lived to the age of ninety-one. So far as I am aware, neither man was described as a problematic social burden due to his age as poorer people were. Nor were general conclusions drawn about competence in later life from the activities of such prominent people.

In the post-war decades older people were widely represented in social research and everyday comment as needy and problematic. This changed from around 2010 when the ageing 'baby boomer' generation (born 1945–65) began to be represented as exceptionally wealthy and selfish, and the interests of older and younger generations were represented as seriously conflicting. This perception was stimulated by a book by David Willetts, then a Conservative government Minister: *The Pinch. How the Baby Boomers Took Their Children's Future – and Why They Should Give It Back*.[48] This poorly researched work argued that the baby boomers constituted 'the biggest, richest generation that Britain has ever known', due to large occupational pensions and savings following high lifetime incomes, plus ownership of property which had risen sharply in value since the 1970s, in contrast with younger generations with relatively low incomes and poorer pension prospects who could not afford to buy their homes. The older generation were accused of selfishly lavishing their money on their own pleasures rather than supporting younger people.[49]

It was true that some older people were and are wealthy, but thousands were and are very poor, most but not all of them women. The independent research institution, the Joseph Rowntree Foundation found that in 2017 1.9m pensioners in the UK, 16 per cent of all pensioners, were living below the internationally recognized poverty line (incomes below 60 per cent of the median), while many thousands lived precariously just above the line because the UK has the lowest state pensions and means-tested supplements in Western Europe.[50]

Willetts and his followers overlooked the fact that inequalities within generations are as significant as inequalities between them. A sensitive indicator of this is the gap in life expectancy between rich and poor. I cannot find figures for this in the post-war decades, but in 2010 a man born in wealthy Kensington in London could expect to live seventeen years longer than a man born in poorer, racially mixed Tottenham, and to remain healthy for a similarly longer period.[51] There was a similar gap among women. The disparities continue. In 2016–18, life expectancy at birth for the most prosperous males in England averaged 83.4 years, for the least prosperous (including many Black and Asian residents) 73.9; female life expectancy varied between 86.3 and 78.7 years. There were similar inequalities in expectation of healthy life.[52] It is likely there was a similar gap in the 1940s and 1950s.

And there is clear evidence that, far from selfishly spending their surplus wealth on expensive cruises and other pleasures while the younger generation pay for their pensions and care, many wealthy older people transfer substantial sums in their lifetimes to younger relatives before passing on their remaining assets at death.

These transfers are not easy to trace because they are not officially recorded, but it was shown in 2005 that 31 per cent of grandparents helped grandchildren to buy a home; 16 per cent in their sixties and one-third in their seventies gave financial help to grandchildren and, increasingly as times got harder, to their children.[53] They gave, and give, in kind as well as cash. One researcher concluded that:

> Generally more Third Age parents were providers than recipients of help ... Parental characteristics associated with higher probability of providing help included higher income, home ownership and being married or widowed rather than divorced ... in contravention of depictions of older adults as 'burdens' on younger generations.[54]

In recent decades growing numbers of older people, male as well as female, have helped their children to work by caring for their grandchildren, sometimes giving up their own work to do so. In 2010 one in three working mothers relied on grandparents for childcare, mostly but not exclusively in poorer families.[55] The number is likely to have increased as the costs of other forms of childcare have continued to rise. Similarly, the stereotype of even prosperous older people as 'burdens' upon younger generations, perpetuated by Willetts and others, overlooks other positive contributions of older people to their communities and families.[56] As well as caring for grandchildren and other younger relatives, increasingly they contribute paid work, many because they need the money, others because they enjoy their work. The number of over-sixty-fives in employment grew by 188 per cent from 1999 to 2019, from 5 per cent of all workers to 11 per cent, or 1.31 million workers.[57] People aged sixty-five to seventy-four are also the most likely age group to engage in voluntary work in the UK, often supplementing the welfare state, with 28 per cent of people in this age group serving as volunteers in 2018/2019.[58] In 2013 (the most recent available estimate), over-sixty-fives contributed sixty-one billion pounds to the UK economy through employment, caring for others and volunteering, considerably more than they cost the budget.[59] This net contribution has certainly grown since 2013, as older people's employment, taxpaying and volunteering has grown.

Conclusion

In 1945 knowledge and understanding of old age was very limited in Britain. It has since grown substantially, and is increasingly described as 'gerontology', a field of study drawing upon a range of disciplines, including sociology, social policy, history, medicine, biology and psychology. The research has challenged many long-established stereotypes about older people, including their representation as dependent 'burdens' upon productive younger people, incapable of useful work and increasingly neglected by their families in the modernizing world. Substantial gaps in our knowledge remain and there is a persistent gulf between scientific and popular and political perceptions of later life which tend to cling to stereotypes and negative representations, encouraging discrimination against older people which has never gone away despite increasing evidence of its reality and injustice. This survives persistent and convincing evidence of the diversity of later life including between rich and poor, fit and frail and of the contributions of older people, rich and poor, to the economy, communities and families through paid and voluntary work and care for family and friends, contributions which continue to grow as their numbers grow and more are fit and active later in life. Far from being dependent burdens it is clear that, overall, older people give more than they receive. This is especially true of better-off elders who have been unjustly castigated for their selfish neglect and exploitation of younger generations. Of course a feature of diversity is that not all are or can be active in these ways. Some older people have always been frail, impoverished, lonely and dependent upon always inadequate public services. The persistent failure of governments of all persuasions to give priority to the needs of these older people is another signifier of persistent negativity and discrimination.

Notes

1. For further details and references on the discussion which follows, see P.M. Thane 'The Debate on the Declining Birth-rate in Britain: The Menace of an Ageing Population, 1920s–1950s', *Continuity and Change* 5, no. 2 (1990): 283–305.
2. Sir William Beveridge, 'Population and Unemployment', in R.L. Smyth (ed.), *Essays in the Economics of Socialism and Capitalism: Selected Papers Read to Section F, the British Association for the Advancement of Science 1886–1932* (London: British Association for the Advancement of Science, 1964).
3. D.V. Glass, *The Struggle for Population* (London, 1936).
4. Sir William Beveridge, *Social Insurance and Allied Services*, Report Cmd 6404 (London: HMSO, 1942), 59.
5. Nuffield Foundation, *Old People: Report of the Survey Committee on the Problem of Ageing and the Care of Old People* (London, 1947).
6. I.M. Richardson, 'Age and Work: A Study of 489 Men in Industry', *British Journal of Industrial Medicine* 10 (1953): 269–84.

7   F. Le Gros Clark with Agnes Clark, *Ageing and Industry* (London: Nuffield Foundation, 1956); also see further work by Le Gros Clark for the Nuffield Foundation: *Ageing Men in the Labour Force* (1955), *Bus Workers* (1957), *Women, Work and Age* (962), *Workers Nearing Retirement* (1963), *Work, Age and Leisure* (1966).
8   Linda McDowell, *Working Lives. Gender, Migration and Employment in Britain, 1945–2007* (Oxford: Wiley-Blackwell, 2013).
9   Sarah Harper and Pat Thane, 'The Consolidation of "Old Age" as a Phase of Life, 1945–1965', in Margot Jefferys (ed.), *Growing Old in the Twentieth Century* (London: Routledge, 1989), 47.
10 Thane, 'The Debate on the Declining Birth-Rate', 294–303.
11 For details and references about this, see Pat Thane, 'Geriatrics', in W.F. Bynum and Roy Porter (eds.), *Companion Encyclopedia of the History of Medicine*, vol. 2 (London: Routledge, 1993), 1092–18.
12 M. Warren, 'Care of the Chronic Aged Sick', *Lancet* (8 June 1948), 841–2; M. Warren, 'Care of the Chronic Sick: A Case for Treating Chronic Sick in Blocks in a General Hospital', *British Medical Journal* 2 (December 1943): 822; M. Warren, 'Geriatrics: A Medical, Social and Economic Problem', *Practitioner* 157 (1946): 384–90; M. Warren, 'The Evolution of Geriatric Care', *Geriatrics* 3 (1948): 42–50.
13 Claire Hilton, 'The Development of Psycho-Geriatric Services in England c. 1940–1989' (PhD dissertation, King's College London, 2014); Claire Hilton, *Improving Mental Health Services for Older People: Barbara Robb's Campaign, 1965–1975* (London: Palgrave Macmillan, 2017).
14 T.H. Howell, *Old Age. Some Practical Points in Geriatrics* (London: HK Lewis, 1975), 101.
15 W. Ferguson Anderson and Bernard Isaacs (eds.), *Current Achievements in Geriatrics* (London, 1964); Pat Thane, *Old Age in English History. Past Experiences, Present Issues* (Oxford: Oxford University Press, 2000), 436–40, 443–9.
16 J. Tunstall, *Old and Alone* (London: Routledge and Kegan Paul, 1966), 272–6.
17 Medical Research Council, *The Health of the UK's Elderly People* (London, 1994).
18 Beveridge, *Social Insurance and Allied Services*, 92.
19 See the Comission's website: https://www.equalityhumanrights.com/en, accessed 4 November 2021.
20 Alan Walker (ed.), *The New Science of Ageing* (Bristol: Policy Press, 2014); Alan Walker (ed.), *The New Dynamics of Ageing, Volume 1* (Bristol: Policy Press, 2018).
21 Peter Townsend and Dorothy Wedderburn, *The Aged in the Welfare State* (London: G. Bell and Sons Ltd, 1965), 135.
22 Peter Townsend, *The Last Refuge. A Survey of Residential Institutions and Homes for the Aged in England and Wales* (London: Routledge and Kegan Paul, 1964), 406.
23 Townsend and Wedderburn, *The Aged*, 1, 25–43.
24 Ibid., 63–8.

25 Carers Week, *Breaks or Breakdown. Carers Week Annual Report 2021* (London: Carers UK, 2021).
26 Ibid., 10.
27 Ibid., 140–3.
28 Brian Abel-Smith and Peter Townsend, *The Poor and the Poorest* (London: G.Bell and Sons Ltd, 1965).
29 J.H. Sheldon, *Social Medicine of Old Age* (Oxford: Oxford University Press, 1948).
30 Townsend and Wedderburn, *The Aged*, 103.
31 Ibid., 301–3.
32 Michael Young and Peter Willmott, *Family and Kinship in East London* (London: Routledge and Kegan Paul, 1957).
33 Peter Townsend, *The Family Life of Old People* (London: Routledge and Kegan Paul, 1957).
34 Peter Townsend, *The Family Life of Old People* (Harmondsworth: Pelican Books, 1963 [abridged ed.]), 228.
35 Ibid., 230.
36 Peter Willmot and Miichael Young, *Family and Class in a London Suburb* (London: Routledge and Kegan Paul, 1960).
37 Ibid., 37.
38 Ibid., 38.
39 Ibid., 79.
40 Ibid., 40.
41 Ibid., 50–1.
42 Ibid., 51–7.
43 UK Office of Population, Censuses and Surveys, *Population Trends* (1991), table 2.
44 Michael Marmot, *Health Equity in England: The Marmot Review 10 Years On* (London: Institute of Health Equity, 2020), 13–33.
45 Townsend and Wedderburn, *The Aged*, 88.
46 Pat Thane, 'The "Scandal" of Women's Pensions in Britain: How Did It Come About?', in H. Pemberton, P. Thane, and N. Whiteside (eds.), *Britain's Pensions Crisis. History and Policy* (Oxford: Oxford University Press, 2006), 77–90.
47 Jose Harris, *William Beveridge. A Biography* (Oxford: Oxford University Press, 1997), 461–77.
48 David Willetts, *The Pinch. How the Baby Boomers Took Their Children's Future – and Why They Should Give It Back* (London: Atlantic Books, 2010).
49 See also E. Howker and S. Malik, *Jilted Generation: How Britain Has Bankrupted Its Youth* (London: Icon Books, 2010).
50 Age UK, '300,000 More Pensioners Living in Poverty', *Age UK website*, 4 December 2017, online: https://www.ageuk.org.uk/latest-news/articles/2017/december/300000-more-pensioners-living-in-poverty/, accessed 4 November 2021.

51 Michael Marmot, *The Marmot Review: Fair Society and Healthy Lives. Strategic Review of Health Inequalities in England* (2010); online: www.marmotreview.org, accessed 4 November 2021.
52 Marmot, *Health Equity in England,* 15–20.
53 GrandparentsPlus, 'Policy Briefing Paper 01. Statistics' (Feburary 2011); Emily Grundy, 'Reciprocity in Relationships: Socio-economic and Health Influences upon Intergenerational Exchanges between Third Age Parents and Their Adult Children in Great Britain', *British Journal of Sociology* 56, no. 2 (2005): 233–55.
54 Grundy, 'Reciprocity in Relationships', 233.
55 Julia Griggs, *Protect, Support, Provide: Examining the Role of Grandparents in Families at Risk of Poverty* (London: EHRC and Grandparents Plus, 2010).
56 Among the growing numbers of publications challenging negative attitudes toward later life, see Yvonne Roberts, *One Hundred Not Out: Resilience and Active Ageing* (London, 2012); Margaret Morganroth Gullette, *Aged by Culture* (Chicago, 2004); Walker (ed.), *The New Science of Ageing.*
57 Labour Market Review, UK: December 2019, UK Office for National Statistics, online: https://www.ons.gov.uk/employmentandlabourmarket/peopleinwork/employmentandemployeetypes/bulletins/uklabourmarket/december2019, accessed 4 November 2021.
58 'Community Life Survey and Taking Part Survey 2017–18: Focus on Volunteering by Age and Gender', last updated 3 September 2019, GOV.UK, online: https://www.gov.uk/government/statistics/community-life-survey-and-taking-part-survey-2017-18-focus-on-volunteering-by-age-and-gender, accessed 4 November 2021.
59 Age UK, '£61 Billion – The Economic Contribution of People Aged 65 Plus', Age UK, 1 July 2014, https://www.ageuk.org.uk/latest-press/archive/61-billion-the-economic-contribution-of-people-aged-65-plus/, accessed 4 November 2021.

Epilogue: Socialist ageing in a global context

James Chappel and Isaac Scarborough

Introductory comments

The ageing of our bodies occurs at the most intimate level of our cells, yet our senescence brings us into contact with much larger narratives. Ageing affects our selves and our families, but it also influences the course of national and international history. Global ageing is without a doubt one of the most important human phenomena of the modern era. While historians are constitutionally allergic to positing historical laws, it does appear that some version of the 'demographic transition' is happening, or has happened, everywhere across the world. The collapse of birth rates, combined with the sometimes dramatic expansion of lifespans, has led to unavoidable questions of financing, culture and care.

These challenges are being met in very different ways. Scholars have paid a great deal of attention to the diversity of responses within the capitalist world. Gøsta Esping-Andersen's famous *Three Worlds of Welfare Capitalism*, for example, could be alternatively read as the *Three Worlds of Caring for Older Citizens*, given that, in most places, this is the largest component of welfare spending.[1] More recently, there has been an emphasis on the influence of ageing models exported from the west to developing nations, but largely within the context of contemporary global capitalism. Significantly less attention has been paid to the socialist world, or to comparisons *between* the capitalist and socialist worlds. One purpose of this volume has been to begin to address this lacuna.

Since the essays in the volume are not, for the most part, directly comparative in nature, we would like to use this epilogue to situate the volume's findings in a broader, global context to discover what is unique, and what is not, about ageing in the Soviet sphere. We have organized our remarks into four sections, reflecting what seem to us to be four major themes in both the historical literature on global ageing and the chapters in this volume: science, the urban/rural divide, gender and race/ethnicity/empire. A truly global focus would be impossible in an epilogue of this length; we have chosen, therefore, to focus our comparative attention on Western Europe and America, which is also the site of the majority of historical research on ageing.

Science

For all of the universality of its shared experience, ageing has remained a niche field of scientific inquiry. This was as true in the USSR as elsewhere in the world: while biological gerontology, the study of the underlying mechanisms of ageing, grew in scope, prominence and scientific result over the twentieth century, its institutional funding and clout paled in comparison to other biomedical fields of enquiry. In the USSR, as the contributions to this volume have shown, important (and indeed field-leading) research was conducted into the endocrinological foundations of ageing, cellular degeneration and regeneration, cancer prevention, and the links between heart disease and age-related dementia, to provide just a few examples. Yet these bodies of scientific research often struggled to find an audience outside of academic circles, were rarely – if ever – taken into consideration by politicians, and funding was restricted to a handful of major research institutions, such as the Institute of Gerontology in Kiev.

In many ways, however, this placed Soviet gerontology on an even playing field with most other countries' bodies of research. While a few Western nations, primarily the UK (see Pat Thane's contribution to this volume), began to emphasize the importance of targeted geriatric medicine in the post-war period, the scientific study of ageing struggled for a foothold worldwide. Money available for cancer research in the United States, for example, was at least fifty times greater than for ageing research.[2] Although the International Association of Gerontology (IAG) was founded in 1950 and initially promoted by a group of biological gerontologists, including the United States' Nathan Shock and the UK's Vladimir Korenchevsky, scientific research into ageing remained limited.[3] As early as the mid-1950s Korenchevsky was complaining about the IAG's increasing focus on social gerontology and geriatric medicine,[4] while in both the United States and the UK the number of scientific research institutes focused on ageing-related work was extremely limited. The founding of the United States' National Institute on Ageing (NIA) in 1974 did increase funding for ageing research, but had a similar centralizing impact, concentrating gerontology into a few trajectories and research centres.[5]

These obstacles did little to lower gerontologists' enthusiasm. As Vladislav Bezrukov and Yurii Duplenko's chapter in this volume shows, Soviet researchers struggled proudly in the face of adversity over the twentieth century, mirroring the 'permanent chip on [their] shoulders, almost a bone spur' of self-righteousness that Stephen S. Hall observed amongst mid-century American gerontologists.[6] Ingenuity reigned across the capitalist-socialist divide. When institutions in the United States were unable to acquire the proper dishes to raise micro-organisms, Hall writes, US researchers bought their own glass lasagne dishes;[7] when universities in the USSR could not find money for Petri dishes, Soviet cytologists made their own from the bottoms of cognac bottles.[8]

When it came to scientific research, moreover, the Iron Curtain was more than just a two-way mirror: it was downright porous. As Bezrukov and Duplenko's and Tutorskaya's contributions to this volume show, Soviet scientists were well aware of Western work in gerontology, and Soviet research was also cited and published in the West. The chapter by Jarosz, moreover, demonstrates the physical overlap of scientific holes in the Curtain, with medical equipment, such as an 'iron lung' finding its way from the West into Soviet medical institutions and museums. Soviet gerontologists and their interlocutors in Europe and the United States, working from similarly disadvantaged positions, sent each other publications, visited each other's institutes and shared findings at conferences. This made Soviet gerontologists an indelible element of the broader scientific field of biological gerontology – reflected in the impact their research has had on recent 'breakthroughs' in the field, such as the ongoing trials of metformin as a drug to alleviate many of the chronic ailments more frequently associated with ageing.

As a field of international scientific enquiry that cut across the capitalist-socialist divide, gerontology also provides an important lens into the work of intergovernmental agencies. Soviet gerontologists were closely engaged with the World Health Organization (WHO), the United Nations (UN), the International Agency for Research on Cancer (IARC) and other European-based intergovernmental and non-governmental organizations. Soviet geriatricians and social gerontologists also had contact with these centres, reflected in the international influences cited in a number of this volume's chapters. Some Soviet doctors and scientists even served as bureau chiefs or directors in these institutions, such as Mikhail Akhmeteli, a Soviet doctor who moved between the European Office of the WHO and the Soviet Ministry of Health in the 1960s and 1970s, or Nikolai Napalkov, who moved from the Oncological Institute named for Petrov in Leningrad to become the assistant director general of the WHO in 1989.[9] Vladislav Bezrukov himself was briefly the director of the United Nation's Programme on Ageing during the final years of the USSR. These intergovernmental organizations provided a conduit for scientific and medical exchange across the Iron Curtain – giving lie to the myth of hermetically sealed capitalist and socialist orders of science and ageing alike.

Rural ageing

One of the most persistent myths in the study of old age across the world has remained the idea that ageing is more successful in rural areas. A number of reasons are frequently suggested to explain why and how this may be. There is less of a housing crisis in rural areas, it is argued, and at least in some areas rural life is composed of large, multi-generational families (affording many possibilities for eldercare). In addition, rural economies are not governed by the logic of waged or industrialized labour. Just as older people are unsuited to overly strenuous physical work, these arguments continue, they are well-suited for rural living, which prizes land tenure, experience and social respect.

It is debatable whether this was ever true in any generalizable way. It is almost certainly not true in the contemporary moment. Across the world, population ageing has coincided with urbanization in ways that have proven particularly challenging to the older people left behind. In China and the United States alike, for example, rural areas have been emptying out over generations as younger workers flock to cities. The parents of those workers, if they remain in their home communities, often lack the kinds of familial care that, across the globe, still constitute the primary form of eldercare. Just as importantly, they also lack access to high-quality healthcare and other services that their children enjoy in more developed urban regions.[10]

Post-Soviet spaces are, relatively speaking, latecomers to this phenomenon both demographically and academically. The discourse on 'population ageing' or 'over-ageing' – along with the rural consequences of this demographic shift – has tended to focus on Western Europe and East Asia. Indeed, before 1990, Eastern Europe was significantly younger than Western Europe, and had higher fertility rates, too. After 1990, this changed: fertility rates cratered in Eastern Europe and in Russia. As a consequence, while it might be true that many areas of the former USSR and the 'Eastern Bloc' are comparatively younger than their

Western counterparts, they are ageing faster.[11] In less urban areas, the shift is even more marked, with previous waves of young generation out-migration compounding the ageing of the remaining population and leaving villages essentially hollowed-out of working-age population.

Rural older persons have been 'left behind' in almost every capacity: as an afterthought for many families, just as for policymakers and experts. When the United States passed Social Security legislation in 1935, agricultural workers were left out, ensuring that millions of rural people could not take advantage of the limited social support and pensions provided by the state. Matters have improved since then, but agricultural workers continue to lag in terms of old-age support. Here, the USSR and post-Soviet space has followed a similar trajectory. The Soviet pension system, when designed and implemented in the 1930s, also denied support to farmers and agricultural workers. This was later changed, but even today the livelihoods of older persons in rural (and semi-rural) Russia leave much to be desired. The British geographer John Round, for instance, spent four months in the early 2000s living in a peripheral Russian city to investigate whether or not older people there were able to cope. He found an astonishing paucity of resources: low pensions could not come close to meeting the relatively high cost of living in the remote region. The lack of material support, Round found, however, was matched by an equally astonishing level of resilience on the part of the older Russians themselves, some of whom had resorted to subsistence agriculture to support themselves and their compatriots.[12]

At the same time, little historical work has been conducted on rural ageing in the (post)-Soviet or (post)-socialist spaces. Most of the scholarship on Soviet agriculture has focused, reasonably enough, on the horrors of collectivization, yet it bears remembering that the USSR was an agrarian society for decades thereafter: a majority of the Soviet population was still rural as of the Second World War and one third of the population remained rural as late as 1970.[13] While not often explicitly articulated in this volume, when taken together the essays collected here clearly show that the Soviet world was surprisingly similar to its capitalist cousin in its treatment and neglect of rural older people.

Most immediately obvious, assuming that the essays in this volume track the interests of Soviet experts themselves, is the urban focus in Soviet research and policy on ageing. There is much to read in this collection about Kiev, and the scientific gerontological innovations developed there (Bezrukov and Duplenko). We read, too, about Moscow, Leningrad and other major Russian cities: their architectural plans (Kassymbekova), their nursing homes (Grant) and these cities' psychiatric hospitals (Brokman). Some of this, to be sure, may be a problem of archives, which in general privilege elite, urban sources over impoverished and rural ones. And yet, given what we know about the urban bias of Soviet thinking more generally, it is likely that planners gave far less thought to the rural aged: their first inclination was to consider ways of improving older peoples' lives in cities, not outside of them.

The most explicit articulation of this trend comes in the contribution by Ewelina Szpak. Her work helps to clarify what may be uniquely *socialist* in the experience of rural ageing. In many places, as in the United States, small and privately owned farms are venerated as bastions of virtue and patriotism. In the Soviet Union and other socialist countries, of course, this was not true: prosperous, private landowners were vilified as saboteurs and enemies of the state. In the USSR, agriculture was overwhelmingly collectivized, but in Poland this never fully occurred. In the Polish case, as Szpak writes, most farmers were considered to be ideological enemies of the state. They were not included in state systems of pensions or healthcare and were heavily taxed. Older rural people, instead of relying on the state, had no choice but to utilize older traditions, according to which they signed a contract with their children, exchanging their land for various kinds of care and support. This system, designed for a departed world of private property and market relations, was not appropriate to the Polish present of socialism, especially given the considerable out-migration of younger people to Poland's growing cities. In Szpak's telling, Poland's Communist Party essentially abandoned rural older persons to their own devices.

Szpak's essay suggests that there was something unique in the situation faced by older people in socialism. The drive to collectivize agriculture was not present in all socialist milieus: what would such a process do to rural older persons whose status prior to any state intervention often depended on their legal ownership of land? Szpak's case study shows us what happened in Poland, a place where collectivization did not go very far. But what about in the Soviet Union itself, where it went so far as to leave everyone 'dizzy with success'? The chapters in this volume do not answer that question, but suggest an important direction for future historiographical investigation.

Gender

One aspect of ageing that the chapters in this volume – and Soviet experts, too – have dealt with directly is the undeniable gender divide. As Pat Thane puts it in her chapter, 'Old Age ... has long been predominantly a female experience'. Across the world, as populations have aged, women have found their life expectancies outstrip men's. The causes for this gap between male and female life expectancy remain a matter of debate, but appear to be a combination of genetics and social factors. Recent biological studies, for example, have demonstrated the relative evolutionary advantage afforded in terms of cellular division to women by their double X chromosomes: the paired chromosome appears in cross-species studies to afford boosts in longevity.[14] Decades prior, the Soviet demographer Boris Urlanis made a similar suggestion, while also highlighting the socio-economic factors that were correlated with increasing female longevity. With the onset of modern medicine, he suggested, mortality from childbirth decreased rapidly, as did the long-term medical complications thereof. At the same time, industrial accidents increased notably, which had a much higher prevalence amongst male workers; men were also more likely to fall susceptible to the harmful social choices associated with urban and industrial living, such as extensive tobacco or alcohol use.[15] It may be, as Anna Ozhiganova highlights in her contribution to this volume, that physical productive labour, broadly speaking, has led to a growth in longevity, but this growth has clearly been uneven, especially for men.

As a result of the uneven growth in life expectancies, older populations across the globe are dominated by women. In the late USSR, as Botakoz Kassymbekova writes in this volume, the population of older persons was in fact two-thirds female, a fact impossible to ignore. As Kassymbekova and other contributors to this volume highlight, these older women had particular interests, needs and social demands, all of which often differed from men their age. Whether or not the Soviet state – the decision-makers of which remained overwhelmingly male – managed to take these needs and interests into consideration was a different question. As Danielle Leavitt-Quist writes in her chapter, by the latter decades of the USSR the state's practical need for older grandmothers (*babushki*) to provide free childcare so that younger women could remain in the workplace ran counter to both Bolshevik ideology of active and independent working lives for women (including older women) and those *babushki*'s own interests. Rather than simply carers for their children and grandchildren, Leavitt-Quist highlights, many older Soviet women saw themselves as workers, leaders, social activists and fulfilling many other roles.

Just like elsewhere in the world, it should be said, Soviet *dedushki* (grandfathers) faced much less of a challenge to their older occupations. Whether they chose to retire to their dachas or remain in government service into their seventies – as did many leaders of the Communist Party – they were never scolded for failing their children and grandchildren. This paralleled the experiences of older men and women across the world in the latter part of the twentieth century. Women lived longer than men; their health spans, along with lifespans, were markedly better; they had greater opportunity, time and capacity to enjoy older age. At the same time, capitalist and socialist states alike struggled not to see them as providers of unpaid care for grandchildren and other relatives, a continuation of the 'double burden' faced by women across the Iron Curtain. Just as women were frequently expected in capitalist industrial and post-industrial society to both participate in the workforce *and* take care of children and the home, so too were *babushki* and many other grandmothers expected to somehow balance social activities and lives with the care of young grandchildren.

The deleterious effects of women's double burden in Western society have been increasingly described, as have the impact of this imbalance into older age.[16] Critical voices have also been raised in relation to the flattening effect of modes of ageing applied to non-industrialized societies, such as India or Africa.[17] There, anthropologists and historians have argued, the role of older women has become one of exclusively unpaid and societally unappreciated care, whether for grandchildren or infirm spouses and relatives. Aspects of paid work or social engagement – the other half of the double burden – were instead subsumed completely into the role of carer. While the contributions in this volume show older Soviet women facing a situation closer to that of older Western women, they too were confronted with an imbalance between their needs and interests and those of the state. As Leavitt-Quist points out, however, this was a state that placed particular importance on labour, and the right to labour in an equitable fashion: its suggestion that older women's labour should be directed towards the unpaid pursuit of childcare was thus especially difficult for many older Soviet women to accept.

Race, ethnicity, empire

International evidence suggests that ageing is an intersectional issue: older people who belong to racial or ethnic minorities also frequently experience greater economic and healthcare challenges (this is sometimes referred to as 'double jeopardy').[18] The inequities of working life persist into later life in all sorts of pernicious ways. For example, if racial minorities are subject to higher levels of incarceration or deportation, older members of the group in question will lack the intact and stable family unit that is a crucial deliverer of care in older age.[19] Populations with endemically lower socio-economic outcomes, such as the majority of racial minorities in most Western societies, also face much greater long-term health challenges: the deprivations of early life come to play out in the prevalence of chronic illness amongst older persons in these groups.

There are, however, countervailing forces, and in some cases social policy helps to make inter-racial disparities less prominent in old age than in other age brackets. In the American case, for instance, the Social Security system is perhaps the most 'colour-blind' part of the country's welfare system. Child and family welfare systems are often means-tested and are often delivered by local welfare agencies, which are likely to be swayed by locally prevailing prejudices. The Social Security system, though, is a federally administered benefit, and accrues in equitable amounts to almost all Americans, regardless of their race.[20] This does not make up for the long-term health effects of economic hardship and discrimination faced by racial minorities in the United States (as elsewhere), but it may at least avoid further exacerbation in older age.

In recent years, scholars have also begun thinking about the role of empire in the construction of old age. In *As the World Ages*, Kavita Sivaramakrishnan has notably explored the attempts in the middle decades of the twentieth century to map and theorize old age in imperial and post-imperial spaces. Western experts encountered many issues in their attempts to identify and ameliorate the 'challenge' of old age in developing nations, Sivaramakrishnan writes, most notably the fact that many non-Western people did not think in terms of a 'calendar' age at all. The models of ageing and older age, brought by Western experts to former imperial holdings, often had little application in local contexts. Sivaramakrishnan shows, however, how these difficulties did not keep experts from conjuring a romantic view of older persons in 'primitive' societies – and how the well-intentioned application of Western ideas of ageing often led to further degradation in terms of older people's standards of living.[21] Colour-blindness (or racial- or ethnic-blindness) and the application of 'universal' models, Sivaramakrishnan suggests, cannot always supersede national borders or even the internal borders of empire.

It remains unclear as to how the dynamics of race and empire can be applied to the case of ageing in Soviet world, or even how this should be theorized. There is an enormous literature on ethnicity and empire in the Soviet Union. While Russians were of course the largest 'nationality' in the Soviet Union, the state itself was a federation that included a wildly diverse group of peoples. Soviet Party workers and planners alike worked exceptionally hard to categorize and learn about the peoples that were under their rule.[22] Partly this was done to find ways of promoting local nationalities under the much-touted heading of *korenizatsiia* (localizing) – but also in order to engage outlying regions and ethnicities in the broader Soviet economic project.[23] While the Soviet Union was not an apartheid state along the lines of South Africa or the Jim Crow American South, it is indisputable that some nationalities were treated better than others. Stalin's attitude towards the Ukrainians is famous, but there are many other examples.[24] Central Asian economies, for example, remained deeply underdeveloped until the Soviet collapse, with many regions remaining agricultural monocultures.[25] In an even more obvious mistreatment of ethnic minorities, moreover, the Soviet state deported more than 3,000,000 representatives of ethnic groups (Koreans, Finns, Germans, Chechens, Meskhetian Turks, Balkars and many others) from their regional home-regions before and during the Second World War because of these groups' suspected lack of loyalty to the Soviet regime.[26]

Curiously, issues of race, ethnicity and empire are rarely mentioned in the chapters included in this volume. Of course, no essay or volume can cover everything, but the absence is striking. Does this indicate that, when it came to gerontological research, Soviet doctors and researchers did not think in 'national' terms? As a point of comparison, it might be noted that gerontological research in the United States was focused on white Americans, without comment, until the civil rights movement of the 1960s. Afterwards, researchers' attention was drawn to the specifically racial components of the issue.[27] Without a similar movement in favour of minority rights, it might seem as though the standardization of Soviet research around models of ethnic Russian behaviour and ageing could have gone unchallenged. It is the case that Soviet research in the 1970s and 1980s had begun to focus on regional and ethnic disparities in terms of longevity – but primarily with a focus on smaller pockets of 'exceptional' longevity in Abkhazia and Azerbaijan, rather than the endemically lower life expectancies in places like rural Central Asia.

Whatever the reason for its absence here, there is certainly room for more research about the role of race in Soviet and socialist ageing. Did the Soviet Union and its researchers 'romanticize' the ageing of ethnic minorities, as was the case in the British Empire? Or, alternatively, did they seek to bring a standardized model of socialist ageing into the Soviet hinterlands? How was older age a factor in the various forms of ethnic repression that marked the Soviet experience? During the Holodomor, for instance, 'old age' was often listed as a cause of death for starvation victims, even relatively young ones.[28] What does such a bureaucratic norm tell us about the relationships between age, ethnicity and violence? This would be a rich vein for future work.

Concluding comments

As these short synopses indicate, it is challenging to draw over-arching conclusions about the particular place of *Soviet* ageing in a global context. In fact, the most persistent finding seems to be that capitalist and socialist models of ageing might not have been so different as one would expect. It is certainly not the case that the Soviet Union or socialist world more broadly was any sort of utopia for older people. Like its twentieth-century capitalist counterpart, the Soviet world was obsessed with labour and productivity as the basic grammar of social relations. Older people, especially those who were disabled, could not contribute and were often treated as an afterthought. Older women, in the Soviet Union as in the United States, were often tasked with performing heroic feats of childcare; and in both places, too, this clashed with the achievements of a women's movement that was urging women towards equal standing in the workplace.

This, though, is in and of itself worth remarking upon. What does it say about global ageing, and its history, if we find such similar phenomena in societies that are as different as the United States, Poland and the Soviet Union? One potential answer has been suggested by Donna Harsch, a historian of gender and public health in modern Germany. In her exploration of infant health in West and East Germany, Harsch has found a gradual convergence, as both regimes came to care about infant mortality a great deal, and in surprisingly similar ways.[29] She is one of several scholars who is now revisiting the 'convergence' thesis, this time in a broader socio-economic scale.[30] As the Cold War recedes further into history, it is becoming increasingly apparent just how much the different regimes had in common. Both the Soviet Union and the United States were desperate to increase their productive powers; both were concerned with the health of their citizens; both were grappling with the consequences of an ageing population. They leveraged many of the same tools to engage with this population, and for that reason the popular culture of ageing, and even of ageism, took on remarkably similar forms, and resulted in remarkably similar sorts of inequities.

The analysis offered here, though, is incomplete. As several of the subsections above indicate, there is a great deal of work to be done on the history of socialist ageing, and of global ageing, too. This strikes us as a particularly important task for historians to take up. The world that we are all ageing into now will be demographically older every year. This raises monumental questions for public finance, popular culture and medicine. Those questions could of course be answered without any historical awareness at all – as they often are – but this will likely result in solutions that reproduce the same degradations and exclusions experienced in the twentieth century and the present moment alike. A historically informed approach to ageing, and to ageing policy, might be a better approach: the chapters in this volume constitute a valuable contribution to that end.

Notes

1 Gøsta Esping-Andersen, *The Three Worlds of Welfare Capitalism* (Princeton: Princeton University Press, 1990).
2 Calculated from the National Institutes of Health appropriations figures: NIH Almanac, 'Appropriations (Section 1)'. https://www.nih.gov/about-nih/what-we-do/nih-almanac/appropriations-section-1. In the USSR, monetary comparisons are more complicated, but never once was geriatrics, ageing or gerontology listed by the Soviet Ministry of Healthcare as a 'priority area' – a classification given to cancer research and paediatrics, for example, and which provided greater access to resources and funding. For an example of an early 1980s Ministry of Healthcare priority list that fails to mention geriatrics, see: State Archive of the Russian Federation (GARF), f. R-8009, op. 51, d. 2166, ll. 11–153.
3 On the founding of the IAG, now officially the International Association of Gerontology and Geriatrics (IAGG), see W. Nathan Shock with George T. Baker III, *The International Association of Gerontology: A Chronicle, 1950–1986* (New York: Springer, 1988).
4 Shock with Baker, *The International Association*, 23.
5 On the limitations to funding for gerontological research in both the United States and the USSR, see Isaac Scarborough, 'A New Science for an Old(er) Generation: Soviet Gerontology and Geriatrics in International Comparative Perspective', *Social History of Medicine* (forthcoming).
6 Stephen S. Hall, *Merchants of Immortality: Chasing the Dream of Human Life Extension* (New York: Mariner Books, 2003), 16.
7 Hall, *Merchants of Immortality*, 127–9.
8 Interview with Dr Alexandre Sidorenko, Vienna, Austria (via Skype), August 2019.
9 On Akhmeteli, see Central State Archive of Supreme Bodies of Power and Government of Ukraine (TsDAVO), f. 4783, op. 1, d. 146, l. 1; 'Mikhail Andreevich Akhmeteli', WHO Employment Record, WHO Archive, Geneva; on Napalkov – V.N. Anisimov, *Gody priveredlivye* (St. Petersburg: Eskulap, 2014), 155; Boleslav Lichterman, 'Nikolai Pavlovich Napalkov', *BMJ* 336, no. 7652 (10 May 2008): 1076.

10 For a nuanced look at the evidence from the American case, see Nina Glasgow, 'Older Rural Families', in David L. Brown and Louis E. Swanson (eds.), *Challenges for Rural America in the Twenty-First Century* (University Park, PA: Pennsylvania State University Press, 2003), 86–96.

11 Laszlo Kulcsar and Cristina Bradatan, 'The Greying Periphery: Ageing and Community Development in Rural Romania and Bulgaria', *Europe-Asia Studies* 66 (2014): 794–810.

12 John Round, 'The Economic Marginalization of Post-Soviet Russia's Elderly Population and the Failure of State Ageing Policy: A Case Study of Magadan City', *Oxford Development Studies* 34 (2006): 441–56.

13 Charles Becker et al., 'Russian Urbanization in the Soviet and Post-Soviet Eras', *United Nations Population Fund, Urbanization and Emerging Population Issues Working Paper 9* (November 2012), 6, available online: https://pubs.iied.org/sites/default/files/pdfs/migrate/10613IIED.pdf, accessed 4 November 2021.

14 For example, see: Zoe A. Xirocostas, Susan E. Everingham, and Angela T. Moles, 'The Sex with the Reduced Sex Chromosome Dies Earlier: A Comparison across the Tree of Life', *Biol. lett.* 16 (2020): 1–6.

15 See B.Ts. Urlanis, *Evoliutsiia prodlzhitel'nosti zhizni* (Moscow: Statistika, 1978), 116–37. Importantly, Urlanis points out that the gap between female and male longevity was not notable until the onset of the industrial revolution and modern medicine – i.e., not until the twentieth century.

16 For an overview, see S. Payne and L. Doyal, 'Older Women, Work, and Health', *Occupational Medicine* 60 (2010): 172–7.

17 Amongst other critical voices, see Lawrence Cohen, *No Ageing in India: Alzheimer's, The Bad Family, and Other Modern Things* (Berkeley: University of California Press, 1998); Anagha Tendulkar, 'Family as Caregiver to Elderly during Lockdown in Urban India', paper presented to the workshop *Old Age Care in Times of Crisis: Past and Present*, London (online), April 2021.

18 This was first deployed in Hobart Jackson, *Double Jeopardy: The Older Negro in America Today* (New York: National Urban League, 1964). For a useful compendium, and critique, of the extant literature, see Sandra Torres, *Ethnicity and Old Age: Expanding Our Imagination* (Bristol: Policy Press, 2020).

19 Corey Abramson, *The End Game: How Inequality Shapes Our Final Years* (Cambridge, MA: Harvard University Press, 2015).

20 Robert Lieberman, *Shifting the Color Line: Race and the American Welfare State* (Cambridge, MA: Harvard University Press, 1998).

21 Kavita Sivaramakrishnan, *As the World Ages: Rethinking a Demographic Crisis* (Cambridge, MA: Harvard University Press, 2018), ch. 1.

22 Francine Hirsch, 'The Soviet Union as a Work-in-Progress: Ethnographers and the Category "Nationality" in the 1926, 1937 and 1939 Censuses', *Slavic Review* 56 (1997): 251–78.

23 Terry Martin, *The Affirmative Action Empire: Nations and Nationalism in the Soviet Union, 1923–1939* (Ithaca: Cornell University Press, 2001).
24 On Ukraine and the ongoing controversy around the 'Holodomor' or mass starvation of Ukrainian peasants under Stalin's rule, see N. Naimark, 'Applebaum, Fitzpatrick and the Genocide Question', *Contemporary European History* 27, no. 3 (2018): 435–9.
25 Isaac Scarborough, 'Central Asia in the Soviet Command Economy', in David Ludden (ed.), *Oxford Research Encyclopaedia of Asian Commercial History* (New York: Oxford University Press, 2021).
26 Eric D. Weitz, 'Racial Politics without the Concept of Race: Reevaluating Soviet Ethnic and National Purges', *Slavic Review* 61 (2002): 1–29. For the most up to date figures, see Viktor Berdinskikh, *Spetsposelentsy: politicheskaia ssilka narodov sovetskoi rossii* (Moscow: NLO, 2005); also Isaac Scarborough, 'An Unwanted Dependence: Chechen and Ingush Deportees and the Development of State-Citizen Relations in late-Stalinist Kazakhstan (1944–1953)', *Central Asian Survey* 36, no. 1 (2017): 93–112.
27 Sandra Edmonds Crewe, 'The Task Is Far from Completed: Double Jeopardy and Older African Americans', *Social Work in Public Health* 34 (2019): 122–33.
28 Hennadii Boriak, 'Population Losses in the Holodomor and the Destruction of Related Archives; New Archival Evidence', *Harvard Ukrainian Studies* 30 (2008): 199–215, here 204–5.
29 Donna Harsch, 'The Fight against Infant Mortality in Cold War Germany: East/West Convergence on Liberal Governmentality', *Journal of Modern history* 93 (2021): 401–32.
30 For another important comparative work in this vein, see Dora Vargha, *Polio across the Iron Curtain: Hungary's Cold War with an Epidemic* (Cambridge, MA: Cambridge University Press, 2018).

Select bibliography

General literature on ageing

Abramson, Corey. *The End Game: How Inequality Shapes Our Final Years*. Cambridge, MA: Harvard University Press, 2015

Achenbaum, W. Andrew. *Crossing Frontiers: Gerontology Emerges as a Science*. New York: Cambridge University Press, 1995

Armstrong, Sue. *Borrowed Time: The Science of How and Why We Age*. London: Bloomsbury, 2019

Aronson, Louise. *Elderhood: Redefining Aging, Transforming Medicine, Reimagining Life*. New York: Bloomsbury, 2019

Binstock, Robert H. and Linda K. George (eds.). *Handbook of Aging and the Social Sciences*. San Diego; London: Academic Press, 1996

Dannefer, Dale and Chris Philipson (eds.). *The SAGE Handbook of Social Gerontology*. London: SAGE Publications Ltd., 2010

De Beauvoir, Simone. *Old Age*, trans. Patrick O' Brian. Middlesex: Penguin Books, 1985 [1970])

Hall, Stephen S. *Merchants of Immortality: Chasing the Dream of Human Life Extension*. Boston: Houghton Mifflin, 2003

Hazan, Haim. *Old Age: Constructions and Deconstructions*. Cambridge: Cambridge University Press, 1994

Jefferys, Margot (ed.). *Growing Old in the Twentieth Century*. London: Routledge, 1989

Katz, Stephen. *Disciplining Old Age: The Formation of Gerontological Knowledge*. Charlottesville: University Press of Virginia, 1996

Shock, Nathan W. with George T. Baker III. *The International Association of Gerontology: A Chronicle, 1950–1986*. New York: Springer, 1988

Sinclair, David A. with Matthew D. LaPlante. *Lifespan: Why We Age – and Why We Don't Have To*. London: Thorsons, 2019

Sivaramakrishnan, Kavita. *As the World Ages: Rethinking a Demographic Crisis*. Cambridge: Harvard University Press, 2018

Walker, Alan (ed.). *The New Science of Ageing*. Bristol: Policy Press, 2014

Soviet, East European and post-Soviet literature on ageing and medicine

Alabovskii, Iu. I. 'Sostoianie zdorov'ia i vnebol'nichnaia meditsinskaia pomoshch' litsam pozhilogo vozrasta (po materialom Stavropol'skogo kraia)'. DMSc diss., Stavropol' Medical institute, 1970

Anisimov, V.N. *Gody priveredlivye*. St. Petersburg: Eskulap, 2014

Arshavsky, I.A. *Ocherki po vozrastnoj fiziologii*. Moscow: Meditsina, 1967

Bogdanov, A.A. *Bor'ba za zhiznesposobnost'*. Moscow, 1927

Bogomolets, Al.A. (ed.). *Starost'. Trudy konferentsii po probleme geneza starosti i profilaktiki prezhdevremennogo strenija organizma*, 17–19 December 1938. Kiev: Publishing House of the Academy of Sciences of the Ukrainian SSR, 1939.

Bogomolets, A.A. *Izbrannye trudy, v 3-x tomakh*. Kiev: Akademia nauk Ukrainskoi SSR, 1956

Borsowa, I., et al. (eds.). *Encyklopedia seniora*. Warsaw: Wiedza Powszechna, 1986

Chebotaryov, D.F., N.B. Man'kovskii, and V.V. Frol'kis (eds.). *Osnovy gerontologii*. Moscow: Meditsina, 1969

Chebotaryov, D.F. and V.V. Frol'kis (eds.). *Gerontologiia i geriatriia. 1977 Ezhegodnik. Geneticheskie mekhanizmy stareniia i dolgoletiia*. Kiev, 1977

Chebotaryov, D.F. and V.V. Frol'kis (eds.). *Gerontologiia i geriatriia. 1979 ezhegodnik. Prodlenie zhizni: prognozy, mekhanizmy, kontrol'*. Kiev: Institut gerontologii AMN SSSR, 1979

Dilman, M. *Chetyre modeli meditsiny*. Leningrad: Meditsina, 1987

Dogel, A.C. *Starost' i smert'*. Petrograd, 1922

Durmanov, V. Iu. 'Tipologiia kvartir dlia semei s pozhilymi roditeliami'. PhD diss., Moscow, 1978

Frąckiewicz, L. *Karta praw człowieka starego*. Warsaw: Instytut Wydawniczy Związków Zawodowych, 1985

Frol'kis, V.V. *Starenie: Neirogumoral'nye mekhanizmy*. Kiev: Naukova dumka, 1981

Frol'kis, V.V. (ed.). *Biologiia stareniia*. Leningrad: Nauka, 1982

Grando, A. *Ochyma khudozhnykiv*: medycyna v ukraïns'komu obrazotvorchomu mystectvi. Kyiv: RVA Triumf, 1994.

Gumowska, I. *Życie bez starości*. Warsaw: Wiedza Powszechna, 1962

Khavinson, V. Kh. *Peptidnaia reguliatsiia stareniia*. St. Petersburg: Nauka, 2009

Krasucki, P. *Praca ludzi starszych*. Warsaw: Instytut Wydawniczy CRZZ, 1979

Mil'man, M.S. *Uchenie o roste, starosti i smerti*. Baku, 1926

Morozova, A. '*Neleninskii bol'shevizm*' A. A. Bogdanova i 'vperedovtsev': idei, al'ternativy, praktika. Moscow: Nestor-Istorija, 2019

Nagornyi, A.V. *Problema Stareniia i dolgoletiia*. Kharkov: KhGU, 1940

Nagornyi, A.V., V.N. Nikitin, and I.N. Bulankin. *Problema stareniia i dolgoletiia*. Moscow, 1963

Pavlovskaia, E. 'Sotsial'no-kul'turnyi aspekt formirovaniia Predmetno-prostranstvennoi sredy otdykha i obshcheniia liudei pozhilogo vozrasta na gorodskikh pridomovykh territoriiakh'. PhD diss., Moscow, 1985

Romashova, M. "'Defitsitnaia Babushka": Sovetskii diskurs starosti i tsenarii starenia'. *Novoe Literaturnoe Obozrenie* 3 (2015): 55–65

Rosseta, E., et al. (eds). *Problemy ludzi starych w Polsce*. Warsaw: PWE, 1974

Różycka, J. *Psychologia zachowań kobiet w wieku starszym*. Wrocław: Ossolineum, 1971

Rudakov, P.G. *Doma-Internaty dlia prestarelykh (arkhitekturno-planirovochnoe reshenie)*. Avtoreferat dissertatsii na soiskanie uchenoi stepeni kandidata arkhitektury, Nauchno-issledovatel'skii institute teorii i istorii arkhitektury i stroitel'noi tekhniki, Moscow, 1962

Rysz-Kowalczyk, B. (ed.). *Społeczne kwestie starości*. Warsaw: Ośrodek Badań Społecznych, 1991

Sachuk, N.N. and N.N. Lakiza-Sachuk. *Pozhiloi chelovek v urbanizirovannom obshchestve*. Moscow: Akademiia Nauk SSSR, 1977

Shapiro, V.D. *Chelovek na pensii*. Moskva: Mysl, 1980

Shmalgauzen, I.I. *Problema smerti i bessmertiia*. Moscow, 1926

Smirnova, O. and L. Barmashina (eds.). *Zhilye doma kvartirnogo tipa dlia prestarelykh*. Moscow: Gosudarstvennyi komitet po grazhdanskomu stroitel'stvu, 1977

Sonin, M. Ia. and A.A. Dyskin. *Pozhiloi chelovek v sem'ie i obschestve*. Moskva: Finansy i statistika, 1984

Stepanova, V.K. (ed.). *Arkhitekturnaia sreda obitaniia invalidov i prestarelykh*. Moscow: Stroizdat, 1989

Szwarc, A. (eds.). *Ludzie starzy i starość na ziemiach polskich od XVIII do XXI wieku (na tle porównawczym)*. Vol 2, 153, Warsaw: DiG, 2016

Tryfan, B. *Problemy ludzi starych na wsi. Studium porównawcze sytuacji w Polsce i we Francji*. Warsaw: PAN, 1971

Urlanis, B.Ts. *Evoliutsiia prodlzhitel'nosti zhizni*. Moscow: Statistika, 1978

Valentei, D. (ed.). *Pozhilye liudi v nashei strane*. Moscow: Statistika, 1977

Valentei, D. (ed.). *Naselenie tret'ego vozrasta*. Moscow: Narodonaselenie, 1986

Vilenchik, V.I., et al. (eds). *Zhilishcha dlia prestarelykh: Potrebnosti i puti ikh udovletvoreni*ia. Minsk: Belorusskii nauchno-issledovatel'skii institut nauchno-tekhnicheskoi informatsii i tekhniko-ekonomicheskikh issledovanii Gosplana BSSR, 1989

Voronov, S.A. *Starost' i omolazhivanie*. Moscow, 1927

Western literature on Soviet, East European and Post-Soviet Medicine and Science

Bauer, Raymond. *The New Man in Soviet Psychology*. Cambridge, MA: Harvard University Press, 1952

Bernstein, Anya. *The Future of Immortality: Remaking Life and Death in Contemporary Russia*. Princeton: Princeton University Press, 2019

Bochen, Antoni, et al. (eds.). *Polish Medicin*e. Bydgoszcz: Quxi Media, 2018

Byford, Andy. *Science of the Child in Late Imperial and Early Soviet Russia*. Oxford: Oxford University Press, 2020

Chappel, James. 'On the Border of Old Age: An Entangled History of Eldercare in East Germany'. *Central European History* 53 (2020): 353–71

Craciun, Catrinel. '(De)Gendering of Older Patients: Exploring Views on Aging and Older Patients in Romanian General Practitioners'. *Actualidades en Psicologia* 30 (2016): 1–9

Dixon, Simon. (ed.). *The Oxford Handbook of Modern Russian History*. Oxford: Oxford University Press, 2013

Filtzer, Donald. *The Hazards of Urban Life in Late Stalinist Russia: Health, Hygiene, and Living Standards, 1943–1953*. Cambridge: Cambridge University Press, 2010

Graham, Loren R. *Science in Russia and the Soviet Union; a Short History*. Cambridge: Cambridge University Press, 1993

Grant, Susan (ed.). *Russian and Soviet Health Care from an International Perspective*. London: Palgrave Macmillan, 2017

Hoffmann, David. L. *Stalinist Values: The Cultural Norms of Soviet Modernity, 1917–1941*. Ithaca, NY: Cornell University Press, 2003

Klots, Alissa and Maria Romashova. 'Lenin's Cohort: The First Mass Generation of Soviet Pensioners and Public Activism in the Khrushchev Era'. *Kritika: Explorations in Russian and Eurasian History* 19 (2018): 573–97

Kremenstov, Nikolai. *A Martian Stranded on Earth: Alexander Bogdanov, Blood Transfusions, and Proletarian Science*. Chicago: University of Chicago Press, 2011

Krementsov, Nikolai. *Revolutionary Experiments: The Quest for Immortality in Bolshevik Science and Fiction*. Oxford: Oxford University Press, 2013

Kulcsar, Laszlo and Cristina Bradatan. 'The Greying Periphery: Ageing and Community Development in Rural Romania and Bulgaria'. *Europe-Asia Studies* 66 (2014): 794–810

Lovell, Stephen. 'Soviet Socialism and the Construction of Old Age'. *Jahrbücher fur Geschichte Osteuropas*, Neue Folge, 51 (2003): 566

Lovell, Stephen. *Generations in Twentieth-century Europe*. New York: Palgrave Macmillan, 2007

Mokhov, Sergei. 'Care for the Dying in Contemporary Russia: The Hospice Movement in a Low-Income Context'. *Mortality* 26, no. 2 (March 2021): 202–15

Mücke, Lukas. *Die allgemeine Altersrentenversorgung in der UdSSR, 1956–1972*. Stuttgart: Franz Steiner Verlag, 2013

Phillips, Sarah D. '"There Are No Invalids in the USSR!", A Missing Soviet Chapter in the New Disability History'. *Disability Studies Quarterly* 29 (2009)

Rivkin-Fish, Michele. *Women's Health in Post-Soviet Russia: The Politics of Intervention*. Bloomington: Indiana University Press, 2005

Rouhier-Willoughby, Jeanmarie. 'Contemporary Urban Russian Funerals: Continuity and Change'. *Folklorica* 12 (2007): 109–26

Round, John. 'The Economic Marginalization of Post-Soviet Russia's Elderly Population and the Failure of State Ageing Policy: A Case Study of Magadan City'. *Oxford Development Studies* 34 (2006): 441–56

Scarborough, Isaac. 'A New Science for an Old(er) Generation: Soviet Gerontology and Geriatrics in International Comparative Perspective'. *Social History of Medicine* 35 2022.

Starks, Tricia. *The Body Soviet: Propaganda, Hygiene, and the Revolutionary State*. Madison: University of Wisconsin Press, 2009

Todes, Daniel Philip *Ivan Pavlov: A Russian Life in Science*. New York: Oxford University Press, 2014

Vargha, Dora. *Polio across the Iron Curtain: Hungary's Cold War with an Epidemic*. Cambridge: Cambridge University Press, 2018

Literature on ageing in the UK and United States

Bynum, W.F. and Roy Porter (eds.). *Companion Encyclopedia of the History of Medicine*. Vol. 2. London: Routledge, 1993, 1092–118.

Hilton, Claire. 'The Development of Psycho-Geriatric Services in England c. 1940–1989'. PhD diss., King's College London, 2014

Hilton, Claire. *Improving Mental Health Services for Older People: Barbara Robb's Campaign, 1965–1975*. London: Palgrave Macmillan, 2017

Howell, Trevor H. *Old Age. Some Practical Points in Geriatrics*. London: HK Lewis, 1975

Le Gros Clark, F. with Agnes Clark, *Ageing and Industry*. London: Nuffield Foundation, 1956

Nuffield Foundation. *Old People: Report of the Survey Committee on the Problem of Ageing and the Care of Old People*. London: Nuffield Foundation, 1947

Pemberton, Hugh, Pat Thane, and Noel Whiteside (eds.). *Britain's Pensions Crisis. History and Policy*. Oxford: Oxford University Press, 2006

Roberts, Yvonne. *One Hundred Not Out: Resilience and Active Ageing*. London: The Young Foundation, 2012

Thane, Pat 'The Debate on the Declining Birth-rate in Britain: The Menace of an Ageing Population, 1920s–1950s'. *Continuity and Change* 5, no. 2 (1990): 283–305

Thane, Pat *Old Age in English History. Past Experiences, Present Issues*. Oxford: Oxford University Press, 2000

Townsend, Peter. *The Last Refuge. A Survey of Residential Institutions and Homes for the Aged in England and Wales*. London: Routledge and Kegan Paul, 1964

Townsend, Peter and Dorothy Wedderburn. *The Aged in the Welfare State*. London: G.Bell and Sons Ltd, 1965

Index

Page numbers in italics refer to figures and tables.

Abel-Smith, Brian 215
abortion 168, 169
Abrikosov, Aleksey Ivanovich 177
Academy of Medical Sciences of the USSR 24–5, 26, 28, 29, 53, 102
Academy of Sciences of the Ukrainian SSR 25, 26
Academy of Sciences of the USSR 25, 27, 28, 29, 62
accessibility
   building 114, 119
   healthcare 12, 79, 200, 211–12, 214, 228
   space and 97, 102
   to x-ray equipment 77–8, 80
active rest 174–5
activism of older people
   archiving 149–50, 152, 157–8
   for communism 6, 11
   modern *babushki* 133, 146 n.7
adaptational theory of ageing 22–4
adult dependents 138
Agamben, Giorgio 83
age discrimination 12, 211–12, 220
ageing, global. *See* global ageing
ageing process
   background and overview 2, 7, 225
   classifications 27, 34 n.34
   dementia 74, 87 n.3
   physical-chemical studies 18–22
   premature 51, 57, 66 n.3
   visionary biology 51–3
'Age-related Variability as a Result of the Laws of Mutual Interaction of Organismal Elements' (Belov) 22
age shifts. *See* demographic shifts
age thresholds 124 n.1, 134, 146 n.11
agriculture. *See also* farmers
   global 229–30
   Poland 187, 193–5, 202 n.7
Akhmeteli, Mikhail 227–8
alcoholics 76

All-Union Conference on Ageing, the Genesis of Old Age and Preventing Premature Ageing 24
All-Union Institute of Experimental Medicine (VIEM) 53–4
All-Union Society of Gerontologists and Geriatricians 27
All-Union Society of Old Bolsheviks 152, 163 n.17
All-Union Symposium on 'Neurohormonal Regulation in Ontogenesis' 27
All-Union Task Force 24, 28
All-Union Television 61
Alpatov, Vladimir 54
Al'perovich, Mikhail 160
'American Nursing Home is a Design Failure, The' (Davidson) 92
Amosov, Nikolai 56
'Amphibian Girl' (Charkovsky) 61
anaemia 175
Anderson, W. Ferguson 211
Anichkov, Nikolay Nikolaevich 177
animal experiments
   Arshavsky 53, 55, 56–7, 58, 61
   Charkovsky 61, 62
   museums 173
animal transplantation 41–3, 45, 49 n.28
annuities 187, 193–4, 195, 202 n.8
anti-ageing treatments 8, 17, 52. *See also* rejuvenation
apartment housing
   age-specific distribution 119
   background and overview 114
   living conditions 94
   research 97
   room counts 118
   service accommodation 96, 108 n.21
   sports training 60
   types 97, 109 n.45, 115–17, 118
Apgar, Virginia 58

Apgar Score 58
Aquaculture 59, 61, 62–4, *63*, 65
Archive of Perm Oblast 157–8
Archive for Private Persons 153–5
archives, state 151, 157–8, 164 n.33, 230
archiving Soviet pensioners 149–61
    background and overview 149–51
    local history museums 151
    mobilization of older citizens 151–3, 160
    personal legacies 153–61, 164 n.33
Aronson, Louise 2
Arshavsky, Ilya
    about 9, 53, 54–5
    alternative practices of child development 59–61, 62–4, *63*
    contributions overview 64–6
    energy principle of skeletal muscles 53–6
    infant immaturity 56–9
Ashwin, Sarah 137
assimilation limit 19
As the World Ages (Sivaramakrishnan) 233
atheism 11, 38, 52, 155
Atrophy of the Heart, The 196–8
attitudes to and perceptions of older people 7–8
autobiographical texts 153, 162 n.6
autonomy 115, 124
autopsy 176
auto-transplantation 45, 49 n.28
Azerbaijan Medical Museum 171, 173, *176*, 176–7

babushki
    background and overview 6, 7, 10–11, 131–3
    gender and family 133–8
    grandchild care 122–3, 131, 133–7, 139–41, 196, 231
    sociology 141–5
    state and labour in the household 138–41
baby boomer generation 218
Baranov, Anatoly 3
Baranskaya, Natalya 135
Bauer, E. 18, 19–20, 24, 31 n.9

Becker, Ernest 179
Belov, N. 21–2
Bergauer, V. 19
Bernstein, Seth 142
Bethnal Green, studies on 215–17
between life and death 83–5
Beveridge, William 207, 208, 209, 212, 217
Bezrukov, Vladislov 3, 28, 228
Bidder, J. 21
'big history' 150, 162 n.6
biological gerontology, about 8–9, 226, 227
'Biological and Social Foundations of Ageing' council 25
biopolitics 186, 201 n.3
biopower 201 n.3
biosocial death 85
birth control 35, 168, 169, 208, 211
birth rates
    British 207–8, 211
    global 5, 225
    Soviet 135, 141, 152, 168
Black Eagle Pharmacological Museum 175
Blagoveshchenskii, A. 18
bloc style housing 100, 101, 109 n.45, 110 n.78
blood donation 175
blood-related illnesses 175
blood transfusions 17, 22, 33 n.21, 38, 52
BMA (British Medical Association) 210, 211
Boddington, Paula 81–2
Body Soviet, The (Starks) 37
Bogdanov, Alexander 22, 32–3 n.20–1, 38, 52
Bogomolets, Aleksandr 20, 24–6, 32 n.10, 45–6, 51
Bolsheviks 9, 36–7, 53, 151–2
breast cancer 212
breastfeeding 54, 59, 60, 61, 171
Brezhnev, Leonid 6, 107 n.14, 113–14, 190
Britain's ageing population 207–20
    age discrimination 12, 211–12, 220
    background and overview 207–8
    geriatric medicine 12, 210–11
    later life diversity 217–19, 220
    research 215–17, 226

social care 213–14
work 208–9
British Geriatrics Society 210
British Medical Association (BMA) 210, 211
British Regulation and Quality Improvement Authority's Care Standards for Nursing Homes 102
building access 114, 119
building styles 95–7, 101, 103, 108 n.21, 109 n.45, 110 n.78. *See* also specific styles
Bulankin, I. 22–3
Bulgakov, Mikhail 41, 47

Calasanti, Toni 6
Campbell, David 177
cancer 19–20, 211–12, 226
care homes 91–104
    built environment 96–9
    Covid-19 pandemic 212
    demographics 2, 91, 95, 105–6 n.3–4, 108 n.25, 214, *214*
    design and construction 93–6, 103–4
    design background and overview 10, 91–3, 106 n.6
    hospital transfers to 86
    interiors 99–101, 102–3
    outdoor spaces 101–2
    preference 86, 116, 123
    self-contained 96–7, 109 n.40
    small scale 94, 104
    styles 95–6, 99–101, 110 n.78
care of grandchildren. *See* grandchild care
cells 18–19, 20, 23, 31 n.8, 32 n.16, 231
cellular metabolism 34 n.35, 55
centenarians 178
Central Council of Trade Unions (VTsSPS) 104
Central Scientific Research and Design Institute of Standard and Experimental Accommodation Design (TsNIIEPzhilishcha) 95, 99, 100, 103
centralized building style 110 n.78
Charkovsky, Igor 59, 61–3, *63*, 65
Chebotarev, D. 25, 26–7, 28
Chekhov, Anton 176
chelation 23, 33 n.24
childbirth *170*, 170–1, 231. *See* also pregnancy

child development 59–61, 62–4, *63*, 171–2. *See also* physiological immaturity
childhood illnesses 59
child-rearing 59–61, 122–3, 169. *See also* grandchild care
cholera 173
chromatin 18, 23, 31 n.8, 33 n.24
chromosomes 231
Churchill, Winston 217
class hierarchies 94, 159
classifications of ageing 27, 34 n.34
Clinical Medicine Division of the Academy of Medical Sciences 26
cold strengthening 59, 61, 63, 64–5, 68 n.58
collectivism 136, 187, 229, 230
colloids 18, 19, 20, 31 n.3, 32 n.10, 33 n.22
commemorative campaigns. *See* memory politics
Commission for the dissemination of hygienic knowledge 35
communal apartment housing 114, 115–17
communism
    activism 152
    labour 11, 139
    men 137–8, 147 n.30
    Poland 187
    propaganda 35, 37
    values and morality 133, 140–1, 145
    women 6, 133, 137–8
conferences and symposiums on gerontology 24, 27–8, 54
Conservative government of Britain 209, 214
consumerism 132, 136
continence care 77, 81–2
contraception 35, 168, 169, 208, 211
convergence thesis 235
coronavirus pandemic 91, 212
Council of Ministers 104, 151
Crawford, Robert 84
creativity hypothesis 59
Crisis of Endocrinology, The (Bogomolets) 45–6
cryonics 8, 52
'Cultivating National Health' exhibit 36
'cultivation of public health is the work of the working class' slogan 38, *39*

cultural activities 81, 97–8, 104
cybernetics 22, 32–3 n.20

Davidson, Justin 92
Davitashvili, Eugenia 62
day care centres 134, 171
dead body disposal 82
death
    concept 37
    Gannushkin Hospital 82, 83–4
    medical museums 11, 175–9
    natural 175–6, 177, 178–9
    pure 176
    social 85
death decade 37
de Beauvoir, Simone 7
dedushki 154, 231–2
dehumanization 81–3, 84–5
dementia 74, 81, 83, 84, 87n3
demographic shifts
    Britain 207
    global 225, 228–9
    Poland 186–7, 196, 202 n.9
    Soviet 1–3, 25
Denial of Death (Becker) 179
Department of Health Enlightenment 38
Department of Maternal and Child Health 168
de-Stalinization 188, 192, 200
developmental physiology 53–6
Dilman, Vladimir 21, 32 n.16
diorama of dying soldiers *176*, 176–7
disposable soma 32 n.14
DNA 23, 31 n.8, 33 n.24
Doerr, Wilhelm 176
Dogel, A.C. 24
dolphin babies 61
Doronina, L. 135
Dresden glass man 174
Dresden Museum of Hygiene 174
duality concept of ageing 36
Durmanov, Dmitry 118

East Germany 186, 235
education, health. *See* health education; museums of medicine
education and training, medical 41, 210–11
EHRC (Equality and Human Rights Commission) (Britain) 212
Ehrlich, Paul 40, 48 n.14

elder care
    body management 80–3, 84–5
    conclusions 85–6
    Gannushkin Psychiatric Hospital overview 75–8
    between life and death 83–5
    overcrowding and staff shortages 79–80
elderly population rates. *See also* demographic shifts
    British 207
    Polish 186, 193, 204 n.38
    Soviet 92, 95, 108 n.27
    urban 115, 117
elevational ageing mechanisms 21, 32 n.16
elevators 78, 99, 101
'On the elimination of illiteracy in the RSFSR' decree 38
empire, role of 233–4
employment of elderly 137, 138–9, 212, 219
Endocrinological Museum 41
endocrinology 36–7, 41–3, 44–7
energy funds 54, 55–6, 60, 62, 65
Energy Principle of Skeletal Muscles 55–6, 60, 65
Energy Principle of Skeletal Muscles (Arshavsky) 60, 65
Engels, Friedrich 55
Equality Act (British) 212
Equality and Human Rights Commission (EHRC) (Britain) 212
Ermakova, L. 136
Esping-Andersen, Gøsta 225
ethnicity 232–4
experimental science, defined 52–3
experiments with animals. *See* animal experiments
'Extending Life' programme 25, 29–30
extrasensory phenomena 61–2, 63

fairy tales 17, 30 n.1, 40, 46, 48 n.16
families
    archives 154, 156–7
    British elderly 213, 214, 215–17
    global ageing 228–9
    housing 115, 116, 117, 118–19, 124
    multigenerational 117, 118, 134
    Polish elderly 194, 196–9, 204 n.46
    power dynamics 141–2
Family and Kinship in East London (Young and Wilmot) 215–17

Family Code 5, 13 n.11, 118
Family Life of Old People, The (Townsend) 216
For Family Reasons 137
farm handovers to state 194–5
farmers
   global 229, 230
   Poland 187, 193–5, 202 n.7–8, 230
fashion 142, 148 n.49
Featherstone, Katie 81–2
Fedorov, Nikolai 52
Feldsher and Midwife 169
feminism 208, 211, 235
fertility 5, 228
Fight for Life and Health, The (Bogdanov) 22
financial independence 141–2
Firsov, Zaharii 59, 61
Five-Year-Plans 96, 103, 173
foetuses 57, 62
Fomin, G.N. 96
Foucault, Michel 201 n.3
free energy 19, 55, 56
free medical care systems 172, 187, 211
Frolkis, Vladimir 23–4
Fundamentals of Endocrinology 44–5

Gaidukov, N. 18
ganglia 24, 33 n.26
Gannushkin Psychiatric Hospital
   body management 84–5
   conclusions 85–6
   elder care overview 75–8
   between life and death 83–5
   overcrowding and staff shortages 79–80
gardens 101–2, 122, 139–40, 147 n.34
Gebhard, Bruno 174
gender. *See also* women and ageing
   care homes 94, 107 n.17
   disparity 5, 117
   elder care 85
   housing 117, 121
   roles 137–8, 147 n.30, 231–2
genetic-regulatory theory of ageing 23
geriatric cabinets 119, 127n51
geriatrics
   background and overview 1, 4
   Britain 12, 210–11
   global 226–7
   Soviet Union 26–7, 73, 236 n.2
German Democratic Republic 186, 235

German population in People's Republic of Poland 188
gerontology
   background and overview 4, 8–9, 17–18
   biological pre-history 18–22
   Britain 219–20
   funding 1, 226–7, 236 n.2
   growth 24–30
   life expectancy 51–2
Gerontology Branch of the National Institutes of Health 25
geropsychiatric care. *See* Gannushkin Psychiatric Hospital
gestational dominance 57
Gierek, Edward 190
Gilgamesh, legend of 17, 30 n.1
Giprogor (Russian Institute for Urban Planning and Investment Development) 100, 110 n.70
Glass, David V. 208
glass man 174
global ageing
   background and overview 225–6
   conclusions 235–6
   gender 230–2
   race, ethnicity and empire 232–4
   rural 228–30
   science 226–8
Goldshtein, B. 23
Gomułka, Władysław 190
Gorbachev, Mikhail 104
Gorer, Geoffrey 178–9
Gorev, Nikolai 25, 26
Gorky, Maxim 53
Gosstroi USSR (Ministry of Construction and Architecture) 95, 96, 99
government support for mothers 170
Graham, Loren R. 167
grandchild care
   Britain 215, 216, 219
   Soviet Union 122–3, 131, 133–7, 139–41, 196, 231–2
grandfathers 154, 219, 231–2
grandmothers. See *babushki*
Grando, Alexander 167
Grandparents' financial help to younger generations 219
Grant, Susan 167, 179
gravidan therapy 52

gravitational shock 62
Great Patriotic War 5–6, 117, 149, 234
Green House home 104
Gudiene, Velma 167

Hall, Donald 2
Hall, Stephen S. 227
hardening the body 59, 61, 63–5, 68 n.58
Harsch, Donna 235
Hazan, Haim 7, 8
health education 35, 38, 41. *See also* museums of medicine
'Healthcare of Russia -1917' exhibit 36
Heart of a Dog (Bulgakov) 41
heart rates 56
Herald of Endocrinology 41
hetero-transplantation 41–3, 45, 49 n.28
Hilton, Claire 210
historical turn 149–50, 161
history of medicine 165, 166–7.
  See also museums of medicine
Hoffmann, David L. 84
Holodomor 234
Holquist, Peter 84
home visitation system 171–2
homo-transplantation 45, 49 n.28
hormones 32 n.16–17, 48 n.17
'Hormones and the Bolsheviks' (Kremenstov) 36
household labour 135–8, 140–1, 142
housing. *See also* apartment housing
  background and overview 2, 4, 10
  British 213–14, *214*
  family 115, 116, 117, 118–19, 124
  micro-districts 115–16, 119, 120–3
  policy 113–14
  sociology 114–15
  types 97, 115–17, 140
Housing Maintenance Offices (*ZhEK*) 139
humanization 10, 120
Husemann, Friedrich 176
hygiene 38
  museums 35–6, 168, 172–3, 174
  social 26–7, 35, 46, 171, 172
hypothalamus 28, 34 n.35
hypoxia 53, 57, 58
hysteresis 18, 19, 20, 31 n.8

IAG (International Association of Gerontology) 28, 226
'ideal' Soviet 9–10, 74, 83–4, 143
identification of hospitalized elders 85
illiteracy 38, 158
imbalance of living systems 19, 31 n.9
immaturity, physiological 57–9
immaturity, social 193, 198, 200–1
immortality
  fairy tales 17, 40
  Soviet pursuit of 7–8, 37–8, 52
incentives to have children 5, 207–8
individual, place of the 3–5
individual development, theory of 54–5
individualism 74, 132, 136, 145
industrialization 187, 190, 237 n.15
inequalities 6, 189–90, 218, 232–4, 235
infants 52, 54, 56, 57–61, 62, 64, 235
Inglot, Thomas 190
Institute of Blood Transfusion 33 n.21, 38
Institute of Experimental Endocrinology 41
Institute of Experimental Pathology and Therapy of the Academy of Sciences of Abkhazia 173, 178
Institute of Gerontology and Experimental Pathology 54
Institute of Gerontology in Kiev
  ageing classification 34 n.34
  care home design 102–3
  funding 226
  research 4, 9, 23, 25–30, 143
Institute of Labour and Social Policy 191
Institute of Radio Engineering and Electronics 62
'Instructions for designing homes for the elderly and disabled people' 103
intergovernmental agencies 227–8
International Agency for Research on Cancer (IARC) 227
International Association of Gerontology (IAG) 28, 226
iron lung 174, 181 n.23, 227
Iron wine 175
Ivanov, Porfiry 63, 68 n.58
Ivanov, V. 26
Ivanova, Tatiana 157
Ivan Pavlov (Todes) 44

Joseph Rowntree Foundation 218

Kadzhaia, Valery 135
Kashikhin, Leon 159
Kaup, Migette 104
Keynes, John Maynard 207
Khan-Magomedov, Selim 120
Kharkov school of developmental physiology and biochemistry 19, 20–1
Kholodkovskii, N. 18
Khrushchev, Nikita 5, 6, 13 n.11, 107 n.14, 113–14
Kiev 25, 114, 115, 117
Kiev Zonal Scientific-Research Institute for Standard and Experimental Design 97, 103
Kizel, A.A. 18–19
Koltsov, Nikolai 46–7
Komarov, Lev 51, 52, 54
Kommunist 138–9
Komsomol (organization) 151, 157–8, 164 n.35
Komsomol (village) 158
Korenchevsky, Vladimir 226
Koriakov, S. 96
Kostukijukievicus, Anatloiiu 167
Krasnaia Zvezda 134
Kravchenko, A.T. 173
Kravkov, Nikolai 40
Krementsov, Nikolai 36–7, 43–4, 52, 167
Krokodil 144, 144–5

labour
  Britain 208–9
  gender 5–6, 231, 232
  household 135–8, 140–1, 142
  modern *babushki* 131–2, 133, 134, 145
  Poland 189
  rejuvenation and life expectancy 37, 55–6
  therapy workshops 92, 100, 101
Labour government of Britain 208, 209, 211
Last Refuge, The (Townsend) 213–14, *214*
Latvian Medical Exhibition 169, *170*, 170–1
Latvian Society for the Promotion of Health and Education 169
Latynina, A. 154, 160–1
Lawton, Julia 82–3
Leibing, Annette 85

leisure 120, 132, 133–4, 139, 142–5
Leningrad 27, 101, 103, 114, 115–16, 117
Lepeshkin, V. 18
'Life, Ageing, and Death' (Nagornyi) 20
life cycle. *See* ontogenesis
life expectancy 146 n.6
  Arshavsky 54, 55–6, 57, 58, 60
  Britain 207, 217, 218
  gerontology history 19, 20
  global 231, 234
  rejuvenation 37, 55–6
  women 6, 132–3, 152, 217, 231, 237 n.15
lifts, building 78, 99, 101
'Like a Fish in Water' 61
Literary Gazette 152, 154, 155, 160–1
living alone 215, 216
living death 83–4
living water 40, 48 n.16
location and housing 116–17
loneliness 135, 196, 215
longevity 178, 231, 234, 237 n.15. *See also* life expectancy
Lovell, Stephen 74

magic 40, 46
'March of the Pilots' (Herman) 36, 47 n.3
Marchuk, P. 25
maternity 168–71, 170
maternity hospitals 54, 60
maternity houses 170, 170–1
Matryona's Home (Solzhenitsyn) 131
Mechnikov, Ilya 18, 25
medical education and training 41, 210–11
medical equipment shortages 77–8
'Medical exhibition with an exposition of birth control items' 169
medical museums. *See* museums of medicine
Medical Research Council (Britain) 211
Medvedev, Zhores 54
Mekas, Taurus 167
memory politics 149–50, 151–2
mental health. *See also* Gannushkin Psychiatric Hospital
  background and overview 73–5
  dementia 74, 81, 83, 84, 87 n.3
  home care design 102, 104
metabolism 19–20, 21, 55, 56

Metchnikoff, Elie 51
metformin 227
metro stations 119
MG-03-1 care home plan 100
micelles 20, 32 n.10
micro-districts 115–16, 119, 120–3
mind-body dualism 76, 88 n.19
Ministries of Social Security 179
Ministry of Construction and Architecture (Gosstroi USSR) 95, 96, 99
Ministry of Health (Britain) 210
Ministry of Healthcare of the USSR 28
Ministry of Internal Affairs 151
Ministry of Social Welfare 94, 96, 99, 103
Mitchell, Timothy 4
mobility 99–100
modern *babushki*. See *babushki*
molecules 18, 19, 20, 23, 33 n.22
Molkov, Alfred 35
Monty Python 179
Moscow 98, 100, 103, 108 n.27, 115
Moscow Society of Naturalists (MOIP) 54
Moscow University Surgical Clinic 41–3
Mother Heroines 170
mother-in-law apartments 140
mothers, government support for 170
multigenerational apartment housing 118
multigenerational families 117, 118, 134
Murzilka 156
Museum of Healthcare in Tashkent, Uzbekistan 168–9, 171, 172, 173, 174
Museum of Medicine of Azerbaijan 171, 173, 176–7, 177
Museum of Social Hygiene 35–6
Museum of the Institute of the Sanitary Enlightenment 35
Museum of the Sklifosovsky Institute 36
Museum of Traditional Medicine in Isfara, Tajikistan 175
museums of medicine. See also *specific museums*
  background and overview 165–6
  child development 171, 172
  conclusions 179–80
  hygiene 172–3
  methodology of analysis 166–7, 180 n.2
  old age and death 176–9
  as propaganda 35–6

prophylactic healthcare 173, 174, 175
reproduction 168–71

Nagornyi, A.V. 19, 20–1, 25
Napalkov, Nikolai 228
Narkomzdrav (People's Commissariat of Health) 35, 38, 47, 74, 169
National Health Service (NHS) (Britain) 210, 211, 212
National Institute on Ageing (NIA) (U.S.) 226–7
National Museum of Abkhazia 178
National Museum of Medicine of Ukraine 167, 169, 171, 172–3, 175, 176
natural death 175–6, 177, 178–9
Nedelia 131, 135, 136, 142, 143
neighbours 115, 117, 120, 121
nervous systems 33 n.26, 55, 57
neurohormonal regulation 21, 27, 29–30, 32 n.17
neurology and psychiatry convergence 76, 88 n.19
new wallet 188–9, 203 n.23
newborns 52, 54, 56, 57–61, 62, 64, 235
NHS (National Health Service) (Britain) 210, 211, 212
NII (scientific-research institutes) 29, 34 n.37
Nikitin, Boris and Elena 59–60
Nikitin, V. 22–3
Nuffield Foundation 208, 215
nursery schools 134, 171–2
nursing homes. See care homes

objective-management method of planning 29, 34 n.36
'Old Communist's Story, An' (Sokolov) 156
old wallet 188, 189, 202 n.23
ontogenesis
  about 21, 22–4, 32 n.12, 32 n.16
  Arshavsky 54, 56–7, 65
  child development 171–2
  conclusions 179–80
  hygiene 172–3
  methodology of analysis 166–7
  museum narratives overview 165–6
  old age and death 175–9
  prophylactic healthcare 173, 174–5
  reproduction 168–71

Oppel, Vladimir 45
organic psychoses 76, 88 n.14
outdoor space 101–2, 121–3
overcrowding, hospital 77, 79, 82

P-03-2 care home plan 100–1
paint colours for care homes 102–3
pansionats 94, 97, 107 n.17, 108 n.25
Paperno, Irina 162 n.6
parallel-crossed organismal construction 22
paranormal phenomena 61–2
para-science 63, 65
Party Central Committee 104
pathogenesis 26, 86, 177
patient expectations 43
Pauls Stradins Museum of the History of Medicine *170*, 170–1, 173–4, 175
pavilion style care homes 101, 110 n.78
Pavlov, Ivan Petrovich 24, 44, 51, 64, 177
Pavlovskaia, Elena 120–3
peasants 46–7, 187. *See also* farmers
pensioner's homes, Polish 199, 204n54
pension policy in People's Republic of Poland
  conclusion 200–1
  discourse 191–3
  legal framework 187–91, 202 n.17, 202 n.23, 202 n.28
  rural ageing 193–6
  urban ageing 196–200, 204 n.46
pensions
  British 208, 209, 216, 218
  global 229
  labour 137, 138, 142, 208
  pension age 124 n.1, 134, 146 n.11, 207, 209
  Polish (*see* pension policy in People's Republic of Poland)
  reform 6, 146 n.11, 152, 229
People's Commissariat of Health (Narkomzdrav) 35, 38, 47, 74, 169
People's Republic of Poland and old age
  background and overview 185–7, 202 n.7–9
  conclusions 200–1
  discourse 191–3
  legal framework for pension policy 187–91, 202 n.17, 202 n.23, 202 n.28

rural ageing 193–6, 230
urban ageing 196–200, 204 n.46
perceptions of and attitudes to the elderly 7–8
perestroika 104
Peri, Alexis 142
Perm City Women's Soviet 157, 160
personality 150
personhood 83–4, 85, 86
Pfluger, E. 19
PGRs (State Agricultural Farms) 187, 193
Pharmacy Museum 36
phenotypes 58, 60–1
physical activity 9
  Arshavsky 54, 55–7, 58–9, 61, 65
  child rearing 59–61
physical-chemical study of ageing process 18–22
Physical Culture and Sport 60, 61
physiological collectivism 38, 52
physiological immaturity 57–9
Physiological Mechanisms and Patterns of Individual Development (Arshavsky) 55
physiological self-regulation 21
Pinch, The (Willetts) 218
Pioner 156
Pirogov, N.I. 35, 47 n.2
Pirogov Society 47 n.2
place of the individual 3–5
playgrounds 122, 123
Poland, People's Republic of. *See* People's Republic of Poland and old age
polio 173, 174, 181 n.23
Polish United Workers' Party (PZPR) 190, 192
Poor Law 210, 213
Popov, Gavriil 46
poverty in Britain 215, 217, 218
power dynamics of family 141–2
pregnancy 57, 61, 62, 168–71
premature ageing 51, 57, 66 n.3
preventative medicine 36, 38, 73–4, 80–1, 174
private plot gardening 139–40, 147 n.34
privileges, social 94, 100, 188–9, 190, 203 n.23
Problem of Ageing and Longevity, The (Nagornyi) 21, 23
Prokin, Alexander 41–3, 45, 49 n.21

pro-natalism 5
propaganda, medical
   background and overview 35
   museums 35–6, *39*, 47
   publications 43–5, 46
   'radical' science 38, 40–3, 44–7
   rejuvenation 36–8, 40–1, 43, 47
   reproduction and child rearing 168, 169
prophylactic healthcare 74, 173–5
proteins 18–19, 20, 23, 31 n.8
protoplasmic hysteresis 18, 19, 20, 31 n.8
pseudoscience 65
psychiatric care. *See* Gannushkin Psychiatric Hospital
psychiatry and neurology convergence 76, 88 n.19
psychics 61–2
psychotropic medication 81
public hygiene 26–7, 35, 46, 171, 172–3
pure death 176
PZPR (Polish United Workers' Party) 190, 192

queuers 196
quiet archival revolution. *See* archiving Soviet pensioners

race 207, 232–4
Rakitin, Vasilii 158
rate-of-living theory 55
'Reactive Capacities of the Ageing Organism' symposium 27–8
Red Cross Infant Nursery 169
rejuvenation 7
   life expectancy 37, 55–6
   medical propaganda 36–8, 40–1, 43, 47
Rejuvenation (Vasilevsky) 40
reproduction 5, 168–71
research, scientific
   Aquaculture 59, 61, 62–4, *63*, 65
   British 211
   death 37–8
   developmental physiology 54–8
   endocrinology 44, 45
   global 226–7, 234
   infant development 59–64, *63*
   Institute of Gerontology 24–30
   life extension 40–1, 51–2, 60
   ontogenesis 22–4

paranormal phenomena 61–2, 65
popularity 52–3
pre-gerontology history 18–22
psychiatry 73–4, 76, 87 n.3
scientific-research institute 29, 34 n.37
urban ageing 113, 114, 116, 120–3
research, social
   British 215–20
   care homes 92, 97–8, 103
   work 208–9
retirement
   age 124 n.1, 134, 146 n.11
   Britain 209
   modern *babushki* 133–4, 139
   Poland 188, 189–90, 191, 202 n.8
Revolutionary Experiments (Krementsov) 35–6
revolution in sciences 37, 44
roentgen equipment 78
roles, gender 137–8, 147 n.30, 231–2
Round, John 229
Rozanov, Vladimir 45, 49 n.27–8
Rubanenko, Boris Rafailovich 95, 108 n.28
Rubner, Max 19, 55
Rudakov, P.G. 95, 97–8, 99, 100, 102
Rudeiko, V.A. 109 n.41, 110 n.78
rural ageing 193–6, 228–30
Russell, Bertrand 53
Russian Folk Medicine (Popov) 46
Russian Institute for Urban Planning and Investment Development (Giprogor) 100, 110 n.70
Russian Medical Museum 35, 36, *39*, *42*, 47
Russian Society of Neuropathologists and Psychiatrists 73
Ružička, V. 19

Saltykov, R.A. 173
Samarina, A. 103
sanatoria 141, 174–5
sanitation 171, 172–3
Sarkizov-Serazini, Ivan 64–5
schizophrenia 76
science and story of ageing 3–4
science revolution 37, 44
Scientific Council on Applied Human Physiology 28
Scientific Council on Gerontology and Geriatrics 24–5, 28

Scientific Outlook, The (Russell) 53
scientific-research institutes (NII) 29, 34 n.37
Scotland 211
Second World War 5–6, 117, 149, 234
'second youth' 134, 135, 142, 143
self-contained care homes 96–7, 109 n.40
self-fulfillment 133–4
self-improvement 9–10, 74–5, 83–4
Semashko, Nikolai A. 38, 46, 74, 173
semi-alternative science 65–6
senility 42–3
Seventeenth International Congress of Medicine 40
sexuality 168–9
Shapiro, V.D. 140, 141
Shereshevskii, N. 24
Shervinsky, Vasily D. 41, 44–5
Shibaeva, A.N. 169
Shmalgauzen, I. 21, 24, 25
Shock, Nathan W. 28, 226
Shumeiko, Elena Vladimirovna 153
Sidenbladh, Erik 61
sidewalks 119
Sina, Ibn 168
single-family apartment housing 115, 116
Sivaramakrishnan, Kavita 233
skeletal muscles principle 55–6, 60, 65
Skripalev, Vladimir 59, 60
smallpox 173
small-scale care homes 104
Smirnova, Ol'ga 109 n.45–6
social conscience 198
social death 85
social hygiene 26–7, 35, 46, 171, 172–3
social immaturity 193, 198, 200–1
socialism
    babushki 131–2, 133, 140
    capitalism 225, 227, 232, 235
    care homes 93, 97, 98, 100, 101
    medicine 37, *42*
    memory 150, 153, 155, 160, 161
    Poland 190, 191–2
    race and ethnicity 234
    rural ageing 230
Social Security (U.S.) 229, 233
'Social Surveys of Old People' 215
social welfare centres 104, 200
socially useful work 11, 133–4, 136–7, 138, 140

Society of Russian Doctors 35, 47 n.2
Socio-cultural Aspects of the Formation of Material-spatial Leisure Environments and Older People's Interaction in Urban Near-house Territories (Pavlovskaia) 120–3
sociology 114, 141–5
Sokolov, Grigorii 156
Sokolova, Anna 37
Sokolova, Galina 155–6, 159, 160
Sokolova, Valentine Grigor'evna 149, 150, 155–61, 163 n.26
Solzhenitsyn, Alexander 131
Soviet Academy of Medical Sciences 24–5, 26, 28, 29, 53, 102
Soviet Academy of Sciences 25, 27, 28, 29, 62
Soviet Commissariat of Health 173
Soviet Council of Ministers 104
Soviet Woman 142
specialists, medical 25–6, 29, 79
sports training 59, 60, 61
stable imbalance of living systems 19, 31 n.9
'Stadium in an Apartment' column 60
staff shortages, hospital 79–80, 82
Stańczak-Wiślicz, Katarzyna 192
standard of living 6, 142, 233
standardization 4, 96, 234
Starks, Tricia 37, 167, 171–2
State Agricultural Farms (PGRs) 187, 193
State Archival Regulations of 1941 164 n.33
State Archive of the Perm Oblast 149, 157
State Committee for Civil Construction and Architecture 96
'state effects' 4
State Institute of Social Hygiene 35
Steinach, Eugene 40, 48 n.17
stereotypes 7, 217, 219, 220
stories, about 165–6
Strazheskii, N. 26
streets 119
stress response 61, 65
stressful stimulation 58
styles and types, building. See also *specific building styles and types*
    apartment housing 97, 109 n.45, 115–17, 118
    care homes 95–6, 99–101, 110 n.78

supernatural 65
surveys
    British 215–17
    care home design 93, 97–8, 99, 109 n.46
    grandchild raising 134, 143
    housing 120–1
swimming 59, 61, 62–4, *63*, 65
'Swimming before Walking' (Charkovsky) 61
syphilis 40, 168–9
systems theory 22, 33 n.20
Szpak, Ewelina 230

Tallinn school of urban sociology 120
tank respirator 174, 181 n.23, 227
Tarkhanov, Ivan 51
technological revolution 135–6
teen obligation to grandparents 143–5, *144*
tektology 22, 32–3 n.20
testicle transplantation 41, 43
theory of conditional reflexes 64
theory of dominant focus 57
theory of individual development 54–5
Three Worlds of Welfare Capitalism (Esping-Andersen) 225
tipizatsiia 96
tipovoe building style 95–6, 100, 103, 108 n.24, 110 n.78
Todes, Daniel P. 44
'Towards the Causes of Ageing' (Bauer) 19
Townsend, Peter 213–15, *214*, 216, 217
transfer of farms to state 194–5
transparent man 174
transplantation 41–3, 45, 48 n.17, 49 n.28
transportation 116, 119
transporting patients 78–9, 82
treatment exclusion of elderly 211–12
Trzebiński, Jerzy 166
TsNIIEP zhilishcha (Central Scientific Research and Design Institute of Standard and Experimental Accommodation Design) 95, 99, 100, 103
types and styles, building. *See* styles and types, building

Ukhtomsky, Alexei 53, 57
Ukrainian National Medical Museum 175, 177

United Kingdom 102. *See also* Britain's ageing population
United Nations (UN) 227, 228
United States
    care homes 104
    research 226–7, 234
    rural ageing 228, 230
    USSR comparison 235
    welfare 229, 233
urban ageing
    background and overview 10, 113–15, 125 n.8
    built environment 120–3
    global 230
    housing types 115–17
    infrastructure 118–23
    in Poland 187, 196–200, 204 n.46
    scientific research 113, 114, 116, 120–3
    urban sociology 114, 120
Urlanis, Boris 231, 237n15
useful work 11, 133–4, 136–7, 138, 140

vaccines 173
Vasilevsky, Lev 40–1, 43
venereal diseases 40, 107 n.17, 168–9
VIEM (All-Union Institute of Experimental Medicine) 53–4
visionary biology 51–3
voivodeships 191, 203 n.30
volunteering 151, 152, 219
Voronov, S.A. 24

walking 119, 123
Warren, Marjorie 210, 211
war representations 177
We and Our Children (Nikitin and Nikitin) 60
Wedderburn, Dorothy 213, 214, 215, 217
Week Like Any Other, A (Baranskaya) 135
welfare, social
    British 217, 219
    global 225, 233
    Polish 190, 195–6, 200
    reforms 6, 13 n.15
West Germany 235
Western urbanist thought 114, 125 n.8
WHO (World Health Organization) 34 n.34, 58, 170–1, 175–6, 227–8
Willetts, David 218, 219
Wilmot, Peter 215–17

women and ageing 5-6
    activism 6, 133, 146 n.7, 149, 152
    Britain 209, 217, 218
    communism 6, 133, 137-8
    double burden 135, 142, 232
    global ageing 230-2
    life expectancy 6, 132-3, 152, 217, 231, 237 n.15
    Poland's pension policy 198-200
Women's Soviet 157, 160
Women's Voluntary Service (WVS) (UK) 213
Wonderful Achievements of Science, The (Koltsov) 46
Woodford, study in 216-17
work efficiency 208-9
workhouses (UK) 213-14
working on oneself 9-10, 74-5, 83-4
World Health Organization (WHO) 34 n.34, 58, 170-1, 175-6, 227-8

x-ray exams 78, 80

yards 121, 122
Young, Michael 215-17
youth obligation to grandparents 143-5, *144*

Zamkov, Alexey 52
Zavadovskii, M. 24
ZhEK (Housing Maintenance Offices) 139
Zumrad 175

www.ingramcontent.com/pod-product-compliance
Lightning Source LLC
Chambersburg PA
CBHW062124300426
44115CB00012BA/1803